An Introductory Guide for Professionals
Working with Deaf and Hard of Hearing Clients
in Clinical, Legal, Educational and Social Care Settings

Edited by:
Dr Sally Austen
Dr Ben Holmes

First published 2021

© 2021 Dr Sally Austen and Dr Ben Holmes

All rights reserved. No part of this book may be reprinted or reproduced without permission in writing from the publishers unless otherwise stated in the text.

ISBN: 9798520594826

Imprint: Independently published

Editors

Dr Sally Austen is a Consultant Clinical Psychologist with 30 years experience in deaf mental health care and audiology services. She is the co-editor of 'Deafness in Mind. Working Psychologically with Deaf People Across the Lifespan', Austen and Crocker (2004), and of 'Deafness and Challenging Behaviour. The 360° Perspective', Austen and Jeffery (2007).

In her private work, as Austen Psychology, Sally is involved in training, supervision, writing, Expert Witness court work and occasional media work.

Dr Ben Holmes is a Clinical Psychologist working in specialist deaf mental health services and is the current Chair of the specialist interest group for applied psychologists working in deaf mental health care. He has additional training and expertise in clinical neuropsychology and trauma informed care.

In his independent practice, Ben lectures on university clinical psychology training programmes and works as an Expert Witness for the courts.

> Amber, thank you for being one of these people. I am so grateful
> Sally x

To M and H, for making every day a gift. And to all those who 'have my back', Thank You!

Sally

To B for your patience, support and love. To K for your fun and energy, and for giving me a helping hand!

Ben

Contents

Editor biographies and list of contributing authors   7

Acknowledgements   10

A Introduction
   1. How to use this book   12
   2. Your deaf and hard of hearing clients are missing!   14
   3. Terminology   15

Before you assess or treat
B The Importance of language
   1. Language deprivation   20
   2. Nodding   29
   3. Literacy in deaf and deafened people. Using writing to communicate   31
   4. Fund of information and access   34
   5. Theory of Mind   37
   6. Timelines   39
   7. Abstract thought   42
   8. Locus of control   46

C Communication and identity
   1. Communication and language - some definitions   50
   2. Language acquisition   53
   3. Newborn hearing screen   56
   4. Children with deaf parents   60
   5. Oral v manual debate   65
   6. Deaf education: past, present and future   67
   7. Bi- and multi-lingualism: how it can aid cochlear implantation   73
   8. British Sign Language   76
   9. BSL alphabet   82
   10. Being hearing, cultural naiveté and some audist assumptions   84

D Maximising access
   1. Interpreters and communication professionals   90
   2. Working with sign language interpreters (SLIs)   94
   3. Using interpreters with non-fluent or language deprived sign language users   99
   4. Deaf relay interpreters   105
   5. Booking a sign language interpreter   109

6. NUBSLI: checklist for booking a BSL/English interpreter	111
7. Video Interpreting	112
8. Oral communication: lipreading	115
9. What is a lipspeaker?	120
10. Oral communication: improving the effectiveness of communication using residual hearing	122
11. Communication with deafblind people	130
12. Deafblind alphabet	136
13. Non-native BSL users	138
14. Checklist of your client's communication needs	141

Assessments and interventions
E Cognitive and neurodevelopment

1. Diagnostic overshadowing	146
2. Cognitive assessments	147
3. Deaf and hard of hearing people with intellectual disabilities	154
4. Autism Spectrum Disorders in deaf children and young people	160
5. Autism Spectrum Disorders in deaf adults	167
6. ADHD	172
7. Deaf older adults	176
8. Assessing cognitive functioning remotely	183

F Mental health

1. Depression and anxiety in sign language users	192
2. Deaf people and trauma	198
3. Adjustment to hearing loss	204
4. Deaf people and psychosis	210
5. Do deaf people hear voices?	217
6. Pressure of speech or sign	223
7. Psychological therapies	225
8. Group therapy	231
9. Telemental health (TMH)	234
10. Medication and deaf, deafblind or hard of hearing people	239
11. Nursing/care coordinating with deaf service users: examples of good practice	245
12. Challenging behaviour in deaf and hard of hearing children and adults	252
13. De-escalation of aggression	257
14. Restraint	263

G Health service provision
1. The Deaf community and systemic failings in health care — 270
2. Prevalence of mental health problems — 273
3. National deaf child and adolescent mental health services — 274
4. Specialist mental health services for deaf adults — 282
5. Length of inpatient stay and delayed discharge — 287
6. Deaf research hubs - past and present — 289
7. Using standardised assessment measures with deaf people — 292
8. Media walls — 298

H Physical health
1. Aetiology does matter: causes and consequences of deafness — 302
2. Tinnitus — 308
3. Balance and dizziness in people who are deaf and hard of hearing — 315
4. Genetic counselling — 319
5. ENT multidisciplinary working and onward referral — 320
6. Non-organic hearing loss (NOHL) — 323
7. Deaf Wannabees — 329
8. Sleep disturbance — 332

I Legal
1. Deaf people in the Criminal Justice System: guidelines — 336
2. Forensic mental health services for deaf people — 342
3. Capacity to parent assessments with deaf clients — 348
4. Mental Capacity Act assessments — 355
5. Mental Health Act assessment, sectioning, Tribunals and Lay Managers' Hearings — 360
6. Representing a deaf person in court — 363
7. Safeguarding vulnerable adults — 369
8. Deaf registered intermediaries for vulnerable deaf clients — 376
9. Discrimination laws — 379

J Conclusion
What we know we don't know (e.g. future research areas needed) — 386

K Appendices
Working with a deaf or hard of hearing (DHH) young person in CAMHS — 390

L Index — **398**

Authors

1. ***Dr Kevin L. Baker*** (Chapters E3, F1 & G7) Consultant Clinical Psychologist working with deaf adults, families and children, and people with complex needs

2. ***Chris Bojas*** (Chapter I8) Deaf Intermediary, and Psychological Wellbeing Practitioner. working with Deaf adults

3. ***Cath Booth*** (Chapter F3) Head of Service Wales and South West Community, RNID: 31 years working with people who are profoundly Deaf with additional, complex needs and mental health issues

4. ***Grant Budge*** (Chapters F13 & F14) Specialist Deaf service inpatient ward manager

5. ***Dr Steve Carney*** (Chapters F4, F10 & I5) Consultant Psychiatrist in Deaf mental health care

6. ***Adele Cockerill*** (Chapter G5) Assistant Psychologist

7. ***Dr Andy Cornes*** (Chapter I3) Consultant Psychologist, Family and Systemic Psychotherapist

8. ***Jackie Dennis*** (Chapter D2) Registered Sign Language Interpreter

9. ***Dr Anne Easson*** (Chapters H3 & H5) Consultant Audiovestibular Physician

10. ***Dr Lindsey Edwards*** (Chapter H1) Paediatric Clinical Psychologist

11. ***Craig Flynn*** (Chapter I8) Deaf Intermediary

12. ***Lindsey Gagan*** (Chapter D14) Speech and Language Therapist, working with deaf adults in a mental health setting (JDU, Manchester)

13. ***Dr Hannah George*** (Chapters E4 & E8) Consultant Clinical Psychologist and Clinical Lead of the northern arm of Deaf CAMHS, working with deaf children, young people and families, and hearing children with deaf parents

14. ***Neil S. Glickman Ph.D.*** (Chapter C10) Licensed psychologist, University of Massachusetts Medical School and Private practice of psychology/psychotherapy

15. ***Abigail Gorman*** (Chapters G1 & I9) Policy and Public Affairs Manager for Deaf health charity

16. ***Dr Mary Griggs*** (Chapter F2) Clinical Psychologist, working with deaf adults

17. ***Louise Harte*** (Chapter I8) Registered Intermediary/Qualified Translator, working with Deaf adults and children

18. ***Dave Jeffery MSc. BSc. (Hons.), RMN, SPMH*** (Chapters F13 & F14) Deaf Community mental health nurse (now retired). Advanced Nurse Practitioner in violence reduction and aggression management. Co-edited (with Sally Austen) Deafness and Challenging Behaviour: 360 Degree Perspective

19. ***Maria Kilbride BA (Hons.) PGDip*** (Chapter D3) Registered Sign Language Interpreter (NRCPD), working primarily in secure mental health with inpatients and their associated Multi-Disciplinary Teams

20. ***Herbert Klein*** (Chapters C8 & D7) Independent Deaf Advisor in mental health

21. ***Dr Rachel Lever*** (Chapter G8) Clinical Psychologist, working with deaf adults in mental health services

22. ***Hellen McDonald*** (Chapter D8) Support worker with Deaf adults

23. ***Jennifer Meek*** (Chapter F11) Deaf Recovery Community Nurse with Deaf adults

24. ***Dr Constanza Moreno*** (Chapters A3, G3 & Section K) Clinical Psychologist, working in National Deaf CAMHS (London team)

25. ***Professor Jemina Napier*** (Chapter C4) Chair of Intercultural Communication, specialising in sign language interpreting and brokering

26. ***Lenka Novakova*** (Chapters D4 & D13) Deaf advisor, National Deaf Mental Health Service based in South West London and St. George's mental health trust. Prior experience in deaf education and as a child mental health worker, National Deaf CAMHS Corner House

27. ***Jayne Oakes*** (Chapter D11) Deafblind specialist Interpreter working with Deafblind people

28. ***Dr Sue O'Rourke*** (Chapters I1 & I2) Consultant Clinical Psychologist

29. ***Dr Sarah Powell*** (Chapter F9) Highly Specialist Clinical Psychologist, working with deaf adults in primary care

30. ***Paul Redfern*** (Chapter F1) Senior manager, working part-time with British Society for Mental Health and Deafness

31. ***Dr Sara Rhys Jones*** (Chapter E3) Highly Specialist Clinical Psychologist, Learning Disabilities Directorate, Swansea Bay University Health Board

32. ***Dr Katherine D. Rogers*** (Chapters G7) NIHR Post-Doctoral Research Fellow, University of Manchester

33. ***Dr Kate Rowley*** (Chapters C2, C3, C6, C7 & G6) Lecturer in Deaf Studies and Interpreting, University of Wolverhampton, and Director of Language Wise

34. ***Nikki Stephens*** (Chapters D10 & H2) Hearing Therapist, working in the NHS and privately with tinnitus, hyperacusis, misophonia and cochlear implant patients, and also providing generic hearing therapy

35. ***QC Clare Wade*** (Chapter I6) Barrister, Garden Court Chambers

36. ***Dr Elizabeth Wakeland*** (Chapter F5) Clinical Lead, Forensic and Clinical Psychologist

37. ***Dr Rob Walker*** (Chapter E6) Consultant Child and Adolescent Psychiatrist & Clinical Lead, National Deaf CAMHS (Central England)

38. ***Jackie Wan Brown*** (Chapter F11) Community mental health nurse

39. ***Christian Wasunna*** (Chapter I6) Barrister, Garden Court Chambers

40. ***Lesley Weatherspoon*** (Chapter D9) Lipspeaker and British Sign Language/English Interpreter

41. ***Hannah Whalley*** (Chapter F11) Occupational Therapist in deaf mental health care

42. ***Asher Woodman-Worrell*** (Chapter I7) Sensory Adults Social Worker

Acknowledgements

So many people have supported us in the production of this book, for which we are truly grateful.

The work of the 42 contributing authors demonstrates how amazing they are. We have been so pleased and thankful to be able to work with them.

Our work is informed by the influence and collaboration of generations of brilliant clients, researchers and colleagues too numerous to mention.

Many of the contributing authors also supported us by consultation or proofreading other chapters. We particularly thank Herbert Klein, Dr Constanza Moreno, Professor Jemina Napier, Lenka Novakova, Dr Sue O'Rourke, Dr Kate Rowley, Nikki Stephens.

To others who have been available for consultation and proofreading we are immensely grateful for your generosity and skills: including Madeleine Bedford, Dr Jim Crowell, Vicki Carrabin, Dr Emma Ferguson-Coleman, Rachael Hayes, Dr Andy Holwell, Dr Nicoletta Gentili, Jeff McWhinney, Dr Sodi Mann, Clare Myatt, Dipti Patel, Dr Omar Nasiruddin, Helen Rae, Anita Winfield, Professor Barry Wright.

Our illustrators, Shanee Buxton and Ashley Kendall deserve a special credit. Thank you for sharing your amazing skills.

Thank you also to Phil Boswell of Connevan's, Jeff McWhinney of SignVideo, National Registers of Communication Professionals Working with Deaf and Deafblind People (NRCPD), National Union of British Sign Language Interpreters (NUBSLI) and Dr Joanna Atkinson for allowing us to use their photos and illustrations.

Section A

A1 How to use this book
Dr Sally Austen and Dr Ben Holmes

Introduction

Thank you for reading this book. We very much hope it meets your needs and that of your clients.

Who is this book for?

This book is written for people who are experienced professionals in their own field: lawyers, doctors, employers, psychologists, social workers, nurses, care workers, teachers, trainers, managers, administrators and so on.

You may have little or no experience of working with deaf or hard of hearing (HOH) clients.

You may not even know where to find these clients! (see Chapter A2).

What we provide

We hope to provide information (through research and/or professional experience) that helps you adapt your existing knowledge and skills to the needs of deaf or HOH client(s).

Each professional will value different sections of the book. However, we recommend all make use of the printable chapter D14 - 'Checklist of your client's communication needs'.

We would also direct all readers to Sections B and C to consider important background issues that may be pertinent to your deaf or hard of hearing client(s).

To reduce chapter over-lap, bracketed references to relevant other chapters are included throughout the book. Please make use of these links as some chapters should be read in the context of others.

We need your discernment please
Different chapters cover clients with a range of presentations (some deaf, some hard of hearing; some with cognitive, behavioural or mental health problems; and some who are only limited by the barriers created by society). Rather than us repeat this in each chapter, please remember that not all information is relevant to all people who are deaf or HOH.

The use of terminology within this field varies between clients, specialisms, and authors (nearly half of whom in this book are deaf, Deaf or HOH). In order to respect this diversity, we have not standardised its use but chosen to respect each author's preference. We acknowledge this may mean that some people would use different terminology. Future editions of this book may reflect changes in authors' preference over time.

Irrespective of the terminology used in these chapters, it is important that interactions with your client always reflect **their** preferences.

Chapters A3 'Terminology' and C1 'Communication and Language – Some Definitions' are there as a general guide.

This book is not
This book is not a diagnostic manual. References to features of an illness or condition are not in any way a list of symptoms to be ticked off and collated into a diagnosis.

This information is not a replacement for seeking support from specialist professionals (particularly deaf and hard of hearing professionals) who have expertise in your field.

Future editions
We have deliberately self-published to keep the price low so that more people can access this book and so that we can consider an upgraded 2nd Edition in a few years' time. We aim to scrutinise the research and experiential evidence base to keep this book relevant throughout the years.

Constructive contributions on additions or adaptations (including typo-spotting) for the second edition, would be very welcome. Please do so via Email: AustenandHolmes@gmail.com

A2 Your deaf and hard of hearing clients are missing!
Dr Sally Austen

Whether it be by a solicitor, GP, manager or teacher, it is very common for deaf specialists to be told...

'I don't have any deaf or hard of hearing clients.'

This is peculiar because being deaf or hard of hearing (DHH) is extremely common:

- 1 in 5 of the population has some degree of deafness or hearing loss.
- This rises to 1 in 3 in those over 65 years.

- 1 in 1000 babies is born significantly deaf.
- But 150 in 1000 babies born prematurely will be deaf.

- 40% of those with a global learning disability (Intellectual Disability) are significantly deaf or HOH.
- This rises to 90% in people with Down's Syndrome.

- 40% of the UK prison population have some deafness.
- This rises to a shocking 90% where there are multiple limitations in access to services, such as in Australia's Aboriginal prisoner population.

Many specialists and service providers will report having no DHH clients. Having no DHH clients appears to justify having no staff trained to work with DHH people or having minimal facilities that award equal access to these clients: visual fire alarms, sign language interpreters, working loop systems; video doorbells etc.

Maybe it is true that your service requires no adaptations because you have no DHH clients. Or maybe you have no deaf or hard of hearing clients because your service is inaccessible!

- Based on these stats, how many deaf and hard of hearing clients should you have?
- Do these clients know about your service?
- When you find each other, is your service accessible to them?

A3 Terminology
Dr Constanza Moreno and Dr Ben Holmes

You may encounter many terms in literature, or professional work, relating to a person's audiological or cultural status. These terms have varied greatly over time and will continue to evolve. We recommend you ask your client what terms they prefer to use. Their preference may not align with others and may change throughout their life.

This chapter provides definitions that will be used throughout this book. It also makes readers aware of terms that may be found elsewhere, highlighting some that are no longer considered acceptable.

deaf (1)
The uncapitalised word 'deaf' refers to a person that has a reduced level of hearing on tests of audiometry.

Deaf
When deliberately capitalised, the word Deaf indicates membership of the Deaf community. The majority of Deaf people use sign language. The capital D represents pride in a shared linguistic and cultural identity.

deaf (2)
Some, particularly in USA, recommend using 'deaf' in all instances to respect the non-binary nature of the fluidity and variety of an individual's identity, cultural and language experience. This may be particularly relevant to younger deaf people (Woodward & Horejes, 2016). Older, late deafened people may not agree to the use of this term.

d/Deaf
In written text, d/Deaf has been used to cover both those who do, and do not, identify as culturally deaf. It is becoming less commonly used.

deafened
Refers to a person that has lost some or all of their hearing later in life, either suddenly or gradually.

Hard of Hearing (HoH)
Although initially used to describe mild hearing loss in older people, this term is also sometimes used by people who are deaf and have a sense of shared community with other non sign language users.

DHH
The abbreviation DHH is sometimes used to refer to people that are Deaf or Hard of Hearing without making reference to cultural or linguistic identity.

Hearing loss
Refers to someone that was able to hear but has lost some or all of their auditory perception. People with hearing loss may experience this as an emotional and functional loss. Those who identify as culturally deaf may find this term offensive.

Hearing impaired
A term often used medically at a time when 'deaf' was considered derogatory (particularly by non signers). Some people find the term offensive now because it identifies a person by one impairment rather than their many strengths. Those people who do choose to use this term prefer its use as a noun rather than an adjective (i.e. 'I have a hearing impairment', rather than 'I am hearing impaired').

deafblind
This refers to a person who has varying degrees of reduced vision and reduced hearing. They may or may not identify as culturally deaf. Preferred communication style will differ depending on onset and degree of both vision and hearing (see Chapter D11).

Dual-sensory loss/multi-sensory impairment
Similarly to 'deafblind', these terms are sometimes used when someone has varying degrees of reduced vision and hearing, and does not have a deaf cultural identity.

Clinical terms
Presbycusis
Age related hearing loss.

Congenital
Refers to a cause of deafness that is due to genetic, or other, factors that affected the foetus in utero (e.g. infection).

Acquired deafness
Deafness not present at or around birth and that is not congenital.

Prelingual deafness
When a person is either born deaf or becomes deaf within the first few years of life - specifically, the person was deaf before the usual age at which language is established (typically around 2-3 years old).

Postlingual deafness
When a person becomes deaf after they have established language.

Degrees of hearing loss
These are measured in decibels (dB) as an average for the person's better ear on tests of audiometry across different frequencies.

> *Mild*: Sounds start to be heard between 25 and 34 dB. There may be some difficulties following spoken conversations, especially in noisy surroundings.
>
> *Moderate*: Sounds start to be heard between 35 and 49 dB. There will be difficulties following spoken conversations.
>
> *Moderately-severe*: Sounds start to be heard between 50 and 64 dB. There will be difficulties hearing in most situations when not using hearing aids.
>
> *Severe*: Sounds start to be heard between 65 and 79 dB. Powerful hearing aids, lipreading and sign will be needed to follow conversations.
>
> *Profound*: Sounds will not be heard below 80 dB. Sign language and lip reading will be needed to follow conversation. Some sound may be gained from very strong hearing aids or implants.

Non-Organic Hearing Loss (NOHL)
Medically unexplained, the person reports a loss or lack of hearing that is not observed on audiometry assessments. There may be psychological or functional reasons for this (see Chapter H6).

Partially deaf/partially hearing
Historically, this term has been used by education authorities to distinguish between children who may have had sufficient hearing to access speech and those who were profoundly deaf.

Offensive terms
Terminology changes over time. What was once acceptable is now offensive. What is now acceptable may be offensive in the future. We must be willing to adapt to this.

'deaf and dumb'/'deaf mute'
Historically, these terms referred to people who were both deaf and who did not have useful speech. These terms are out of date and are considered offensive. They should not be used.

Some older Deaf people still refer to themselves using the signs for Deaf and Dumb, but the appropriate translation into written or spoken English is simply 'deaf'.

'deafness'
This term is becoming increasingly unpopular as it is often used incorrectly to describe an individual's experience rather than solely as a description relating to their hearing. For example, 'John's deafness meant he missed out on family trips to the cinema'. The term 'deafness' does nothing to explain whether the limiting factor was John, his family or the cinema.

Disability
Many people in the Hearing majority, and many who lose their hearing, often regard deafness as a disability. Most Deaf people do not. Instead they may regard the restrictions they experience as being caused by the failure of the hearing majority to engage with Deaf people, rather than because of a medically identified difference.

The concept of disability is more relevant where language deprivation is present (see Chapter B1) or where the person has associated conditions (see Chapter H1).

Audism
Audism is discrimination or prejudice against a person or group of people based on their ability, or lack of, to hear (see Chapter C10).

References
James Woodward & Thomas P. Horejes (2016) 'deaf/Deaf: Origins and Usage' The SAGE Deaf Studies Encyclopedia

Section B

B1 Language deprivation
Dr Ben Holmes

Language deprivation is a significant neurolinguistic condition resulting from inadequate access to language. The effects are chronic and have a profound impact on a person's life, beyond just communication. It is also completely preventable.

All that is required for language acquisition is a rich, accessible linguistic environment. It does not matter what form this language takes - speech, sign language, or both - **as long as it is accessible to that person** (Hall et al., 2019).

Incidences of language deprivation in hearing people are incredibly rare and generally limited to extreme cases of neglect or abuse[1]. Yet, shockingly, language deprivation affects a significant number of deaf people.

Deaf children will develop fluent language at the same rates as hearing people, provided they have sufficient exposure to accessible language in a developmentally appropriate timeframe (see Chapter C2). However, in one study, as many as 1 in 7 deaf children could not be interviewed in any language despite normal non-verbal IQs (Gregory et al., 1995).

Causes of language deprivation
Late diagnosis
Ninety-five percent of deaf children are born to hearing parents, with little or no experience of deafness. Parents might not notice their child's deafness until later, when a lack of response or engagement with spoken language is observed. In UK this is now much less of a contributing factor because of changes in early assessment of hearing (see Chapter C3).

Hearing professionals often have little experience of working with deaf children and so they may also miss a child's deafness. Consequently, without early intervention to provide access to language, through sign

---

[1] Language deprivation differs from language delay, where fluency is attained; albeit later. Where chronic, incomplete mastery of a first language is observed despite appropriate early access to language, this is likely to result from an underlying language disorder, whether the child is hearing or deaf.

language, assistive technology, or positive communication behaviours, the child will miss significant opportunities to develop language fluency and the associated social communication and cognitive skills.

Reliance on assistive technologies
Assistive technologies (e.g. hearing aids, cochlear implants) can be hugely beneficial for many people and will provide greater access to sound. For some, they may also provide access to spoken language. However, it is important to note that there are also people for whom assistive technology will be insufficient to prevent language deprivation.

Some people may gain no useful benefit at all, and others may gain greater access to sound but without amplification being sufficient to detect speech sounds (see Chapter D10). There may also be people who do not wish to use assistive technology. Therefore, even with assistive technology, access to language can still be significantly affected.

Discouraging signing
Many older deaf people describe their education with the signed phrase 'they hit my hands if I signed'. For over a century an unproven myth has damaged deaf people's access to language by claiming that signing inhibits the ability to speak and lipread (see Chapter C8).

Some professionals still advise parents not to sign with their children (see Chapters C5 & C6), including when waiting to see if a cochlear implant has worked. However, by using this approach, it may not be until attempts to access spoken language have been unsuccessful that access to sign language is considered. Meanwhile, the richest period for language development (0-3 years) may have elapsed and language deprivation will already have set in.

By not holding sign language in equal regard as an effective intervention to prevent language deprivation, some children are needlessly being stopped from accessing language.

Quality of sign being judged by non-signers
The majority of professionals who observe a signing child have little or no sign language skills themselves. Therefore, they may conclude that a child has linguistic fluency when this conclusion reflects their ignorance, not the child's skills.

Recent research to record and analyse fluent signing, and the subsequent development of psychometric measures (by the Deafness Cognition and Language Research Centre (DCAL), University College London), has ensured that comparisons of language ability are overseen by deaf professionals who are fluent in the languages upon which they comment. Comparisons using validated tools may result in language deprivation being spotted earlier and interventions being put in place.

The cognitive impact of language deprivation
In the first few years of life there are billions of neuronal connections being formed and pruned according to individual experience. Neurological imaging shows that chronic language deprivation causes language to be increasingly processed in areas of the brain other than the language centres. This effect increases linearly with age meaning that the longer language input remains impoverished, the more profound and permanent the effects of language deprivation become (Mayberry et al. 2011).

Language is the precursor to how we learn about and understand the world. Higher order cognitive skills require learning from other people's explanations of events, actions, reasons and emotions. The absence of this information therefore impacts on cognitive development, particularly those functions that fall under the umbrella term of executive functioning.

Many other aspects of cognition are affected by language deprivation, including social cognition, where the effects can be pervasive and profound. Examples include:

Theory of Mind (ToM)
The ability to understand the thoughts, feelings and behaviours of others, ToM difficulties are often associated with Autism Spectrum Disorders (ASD). However, without access to language, and the explanations of the actions and thoughts of others, it is not possible to develop a full understanding of differing perspectives, different experiences and that other people might have an independent emotional response to an event (see Chapter B5 for more information).

Social reasoning
The ability to understand and respond to social or cultural rules and norms is central to social reasoning. Society's rules do not always have an

intuitive logic without explanation, the absence of which can therefore have a profound impact on social interactions and social relationships.

Abstract thinking
Affecting the ability to understand and think about things that have not been directly observed or experienced. Language helps us to group, and generalise, the learning from experiences, aiding the ability to apply solutions in novel contexts. Without this ability to generalise and think in the abstract, further learning is impeded and limited to direct experience. (see Chapter B7 for more information).

Emotional understanding and regulation
Constant barriers to success give rise to a range of emotions (e.g. stress, frustration, anger). Someone who has been language deprived will experience these feelings in the same way as everyone else. However, they will not have had linguistic support to:
- label these emotional responses or understand them as normal
- linguistically communicate these feelings to others
- learn about the consequences of actions and their effect on others
- learn ways to self-sooth or resolve emotional distress

With limited ability to linguistically communicate this distress, and limited opportunity to learn how to self-regulate, it is likely that their most accessible form of communication will instead be through action, or lack of (see Chapter F12, Challenging Behaviour).

The linguistic impact of language deprivation
The earlier access to language is achieved, the less the impact of linguistic dysfluency is likely to be. From clinical experience, even in cases where a client has had no access to formal language before the age of 10 it is still possible to develop linguistic skill that result in only minimal difficulties in day to day interactions.

However, whilst intensive linguistic input might improve an individual's ability to communicate, there will always be features of language that never fully develop.

Example: A deaf woman who moved to UK aged 20, with no access to formal language before this time, is referred for social work support because she is very isolated. Since being in UK she has learned some limited sign language and during assessment frequently signs "Uncle, hit, fall, scared" raising concerns about her safety. Through conversation with the family, adaptation of visual resources and the use of a Deaf Relay it becomes apparent that the client is describing an event that happened 15 years ago in her home country when she was at a busy market and observed her uncle being accidentally knocked over by a stranger, resulting in him falling over and hurting himself. This was her first time at the market and she had felt scared.

Difficulties with language that can be observed when someone has been deprived, include:

Conceptual understanding
With limited language exposure, there are many concepts that may never have been explained. Alternatively, concepts may be more difficult to understand because of the level of abstract thought they require. Some people may be able to make reference to concepts in a contextually appropriate way. However, this does not equate to understanding, and difficulties may be encountered when asked to explain this further.

Professionals can sometimes leave a meeting under the impression that there has been a useful and mutually understood conversation. It is only later that it becomes apparent that this was not the case.

Perceptions of, and references to, time
Language deprivation can impact on the ability to express, and understand, events in relation to the passing of time - referred to as timelines (see Chapter B6). This can then impact on an individual's ability to explain whether something has just happened, happened a long time ago or is desired for the future.

The understanding of cause and effect can also be affected, as the temporal link between events is not always made linguistically (e.g. event x happened because of the preceding factors y and z). This can, not only, impact on how a person understands and relays information about events, but also how effectively they can access supportive interventions, such as therapy (see Chapter F7).

Use of directional verbs
In sign language, the use of directional verbs is indicated by using a sign in the context of who did what to whom. Language deprivation can impact

on the way this is expressed so that verbs are used but without indication of direction. For example, 'I shouted at them' and 'they shouted at me' both become 'shout'. This can significantly impact on understanding of events and means that care will be needed to clarify meaning.

Lack of context
Contextual information can sometimes be crucial to making sense of what is said. For example, if using just the first initial of a name or abbreviation, these are only useful if the person you are communicating with is aware of what these abbreviations refer to. Equally, describing a place or object by a visual feature only helps if that visual feature is known about.

It is not uncommon for people who have been language deprived to omit this information, which can impact on how easy it is to understand what is being described. Others who do know what these abbreviations mean (e.g. interpreters, family members etc.) can sometimes provide this information in the form of a voice over. Whilst useful, this can also inadvertently give the impression that the person is more linguistically skilled than they are.

Role shift
Role shift is a linguistic device in sign language used in the retelling of events or stories. A change in role is indicated by adaptations in body language, facial expression or style of signing/communicating to mimic each person's actions, character or role in events. Lack of role shift can make it difficult to know who is saying what to whom.

Overcoming linguistic challenges
When working with someone that has experienced language deprivation in professional settings, it is essential to work with experienced interpreters (see Chapters D2 & D3), Deaf Relays (see Chapter D4), or Deaf Registered Intermediaries (see Chapter I8).

Even with experienced professionals there can be a high risk of misunderstanding. Conversations will therefore take more time, require questions to be asked from multiple perspectives and clarification may need to be sought regularly. It is likely that methods of communicating may also require adaptation (e.g. use of visual resources).

The social impact of language deprivation
Isolation
Someone who feels scared by the demands of a social world that may seem confusing and difficult to understand may choose to try and avoid the most stressful parts of it. However, in doing so, this perpetuates lack of access to a sufficiently rich language environment and can also remove access to support. Subsequently, the individual's ability to acquire information is reduced, limiting the fund of knowledge from which to make future decisions (see Chapter F4).

Misunderstanding of needs
When verbal interaction is difficult to understand, there is an increased risk of accidentally agreeing to things or giving incongruous answers to questions (see Chapter B2). Information made available in written form will also be less accessible (see Chapter B3). Both give rise to the risk of conversations taking place at cross purposes leading, ultimately, to an individual's needs or preferences being misunderstood.

Linked with the difficulties with emotional understanding and regulation mentioned earlier, any resulting expression of frustration in response to this could well be interpreted, unfairly, as challenging behaviour instead of communication frustration (see Chapter F12).

Self-worth, self-esteem and self-confidence
People deprived of language are continually exposed to environments where they may struggle to understand what is happening or what is expected of them, affecting their ability to succeed. This impacts on how that person understands themselves in the world they experience.

Frequent exposure to situations where the individual may feel rejected, inhibited or excluded will place them at significant risk of developing low self-worth, self-esteem and self-confidence, aside from any difficulties in linguistically accessing, or contributing to, what is happening (see Chapter F1).

Mental health differential diagnoses
Language is central to our interaction as social beings. The consequences of language deprivation can have a significant impact on mental health because of the impact on social relationships and social functioning.

However, language deprivation does not inevitably lead to mental health problems.

In mental health settings, language is central to the process of assessment. This is true not just in terms of what is said (e.g. giving an accurate history of difficulties) but also the way a person communicates this information and the way they act.

The sequelae of language deprivation (e.g. cognition, emotion regulation and social interaction) can impact on linguistic and behavioural changes that may mimic symptoms of mental health problems such as depression (see Chapter F1) or psychosis (see Chapter F4). For example:
- Unusual descriptions of events
- Difficulty maintaining one topic of conversation
- Slower, more effortful conversation
- Reduced isolation or engagement in activity

However, it is essential that factors such as these are not misunderstood as a mental health problem, which could lead to inappropriate diagnoses and treatment. It is recommended that contact is made with specialist mental health services for support in assessing and working with people with language deprivation (see Chapters G3 & G4)

Language deprivation vs. Intellectual Disability and ASD
It is important to note that the effects of language deprivation are distinct from Intellectual Disability (ID). However, the consequences and effects of language deprivation can significantly limit a person's communication, social and functional skills. This means that someone with normal intelligence can still require significant levels of support without having ID.

Children and adults that experience language deprivation are frequently thought to have ID or ASD because of the social and communication difficulties that exist, even if this is not the case (See Chapters E4 & E5).

Any assessment of ID or ASD must consider the language environment that someone has existed in and should involve professionals fluent in the client's language, otherwise there is a risk of misdiagnosis. Working with deaf professionals is invaluable.

Summary
Language deprivation has a profound effect on many aspects of functioning and is a phenomenon that almost exclusively affects deaf people. Yet it is easily preventable through the provision of an accessible linguistic environment. It is important that professionals are aware of the potential impact of language deprivation so as not to misattribute what they observe to other causes.

References
Gregory, S., Bishop, J., & Sheldon, L. (1995). Deaf young people and their families. Cambridge University Press: Cambridge.
Hall, M.L., Hall, W.C., & Caselli, N.K. (2019). Deaf children need language, not (just) speech. First Language, 39(4), 367–395
Mayberry, R.I., Chen, J., Witcher, P., & Klein, D. (2011). Age of acquisition effects on the functional organisation of language in the adult brain. Brain and Language, 119(1), 16-29

Recommended reading
Glickman, N.S., & Hall, W.C. (2019). Language deprivation and deaf mental health. New York: Routledge

B2 Nodding
Dr Sally Austen

In a broadly hearing world, we associate nodding with agreement. Whilst there are many articulate deaf people who will make it very clear what they have understood, and take responsibility for checking your comprehension, this is not always the case.

Many deaf people, with and without additional disabilities such as language deprivation or learning disabilities, may nod when they have not understood what is being said.

Within the Deaf community this is teasingly referred to as 'The Deaf Nod', but it is far from humorous. Failure to spot erroneous 'nodding' has resulted in dreadful errors: misdiagnosis of psychosis, undetected vulnerabilities, false guilty pleas.

Glossary:
Expressor – the person talking or signing a statement or question
Receiver – the person hearing, lipreading or watching the signed statement or question

Nod means 'I am listening'
When receiving signed information from another, it is polite to nod to show they have your attention. If the presenter is describing a lively subject such as an argument they recently had, the receiver should nod vigorously; if the conversation is about their vegetable patch, the nodding may be gentler.

Nod means 'Tell me more, I am waiting to see if I understand later'
If a deaf person is aware that they do not fully understand, they may wait before admitting this or asking for clarification in the hope that it becomes clearer later. It is quite common for someone to nod all through a description and then, at the end, when asked, say that they have not understood.

Nod means 'I appreciate your efforts'
Whether deaf or hearing; professional or service user, it takes a strong character and a thick skin to repeatedly say 'I don't understand'. The receiver is aware that their lack of understanding may frustrate or disappoint the expressor. To relieve the expresser of this stress it is

common for the receiver to say that they have understood when they have not.

Nod means 'I really want you to stop'
If the receiver is frustrated, tired, confused and so on, they may think that agreeing will bring an end to this situation.

Nod means 'I don't want you to think I am stupid'
Discrimination against deaf people is rife and many deaf people are aware that they are viewed as less able intellectually. Nodding serves to protect them from revealing lack of knowledge – even though the knowledge gap may be entirely conventional.

To counteract nodding
It is alarmingly common to come across deaf people who have been supported by professionals to sign crucial documents or make life changing decisions, based on information that they have not understood. It is the professionals' responsibility to ensure, where at all possible, that this is prevented.

To detect false nodding ask your client to repeat back what has just been said. It provides vital information. If they cannot repeat back what has just been said, it is likely that they did not understand it.

Double check that they are not just echoing your words or signs. To fully check understanding, ask the client a different question that accesses the same information.

Example:
Solicitor to client (First expression): If you contact your ex-wife, you will be arrested and charged, you may go to prison.

Solicitor to client (Check by repetition): Just checking you understood. What will happen if you contact your ex-wife?

Solicitor to client (Check by different question): You have got your wife's number on your phone. Is it okay to text your wife?

It is the professionals' responsibility to check the clients' understanding.

B3 Literacy in deaf and deafened people. Using writing to communicate
Dr Sally Austen

Literacy in deaf people will depend on a number of factors, including how and when they became deaf, their education and their language fluency.

Deafened adults
Someone who had, and then lost, their hearing in adult life (due to an audiological condition) will retain their adult level of literacy.

Reading and other cognitive abilities may be affected if a person's deafness is the result of a condition that is also an assault on the brain (e.g. a head injury, meningitis, encephalitis).

Reading ability may also be affected by deterioration in eyesight.

Deaf adults
Adults who experienced significant deafness throughout their early schooling tend to have lower levels of literacy than their hearing peers.

Whilst the average IQ of deaf people is similar to that of hearing people, the average literacy of deaf adults is less than 9 years (Mayberry, 2002), which is functionally illiterate. This means that writing as a main form of communication, for some deaf people, is extremely unreliable.

Some of the factors that may have contributed to this are:
- having received inappropriate schooling (see Chapter C6)
- possible language delay or language deprivation (see Chapter B1)
- English being their second language.

Language fluency
In hearing people there is a direct relationship between written skills and fundamental language skills. This is not the case with deaf people, who may be language fluent in their native sign language, yet struggle with literacy (Marschark & Hauser, 2011). Language fluency can only be assessed by a deaf specialist in the deaf client's best language.

Using writing to communicate with deaf people
Each professional, in their unique context, must consider whether it is appropriate to use writing as a primary means of communication. This will depend on:

1. The reading level of the deaf person (as above)

2. The availability of alternatives
- Sign language interpreters (see Chapter D2)
- VRS (Video Relay Service) or VRI (Video Interpreting Service) - see Chapter D7
- Lip speakers (see Chapter D9)
- Potential to improve acoustic environment to increase use of residual hearing (see Chapter D10)
- Potential to improve visual environment to increase use of lip reading (see Chapter D8)

3. The context
Importance:
A receptionist asking a deaf client if they would prefer tea or coffee is significantly different from a solicitor asking an accused whether they would like to plead guilty or not guilty.

Timing:
A discussion about chest pain in an Accident and Emergency department, or whether the client wants their next of kin contacted, may need to be started prior to an interpreter arriving (see Chapters D2, G1 & I9).

On the other hand, predictable and longer-term interventions, such as a discussion about pelvic floor exercises in a postnatal patient, should include adequate communication preparation from the start and therefore not include writing unless it is the client's best and preferred language.

Written British Sign Language (BSL) grammar
BSL has a different grammar to spoken English (as do native sign languages internationally). Thus, a BSL user with reduced literacy, may write in BSL word order.

Literacy and word order are not reliable indications of intelligence or mental wellbeing.

There have been extremely concerning cases of hearing mental health assessors, with no experience of Deaf mental health care, diagnosing thought disorder based only on the presentation of a deaf client's writing.

Of course, professionals should react to anything written that concerns them, but the next step must be to facilitate more reliable communication methods and to seek specialist help.

Consequences of poor literacy
People with poor literacy are often blamed or suffer consequences for events they could not have understood, such as:
- Failing to attend appointments
- Not following written court instructions or orders
- Not taking medication or engaging with interventions as instructed
- Failing written exams despite being functionally very able
- Appearing to have forgotten information (that they did not understand in the first place) and thus being considered less cognitively able

Conclusion
We need to check what assumptions we make about a client's literacy and alter our assessment or intervention accordingly. It is the professionals' responsibility to ensure that all the information is accessible: because it ensures we maximise our care, and because it is law (Accessible Information Standard (AIS), 2016).
www.england.nhs.uk/ourwork/accessibleinfo

References
Mayberry, R.I. (2002). Cognitive development in deaf children: The interface of language and perception in neuropsychology. In S. Segalowitz & I. Rapin (Eds.), *Handbook of Neuropsychology* (2nd ed., Vol. 8, pt II, pp. 71-107)

Marschark, M. & Hauser, P.C. (2011). *How deaf children learn: what parents and teachers need to know.* Oxford University Press

B4 Fund of information and access
Dr Ben Holmes and Dr Sally Austen

Lack of knowledge can be easily confused with lack of ability but it is important to recognise the two are very different. When working with deaf people this is of particular importance as the experiences common to many deaf people can lead to reduced access, or opportunity, to acquire information.

A deaf person with above average intelligence may therefore still have gaps in knowledge. However, these gaps will in no way diminish the many skills that person will also have.

It is important to be aware that there may be times where additional information may be required because of knowledge gaps. Where gaps do exist these should be understood within the context of a person's experience and should not lead to global assumptions about ability.

Reduced opportunity
Some deaf people have experienced reduced opportunities to access information or experiences because of factors that may include:
- limited educational opportunity
- reduced opportunities for incidental learning
- over-protection of significant others

Educational opportunity (see also Chapter C6)
Formal learning situations can sometimes put deaf people at a great disadvantage when interpreters, clear lip speakers or adapted material is not available. Classroom environments do not always consider how a deaf person is accessing communication (e.g. how far they are from the person presenting). The difference in social opportunities present at school can also impact on how easily information is obtained.

Incidental learning
Much of what hearing people learn is attained incidentally: by 'overhearing' conversations, watching the TV, hearing it on the radio or through various written pieces. This is not available to many deaf people. Inequality in access to health information can have long term health impacts (see Chapter G1).

A late deafened person may also have a full fund of information from before they lost their hearing, but a lesser fund post deafness.

Overprotection
Many well-meaning family members or professionals may deliberately, or inadvertently, reduce exposure to situations where skills may be learned. Often this is because of an over-exaggerated perception of vulnerability and therefore the risk that person may be exposed to. However, this disproportionate awareness of risk then limits the opportunity to learn.

In later life, the lack of skill acquisition (e.g. being able to independently cook) at an age that would otherwise be expected can, not only, impact on independence but also might mistakenly be taken by others as an indicator of overall ability.

Reduced access
Unfortunately, it is the case that deaf people experience frequent barriers to information access (see also Chapters G1 & I9). Information via public amenities (such as theatres or libraries) can be disparate. Public services can also sometimes fail to provide information in an accessible way; a recent example of which is the lack of provision of a BSL interpreter during Covid-19 briefings by the British government.

However, even when adaptations are made to try and facilitate greater access, difficulties can still be encountered.

Subtitles are a really important inclusion which enable access for many people. However, this does not guarantee access for all people.
- Some people have lower levels of literacy and so reading subtitles at the speed they are presented can be difficult (see Chapter B3).
- Subtitles are not always completely accurate
- There may also be a lag, particularly in live events, between a person speaking and the subtitle being seen - this can impact on the ability to link information together (e.g. if a graph is being presented at the same time as a person speaks).

The effects of fatigue are also frequently under-considered. Hearing people may switch between watching and listening to a speaker without noticing they are doing so. Deaf people are much more reliant on vision for communication and reliance on sustained visual attention alone can be very fatiguing. Without adequate breaks there may be an impact on the amount of information that can effectively be attended to.

Information deprivation
Poor access to information not only affects knowledge acquisition but can also result in Information Deprivation Trauma (IDT). IDT is a relatively new concept that acknowledges that negative emotional responses, such as fear, helplessness or horror, can result from:
- a lack of understanding of the extent/magnitude/consequences/probability of a current or impending meaningful event; and
- an inability to access information about this event that would reasonably allow a person to prepare appropriately (Schild & Dalenberg, 2016)

For further information on IDT see Chapter F2

Reference
Schild, S. & Dalenberg, C.J. (2016). Information Deprivation Trauma: definition, assessment, and interventions. *Contextual features of trauma, 25 (8),* 873-889

B5 Theory of Mind
Dr Sally Austen

Theory of Mind (ToM) describes the ability to:
- understand that others may feel or think differently from us or have different information from us; and
- have the emotional ability to have an appropriately empathic reaction to the experience of the other person

ToM is crucial to cognitive planning, reasoning skills and empathy. Where it does not fully develop, interpersonal relationships and behaviour can be seriously affected.

The impact of good language access
It is well known that ToM difficulties often exist for people with Autistic Spectrum Disorders (ASD). It is less well known that fluent language acquisition creates the pathway to ToM and thus, those deaf children who have not experienced a language rich environment (see Chapters B1 & C2) are at risk of having difficulties with ToM.

Sometimes difficulties with ToM in deaf children or adults are misattributed to ASD (see Chapter E4 & E5). However, in the absence of ASD it is clear that language deprivation, and not being deaf, is linked to underdeveloped ToM. Research shows that deaf children of fluent deaf signing parents develop ToM at the same age as hearing children of hearing parents (around 3-5 years). However, deaf children of non-signing hearing parents often have significant delays in ToM.

Without fluent language access, it is difficult to achieve the degree of social interaction that children need to learn about the mental states of other people and how their behaviour may relate to these.

Where language access is limited, the conversational opportunities that exist can become very pragmatic and limited to functional information being provided. The effect of this is to reduce exposure to disagreements, and different perspectives, understanding how what is said may relate to an individual's emotional response and how they act for the rest of the day.

In order for anyone to develop ToM it is necessary, but not sufficient, for them to have access to this information. Without access to this 'language rich' environment it will be incredibly difficult to appreciate the mental state and behaviour of others: their motivation, emotion and cognitions.

Late Theory of Mind development

In situations where language access is the limiting factor affecting ToM development, the later provision of a good language environment is essential as ToM can still develop, at least to some degree. However, even where rich language access is later provided, and improvements may be seen to ToM, the effects of earlier ToM deficits could still be observed for many more years.

The missed opportunity to develop socially and cognitively owing to earlier ToM difficulties is likely to result in interpersonal difficulties, which could cause increased isolation, difficulties in groups or with authority figures (e.g. teachers), or limited opportunities for romantic relationships. Ongoing support to help with these other aspects of interpersonal difficulties may therefore still be required.

Accessing services

It appears that deaf adults with underdeveloped ToM are disproportionately represented in specialist services such as mental health, probation and forensics. Theory of Mind deficits significantly impact on behaviour (see Chapter F12) and restrict the type of interventions and therapies that are effective (see Chapters F7 & D3).

B6 Timelines
Dr Sally Austen and Dr Ben Holmes

Timelines enable a person to describe when something happened. A timeline is a concept that few people may have considered the importance of outside of clinical or care services. However, for clients that have experienced language deprivation (see Chapter B1), references to, and the use of, timelines can be significantly affected.

Whilst some clients who struggle with timelines may give you very little of the information you are trying to illicit, others cope by telling you their whole story from the beginning. This can be very time consuming and also mask the features of the narrative that are of particular significance to the client.

What timelines do

In English, verbs are adapted (e.g. the addition of -ed for past tense) to describe events through time. In BSL, time is represented by four different visualised timelines that run broadly from behind (past) to in front (future); low (younger) to high (older); and left (earlier) to right (later). Other cultures, in both sign and writing, may illustrate their timelines differently.

A timeline contains many complex pieces of information:
- When did something happen?
- When did it start?
- When did it stop?
- How long did it last?
- Was it concurrent with another event?
- How many times did it occur?
- What was the intensity of the event?
- How does it relate to other events that have occurred?

The ability to understand, recall and relate events is generally associated with cognitive ability. However, this is more complex when working with deaf people as, irrespective of cognitive ability, use of timelines can also be affected by language dysfluency and language deprivation (Chapter B1), poor information access (Chapter B4) and trauma experience (Chapter F2) - all of which deaf people are more likely to experience.

The importance of accurate timelines
Accessing appropriate services
The use of accurate timelines may influence how services are accessed and how help is provided. For example, in mental health settings having an accurate history of one's difficulties may determine diagnosis and influence treatment. Likewise, in legal settings, timelines are crucial to provide a statement about how someone has been mistreated by another.

Understanding consequences
The ability to interlink events through time is also central to understanding cause and effect, which has relevance to empathy, Theory of Mind (see Chapter B5) and consequently successful interpersonal interactions. For example, to understand why someone might be acting or feeling the way they do, comprehension of the potential impact of previous events is important.

Difficulties understanding cause and effect can act as a barrier to accessing psychotherapy where the ability to reflect on events over time is particularly important.

Example
Client: Why won't X talk to me?

Therapist: "Do you think they are still sad because of the things you said last week?"

Client: "That was before"

Therapist: "Maybe they are still sad?"

Client: "That's finished now, why won't they talk to me?"

Overcoming difficulties with timelines
If someone has difficulties with timelines, the information they are providing is not necessarily inaccurate – but you will need to take more time, and make adaptations to your way of working, to clarify information.

Additional preparation
Therapeutic work may require 'pre-therapy', to help develop an understanding of how events over time are connected and can affect oneself and others (see Chapter F7).

Communication adaptations and support
- Rephrase questions to see whether this gives the same, or different responses.
- Try representing things visually or with objects - literally a long drawn timeline, dating events the client can recall and describe.
- Consider using a deaf relay interpreter (see Chapter D4), to adapt information and questions to maximise your and your client's understanding.

Involve others
With consent, collect information from other sources: family, friends, previous professionals. This can help ensure the accuracy of what is discussed but can also aid you in helping your client to understand how events relate to each other.

B7 Abstract thought
Dr Ben Holmes and Dr Sally Austen

Abstract thought is best described in its contrast to concrete thought.

Concrete thinking, at its most extreme, means for a person to take things literally or to only be able to consider what is seen, experienced or physically around them but not what is beyond their view point.

Abstract thought encompasses being able to understand other's emotions, to make sense of consequences, to understand metaphors and to reflect (or think about thinking).

Development of abstract thought
Abstract thought usually develops slowly throughout childhood and into early adulthood. One of the first signs of abstract thought is a young child's ability to think of objects that are not in front of them, known as object permanence. From this develops the ability to consider, hypothesise and make predictions about what is not in front of them.

Most people have some level of abstract thinking. Where difficulties with abstract thought do exist these are normally related to cognitive impairment either through brain injury (see Chapter H1), intellectual disability (see Chapter E3) or autism (see Chapters E4 & E5). However, the continued development of abstract thought is also reliant on good language access. Language deprivation (see Chapter B1) can therefore also disrupt the development of this skill to varying degrees.

The lack of awareness of language deprivation in mainstream services means that when someone has abstract thought difficulties they can be misdiagnosed with other neurodevelopmental difficulties (see Chapter E1) when actually language and communication are the relevant factors that need to be considered (see Chapters B1 & C2).

Consequences
Where difficulties with abstract thought exist significant social difficulties can occur. This is because of the high level of overlap with cognitive skills underpinning socio-emotional functioning (e.g. Theory of Mind, empathy) and the ability to plan and problem solve (e.g. prospective understanding

of events yet to occur, the ability to generalise learning to new situations, an understanding of cause and effect) that are generally considered to fall under the umbrella term of executive functioning.

Client: That man laughed at me so I hit him.
Professional: What would have happened if you had walked away.
Client: I didn't walk away, I hit him.

Abstract thought can also impact on an individual's understanding of what is expected of them in any given situation which may leave them vulnerable to difficulties in other areas of life (e.g. the ability to engage with services, financial planning). This is because the concepts that underpin many skills (e.g. understanding boundaries and social rules, validating or empathising with feelings, predicting that which has not yet happened) are based on abstract reasoning whereas expected or appropriate behaviour for a situation can be rehearsed or learnt.

It is therefore possible for someone with difficulties with abstract thought to function completely independently in a given situation. However, it may be difficult for this same person to adapt to a new situation, or changing expectations, without support to develop a new routine or set of responses that can be learned.

Identifying difficulties with abstract thought
When meeting with a deaf client it is essential that the right interpreters are booked to ensure that communication is accessible (see Chapters D14 & D5). Without this, it is possible that a client's answers may appear limited when the limit is being caused by you failing to provide access to communication rather than the client having any cognitive difficulty.

For example, if a person that uses British Sign Language (BSL) is engaged in an assessment through written English the possibility of BSL word order being used, or lower literacy levels (see Chapter B3), may give the indication of a lower level of ability than is the case because the person is not being assessed in the right language.

However, even with the right communication support in place, identifying difficulties with abstract can still be hard:

Well rehearsed conversations

When you first meet your client, it is likely that you will discuss topics that are well rehearsed and factual. For example, the presenting problem, the history of the presenting problem and what has been tried before.

Although not all clients are good with Timelines (see Chapter B6) many will present their chronology with impressive accuracy. However, when you introduce abstract concepts you may see this ability crumble.

Client: I found out my husband was having an affair, so I kicked him out.
Professional: If your husband had not had an affair, do you think your relationship would have survived?
Client: He did have an affair.

Acquiescence ('nodding')

For many deaf people that have had very negative experiences of (usually hearing) services, or become accustomed to poor communication access, they may be keen to end an interaction so that they can be left alone or wish to hide the fact that they do not understand. This can lead to very brief answers being given that may make it difficult to fully assess the level of abstract thought that person is capable of (see Chapter B2).

Working with interpreters

Many interpreters will be experienced in working with non-fluent signers (see Chapter D3) and clients who struggle with abstract concepts.

Unless told otherwise, the interpreters will 'unpack concepts' for the client, meaning that the non-signing professional may not be aware how much of the translation from English to BSL also included a translation from abstract to concrete. This can lead to professionals overestimating a client's understanding of more complex concepts.

Hearing professional: Did you get into debt because of the monthly car payments?

Interpreter: You bought the car and agreed to pay money every month. Every month did you have enough money or not enough? Not enough money means now you have Debt. Debt means when you get money you have to pay it straight to the car dealer. Is that right?

Client: Yes that is right.

Although the client has ultimately given the correct answer the professional may assume that, prior to the interpretation, the client fully understood the concept of overspending and debt. In some conversations the professional missing this detail may not matter (e.g. a client asking to open a savings account). However, in other situations (e.g. assessing Capacity to independently manage finances) this information is crucial.

For professionals that need to gather factual (concrete) information, as well as understand their client's broader abilities and difficulties, the (usually extremely empathic) interpreter will understand this conflicted position and be willing to work with you to achieve the most informed outcome possible. As such, they will benefit from you being explicit about the detail and depth required within the consultation before starting.

The language fluency of the professional

To assess the fluency or conceptual complexity of a person's language, the professional leading the assessment must have a higher degree of fluency and conceptual complexity in that language than the person being assessed. This may be achieved with the help of language service professionals (see chapters D1 – 13). However, most likely, deaf professionals and professionals with deaf expertise will be required to assess this further (see Chapters G3 & G4).

It is the responsibility of the professional completing the assessment to ensure that the communication and linguistic arrangements are sufficient to make valid judgements about the ability of the person being assessed.

B8 Locus of control
Dr Ben Holmes and Dr Sally Austen

Locus of control describes a person's sense of their own autonomy. Someone with an internal locus of control believes that their decisions and actions will determine the outcome of events. Someone with an external locus of control believes that outside forces determine life's outcomes; for example luck, fate or the intervention of other people.

For all people, there is a spectrum of perceived locus of control. It is something that can change throughout life and may vary in degree according to specific situations faced or the actions and reactions of other people. However, life experiences can have a significant impact on how an individual learns about their degree of personal control.

Unfortunately, many deaf and hard of hearing people have experienced discrimination (Chapter G1), patronisation (Chapters F1 & C10) and overprotection. Through these life experiences, they may learn to expect that:
- decisions are often made by others
- there may be little or no consequence to actions taken (Chapter F12)
- individual power or agency is limited

Additionally, poor educational opportunity (Chapter C6) and poor access to information (Chapter B4) can result in limited understanding of individual rights. This can lead to deaf and hard of hearing people not knowing that they have protected rights in given situations. Even when they express these rights, it does not always lead to those rights being acted on by others (see Chapters G1 & I9).

The impact of locus of control on health behaviours
Locus of control can impact on how people engage with services, their expectation of professionals and what interventions might help.

An individual with an internal locus of control will be more likely to take responsibility for making changes to health behaviours. Someone with an external locus of control will be more likely to project the responsibility onto someone else.

Locus of control is a factor that can have particular relevance to engagement in psychological therapies. Clients with an internal locus of control are more likely to see themselves as an active partner. They may engage more effectively in 'homework' between sessions and seek behaviour change independently.

Example: "I was feeling low in mood recently and so I started walking my neighbour's dog every day to get more exercise - I've always loved being outdoors"

Those with an external locus of control may be more likely to see themselves as a passive 'patient' that is a recipient of treatment.

Example: "I am sad because my flat is too small, and my social worker hasn't sorted it yet."

It is important to be aware of the life experiences that your deaf or hard of hearing client may have been exposed to, that could have influenced their locus of control.

Sporadic attendance or limited engagement are often interpreted as a lack of interest or desire to change, resulting in swift discharge – often before the client has even been seen. Access to health services for many deaf and hard of hearing people is already fraught with enough difficulty (see Chapter G1).

Instead, consideration should be given to whether locus of control may be an additional factor influencing choices made, that requires separate intervention. Providing access to information (e.g. about rights), interventions that build self-confidence and perceived agency, and support to access those services that can facilitate independence may be needed.

Section C

C1 Communication and language - some definitions
Dr Ben Holmes and Dr Sally Austen

Communication refers to the interchange of message or information from one person to another, either verbally or non-verbally.

Verbal communication is the exchange of information from one person to another using spoken, written or signed language[2].

Nonverbal communication includes vocalisation, gesture, body language, facial expression, touch.

Oral refers to something that is spoken.

Aural refers to something that is heard.

Pre-lingual refers to the period before fluent language is attained (approximately 3-5 years of age).

Post-lingual means the period by which fluent language should have been acquired. Insufficient exposure to language during the pre-lingual period reduces the brain's ability to acquire fluent language post-lingually, in line with reduced neural plasticity (see Chapter C2).

Language is a communication tool. It is defined as a system of conventional spoken, manual, or written symbols by means of which human beings, as members of a social group and participants in its culture, express themselves. The functions of language include communication, the expression of identity, play, imaginative expression, and emotional release (Encyclopaedia Brittanica, 2020).

Sign language. As above, in sign languages these symbols may be hand or body movements, gestures or facial expressions.

---

[2] There is debate about whether signed languages are verbal or whether this term should only refer to spoken language. As in many clinical contexts the term verbal is used to refer to information that is presented linguistically (e.g. verbal memory test), and sign language is equivalent to spoken language, the term verbal will be used as defined above in this book.

Preferred language is the language that a person chooses to use. This may be because it is their most fluent, the one that most represents their identity, for political reasons or just because it makes them happy.

First language is an Individual's most fluent language. A client's First Language may not be the same as the professional's (e.g. the client's First Language is BSL; the professional's First Language is English). The professional may not work in their First Language (e.g. the professional's First Language is Urdu; the client's First Language is English).

Native language. The language of the country that someone is born in or native to. The official native minority languages of the UK are Cornish, Irish, Scots, Ulster Scots, Scottish Gaelic, Welsh, Manx-Gaelic and British Sign Language.

The official **Right** to use any of these native languages is not necessarily matched in practice by resources or national acceptance.

Immigrant language
Referring to the languages of non-native people. There is debate as to how long a language has to be in any country before it becomes another distinct 'native' language or has sufficiently morphed into the original language such that the two languages are now one.

'Mother tongue'
A colloquial term for the first language the person learnt as a baby, often because it was the primary language used in the home environment. This term is no longer recommended due to its gender specificity. Additionally, within deaf discussion fora it is contested as it suggests spoken language over sign.

Heritage language user
A heritage language user has acquired the language used at home, that is a minority language compared to that used in surrounding wider society.

Heritage signer
A heritage signer is someone who has acquired sign language as a baby from their deaf parents. They could be deaf or hearing. This term can be used as an alternate to the commonly used term CODA (Child of Deaf Adults) (see Chapter C4), which tended to be applied to hearing children only.

Bilingual
Having two fluent languages, which often requires exposure to both languages in the pre-lingual phase of brain development.

Second language
Usually refers to a language learnt post-lingually that may not quite reach the point of fluency even if the individual can use the language highly effectively. This is because the brain has reduced neural plasticity in the post-lingual phase to allow the full development of certain features of the language that a fluent or native language user would have.

Available language
Two or more people using whatever mixture of shared language they have.

Dialect
A dialect is generally a form of a language that is specific to a region or social group and usually has differences in pronunciation/sign production, grammar, syntax and vocabulary.

Accent
An accent refers to how people pronounce words or produce signs.

References
https://www.britannica.com/topic/language

C2 Language acquisition
Dr Kate Rowley

Most babies are born with the ability to acquire language, with the exception of those with severe cognitive impairments. If exposed to language, any language, most babies will develop both language comprehension and productive skills. However, if a child is deprived of language due to extreme neglect, abuse or the inability to access the language that surrounds them, they will not develop language. Babies and children need to be exposed to language in order to acquire it.

In good language environments (i.e. access to good adult and child models of language), most babies develop language skills following very similar timetables. For example, most babies will produce their first word at around 10 to 14 months of age. By the age of 18 months, they can produce around 70-80 words. At around 2 years of age, most children will start talking about past events, which shows emerging narrative skills (i.e. the ability to tell stories). By the time children are 3 years old, they will understand and produce around 500 words. At 5 years, most children will have mastered the grammar of the language they have been exposed to since birth. Children continue to develop their language skills throughout the primary school years, developing a deeper understanding of grammatical constructions and acquiring more vocabulary.

Several things can influence the ages and stages of language acquisition. For example, the main carer's level of education and socio-economic status (SES) can influence vocabulary acquisition. Children born into families with higher educational qualifications and SES usually develop larger vocabularies. Other things such as early reading, the frequency in which main carers read with their children, also influences language skills in young children. Early exposure to good language models, as well as early reading, are important predictors in the development of good literacy skills (reading and writing) and academic achievement.

Babies born deaf often struggle to develop good language skills. This is because most babies are born to hearing parents (around 90 to 95%) that do not know sign language. Due to the nature of deafness, deaf babies cannot access spoken language fully, even with the support of hearing technologies (see Chapter B1). However, deaf babies exposed to sign language do go on to develop good language skills and do so following a similar trajectory to those acquiring spoken languages.

For example, deaf babies acquiring sign languages will produce their first sign at around 10 to 12 months of age, produce around 70-80 signs at 18 months and be able to understand and produce 500 signs by the time they are 3 years of age. They also develop narrative skills in a very similar fashion to hearing children acquiring spoken languages. Early sign language fluency and exposure are also important predictors for developing good literacy skills and academic achievement.

As with spoken languages, there are several factors that can influence the ages and stages of sign language acquisition including the main carer's level of education and SES. Furthermore, sign language fluency also can impact sign language acquisition. For example, if parents are not fluent in sign language, their child's vocabulary tends to be smaller compared to those who are exposed to fluent models of sign language. They also seem to have less complex phonological and grammatical systems.

As many families of deaf children do not know sign language, there are many alternative communication strategies that families can adopt to ensure their deaf child picks up language. Deaf children need to look at people in order to communicate, whether this is via speech or sign. Thus, in the first year of life, families should spend time establishing eye contact, teaching their deaf babies to look at them as much as possible. This can be done by playing games such as peek-a-boo, tickling games, as well as waiting for your child to look at you before communicating with them. To gain their attention, you can use touch (tap on their body), visual strategies (e.g. wave in their line of sight etc.). If the child has hearing aids fitted and can make use of sound, you can call for their attention but do not try to communicate with them without them looking at you. They need to learn to look to communicate. As deaf children get older, those with a lot of useful hearing may learn to communicate without looking but this is not likely to be for extended periods of time. As mentioned earlier, hearing technologies do not make deaf children hearing. They still need to combine visual and sound based information to make sense of things.

All families with deaf children should also make use of gestures in order to communicate with their deaf child. To do this, you can point at objects and then tell them what it is once they look at you, you can also show objects, use facial expressions and some iconic gestures for 'eat', 'drink', 'hungry' etc. to communicate. It is important for families to learn a few key signs such as signs for 'mummy', 'daddy', 'park', 'sleep' etc. to make sure that deaf children develop an understanding of the relationships between form (words, signs and/or gestures) and the meanings associated with them. Once they have established this relationship, it will be far easier for them to pick up new vocabulary. This will help deaf children to develop spoken language, if they are able, once they are fitted with cochlear implants, should families decide to take this route. A deaf child that knows the sign for 'mummy', the gesture for 'drink' or 'eat', is much more likely to be able to associate the spoken word for those signs and/or gestures compared to a child that does not know them.

However, if for any reason, deaf children are unable to make use of their hearing, if you have used a combination of communication methods as described above, they will have developed some language skills. They can then build upon this and go on to develop full language(s). This will support them in their literacy and education. Families should ensure that their deaf child has regular contact with deaf adult role models, as well as deaf peers. This will give their deaf child more opportunities to develop important language skills. Furthermore, meeting other deaf adults and peers benefits the wellbeing of the deaf child and their families. The deaf child feels as if they are not the only one and families can see other deaf children and adults successfully navigating their way through life, which can be very reassuring.

The take home message here is that, most children will develop good language skills if they are given the opportunities to do so and this includes deaf children. Spoken language is not fully accessible for deaf children thus it is the responsibility of families and practitioners to ensure that deaf children are exposed to a language that is accessible to them. This means exposing them to sign languages and/or gestures in the early years. They also need to adopt effective communication strategies with their deaf child (e.g. eye contact, pointing, gesturing). Doing so will prevent language deprivation, which has severe and long-term consequences on language, cognition and mental wellbeing.

Further reading
Rowley, K. (2020). *Sign Language Acquisition.* In S. Hupp & J. Jewell (Eds.), The Encyclopedia of Child and Adolescent Development. Wiley Blackwell
Rowley, K., Dumbrill, H., & MacSweeney, M. (2019). The brain needs Language. https://www.youtube.com/watch?v=bV7QD2NOS24

C3 Newborn hearing screen
Dr Sally Austen and Dr Kate Rowley

The NHSP (Universal Newborn Hearing Screening Programme) started in 2001 and was available to 100% of the UK by 2006.

What happens?
The test is conducted, either in hospital, home or community clinic, in the first few weeks of life. A small ear bud, put in the baby's ear, records what the baby is able to hear.

There are two objective tests (meaning the baby is not required to indicate that they have heard). The first is called Otoacoustic Emissions (OAE). If the baby does not show any response to this test it may either be repeated or an Automated Auditory Brainstem Response (AABR) test will be carried out.

All babies who have been in a Special Care Baby Unit (SCBU) for 48 hours or longer, or where there is a known risk of them having a hearing loss, will have both tests done.

Early diagnosis
Prior to the newborn hearing screen, the average age of diagnosis of deafness (that was severe enough to compromise speech and language development) was 26 months, with hearing aid fitting at 32.2 months.

Amplification, using hearing aids gave access to sound, but the late start meant that the critical period for good speech and language acquisition was passed. Many of these children did not acquire good speech and oral language due to a lack of access to the surrounding language, and the average reading age of a deaf school leaver was equivalent to that of an 8 year old hearing child.

The effect of NHSP has been to significantly lower the age of confirmation of deafness. The vast majority of congenitally deaf children have their hearing loss confirmed by 6 months of age, with many identified within the first 4 weeks of life.

Early identification and habilitation, in children pre 9 months of age, has been shown to improve speech and language development, and thus later reading age, as well as social-emotional development - with the best results for those identified within the first 2 months of life. However, it is important to remember that many deaf children still struggle to acquire language and good literacy skills as hearing technologies do not provide them with full access to spoken language.

Post screening
The implementation of NHSP included a broader brief to try and ensure identified children were appropriately managed for the first 3 years of life by:
- promoting precise standards of practice and performance
- providing an educational program for involved professionals
- developing a close working relationship with the National Deaf Children's Society that resulted in the development of comprehensive information leaflets and support for parents

At the same time as the inception of NHSP other programs started to take effect:
- MCHA (Modernising Children's Hearing Aids) introduced digital hearing aids into the UK for all children, with consistently high standards of fitting and maintenance of hearing aid care.
- Increasing confidence in, and acceptance of, cochlear implants for children who were diagnosed early reduced the age of implantation. This was to try and maximise opportunities for accessing speech signals for deaf children with severe to profound deafness.
- Consistent investigation into the cause of each child's deafness and related aetiological training for medics.

Again, it is important to note that despite those initiatives, there are still many gaps and improvements to be made. Many deaf children still lag behind their hearing peers and the support families receive vary depending on where they live.

Sign language
The NHSP promotes early identification of deafness. Early identification improves language development in either oral or signed languages. Although the NHSP pathway is an audiological one with success being

measured in speech and hearing ability, some families of early identified children will decide to communicate with their babies using sign language. However, the majority of audiological professionals (and other parent role models) will have knowledge of spoken languages and little experience to impart knowledge of sign language.

Co-working between NHSP and National Deaf Children's Society (a charity, who can offer professional skills in speech or sign) is beneficial. However, there still appears to be an imbalance in this, with signing less well represented.

It is crucial that deaf professionals are employed to advise about sign language. There appears to be a gap in service provision, with no obvious place for families to turn to for advice regarding sign language.

Psychological impact of the test on the parents
When the NHSP test was being developed, consultation with a group of specialist psychologists, who worked with deaf people, recommended the test not be done in the first two to three weeks, to allow the parents time to adjust to life as a parent, recover physically and, most importantly, to bond with the child.

This was not adhered to, partly because maternity hospital offers mass testing availability, reducing the resources needed for community testing or the risk of parents failing to attend assessment appointments; and partly because the tinier the baby, the more likely they are to lie completely still, thus reducing the chance of false positive results.

It is well researched (Kentish, 2007) that diagnosis of deafness, particularly for hearing parents, can be experienced as traumatic and have negative effects on attachment and parenting style. Thus, such early diagnosis, often in the first few hours of life, whilst having audiological and linguistic benefits as described above, the parents' psychological need may not be so well supported.

This may be in part due to the way the news is shared to parents. Many audiologists use negative terms such as, 'I'm sorry' ,'bad news,' 'diagnosed' (a term associated with serious illness) etc. In addition, they may not provide a positive outlook on the child's future. If parents are informed of their child's hearing loss/deafness in a more positive manner, involving deaf role models, parents often feel more positive about their deaf child's future.

For a deaf professional led explanation of the impact of early identification of hearing status, see the following:
https://www.youtube.com/watch?v=h5ZqKMgXciU

It is potentially alienating for deaf people to be labelled as a having 'failed' to hear, and yet, this is the very wording offered in the NHSP literature. The rate of false positives (caused by background noise during the test, the baby moving, or temporary blockage of their ears) is quite common.

Summary
The benefit of very early diagnosis needs to be balanced with the benefit of leaving non life-threatening diagnoses until the parents have had a chance to enjoy and bond with their baby.

For further information see:
Katherine Harrop-Griffiths (2016). The impact of universal newborn hearing screening. https://adc.bmj.com/content/101/1/1

References
Kentish, R (2007). Deafness and challenging behaviour in the young deaf child in Austen, S and Jeffery, Deafness and Challenging Behaviour. The 360° Perspective, 75-88. Wiley

Pimperton, H., Blythe, H., & Kreppner, J., Mahon, M., Peacock, J.L., Stevenson, J., Terlektski, E., Worsfold, S., Yuen, H.M., & Kennedy, C.R. (2016). The impact of newborn hearing screening on long term literacy outcomes: a prospective study. Archives of Disability in Childhood, 101, 9-15

C4 Children with deaf parents
Professor Jemina Napier and Dr Ben Holmes

A common term that is used to describe children with deaf parents is 'Coda', which is short for a Child of Deaf Adult(s) and refers to someone who has either one or two deaf parents but is not deaf themselves. This is an assimilated American term. The less used British equivalent is HMFD (pronounced Her-Muff-Der): replicating the way a hearing child with deaf parents may describe themselves in BSL - 'Hearing me, Mother Father Deaf'. There is also another emerging term: 'Person from a Deaf Family', that captures any person that lives in a family with at least one deaf person and uses sign language at home (parents, siblings, partners, etc.).

It is commonly reported that around 90%-95% of children born to deaf parents are hearing. There are no known recent statistics that confirm this number, but the assumption is made based on statistics that reveal the numbers of deaf children born to deaf parents.

Many Codas have parents that sign, so the primary language used within the home may well be sign language meaning that child will be a 'native' sign language user. Thus, a more recent term used to describe Codas is that of 'heritage signers'. This is to recognise the equivalence between Codas and 'heritage language speakers' who grow up using the language of their parents at home that is not widely used in the society they live in. As such, these children could be considered as bicultural as well as bilingual. Living in both the hearing and deaf worlds brings both advantages and challenges for heritage signers in terms of their identity.

Heritage signer identity
When parents use sign language and identify as culturally deaf, their hearing children will participate in signing Deaf community activities from a young age, and so may be enculturated themselves to deaf cultural norms and behaviours. However, as they start to experience other settings, such as school, and realise some of the differences between themselves and their parents they may also start to identify with aspects of the hearing world and the use of speech.

The fact that having deaf parents is a critical part of the intersectional identity of Coda/heritage signers is not always recognised (especially by hearing non-signers). Consequently, the person themselves may not realise that they have a bicultural identity until quite late on in their life, if at all. For this child, their parents are deaf and that is a fact that they accept without further consideration as it is a natural part of their experience.

I don't think it makes me feel any different from others who have hearing parents. Yeah, it's just normal. I haven't experienced anything else. (Quote from teenage heritage signer, in Napier, 2021)

However, having a shared experience with other heritage signers can be very valuable, which can be facilitated through support organisations, such as CODA UK and Ireland who organise activities to bring young heritage signers together to explore the what it means to have deaf parents and use sign language.

This bilingual-bicultural heritage can create a tension between feeling advantaged as it provides a greater range of access and experiences in life, but also feeling challenged as they may feel they sit 'in-between' worlds, identifying with both but not fully belonging to either.

Heritage signers as brokers
Being bilingual and bicultural means that heritage signers may deliberately or inadvertently find themselves mediating between their deaf parents and hearing non-signers, often through language and cultural brokering; essentially interpreting between their parents and others. Although it is understandable why children may take on this role as it is a natural instinct to help their parents (and they often offer), it is not always age appropriate or in contexts that are appropriate for a child or family member to be involved.

Despite the existence of professional sign language interpreting services, professionals (e.g. teachers, GPs, solicitors) regularly fail to book professional sign language interpreters, either because they do not know that is expected, how to book, or who pays for a professional interpreter (see Chapter D5); instead, they expect family members who can sign to broker for their deaf parent or sibling. When an appointment is for a hearing child, accompanied by a deaf parent, the absence of an interpreter leaves the child to interpret information about themselves to their parents.

Deaf parents may also make brokering requests of their children. Many situations are low-stakes, such as ordering food in a restaurant or passing a message to a friendly neighbour. However, others may involve children in more high-stakes contexts, such as telephone calls about medical, financial or emotional issues. Even if deaf parents acknowledge that their children should ideally not broker for them, it is sometimes inevitable.

Yeah they asked [me to make phonecalls]... make appointments and that. None of it stands out in my mind... you just did it. Just like going to the shops for them, you know... go and make a phonecall. Ring work and tell them I'm not coming in, or whatever... (Quote from adult heritage signer, in Napier, 2021)

Whilst it may be that there at times where these arrangements are acceptable for all, people can make assumptions about whether the child is either willing or able to broker without checking with them. This may leave the heritage signer and/or the deaf parents feeling pressured to accept the arrangement even if either or both parties are not satisfied with it. This assumption ignores the potential for the child to be exposed to information that is cognitively or emotionally inappropriate for their age, or where they are forced to accept conflicted roles.

It is known that heritage signers frequently broker in a range of situations. As such, through early onset and repeat exposure the role may be accepted without question as the experience becomes 'normal'. However, the potential emotional impact of these experiences and the need for support following events where they feel uncomfortable or pressurised is rarely considered. As such, this may result in negative consequences for the child in terms of their mental and emotional wellbeing.

Heritage signers' wellbeing
The emotional burden that can be associated with a brokering role can impact on mental wellbeing. However, the failure of services to recognise the needs of heritage signers means that support can be lacking.

In the specialist National Deaf Child and Adolescent Mental Health Services (see Chapter G3) referrals are accepted for children with deaf parents. This recognises that these children may need specialist expertise from professionals who work with signing deaf people to understand the issues for them, so that the most culturally appropriate care is provided.

Some adult heritage signers prefer to access mental health services with experience of working with deaf people so that a) they do not have to teach their therapist what it means to have a bilingual-bicultural identity because they have deaf parents and b) they may prefer to access that therapy in their first language, British Sign Language (BSL).

The wellbeing of heritage signers may also be impacted by their experience of either witnessing or directly experiencing stigmatising and shaming statements about their parents' deafness or signing. This is particularly acute when the shamer has seen a signing family but fails to appreciate that one of those family members can actually hear what is being said. Many heritage signers describe being teased or bullied at school for having deaf parents. Even when not explicit, stigmatisation results in many children with deaf parents having negative experiences at school or in their peer group (e.g. not being invited to parties or not having their parents access their school plays).

"I remember my daughter when she was younger feeling worried as she was always asked by her friends why I was deaf and why we signed. I tried to encourage her bit by bit that she could be proud of that and it didn't matter that I was deaf." (Quote from deaf mother, in Napier, 2021)

Linguistic and socio-cognitive development
All children are shaped, linguistically, socially, cognitively and emotionally, in part, by those around them. For hearing and deaf children with deaf parents there is positive research showing that the exposure to fluent sign language in the home from an early age enables them to develop rapidly, often faster that their peers, in language, behaviour and Theory of Mind (see Chapters B5 & C2). This is also the case with other bilingual children (with spoken languages). So being bilingual and bicultural, and engaging in brokering, can be an asset that they take with them into their adult lives.

Looking back I feel blessed for several reasons... 1) I know how to solve problems and make good decisions, 2) being truly bilingual has expanded my cognitive and perceptual world, 3) I am comfortable with people from other cultures and support their struggles for justice and equality; 4) I value honesty and direct/clear communication... (Quote from adult heritage signer, in Napier, 2021).

However, for some children (hearing or deaf), language acquisition may be impeded if there is insufficient access to language role models at home (either in signed, spoken or written languages; see Chapter B1). Additional services, such as Speech and Language Therapy and earlier attendance at nursery school, can be provided. However, for some children this is not sufficient or does not last long enough. If deaf parents cannot access the school curriculum, for example, either through lack of interpreters or through having had poor educational experience themselves, then they may struggle to support their child through their education.

Support for heritage signers
Sharing experiences with other heritage signers can be very valuable. This is facilitated through organisations such as CODA UK and Ireland, who organise activities to bring young heritage signers together to explore what it means to have deaf parents and use sign language, as well as to help them understand their bilingual-bicultural identity. The organisations also host conferences and workshops for adult heritage signers to share their experiences. These organisations work alongside deaf parent support groups such as Deaf Parenting UK, to provide opportunities for deaf parents to explore challenges in mixed deaf-hearing families.

Furthermore, there is a growing awareness of the unique needs of heritage signers and some services are starting to provide specific support to promote emotional wellbeing for them.

Resources
CODA UK and ireland - www.codaukireland.co.uk
CODA international - www.code-international.org
Deaf Parenting UK - www.deafparent.org.uk

References
Bishop, M., & Hicks, S. (2008). (Eds.). *Hearing, Mother Father Deaf: Hearing people in deaf families.* Washington, DC: Gallaudet University Press
Napier, J. (2021). *Sign language brokering in deaf-hearing families.* London: Palgrave
Preston, P. (1994). *Mother Father Deaf: Living Between Sound and Silence.* Cambridge, MA: Harvard University Press

C5 Oral v manual debate
Dr Sally Austen

It is a shame that this chapter even exists in the 21st century.

Despite the complex definitions and differences of Language (see Chapter C1) most clinical, educational and commissioning decisions on how to enable and educate deaf children take a binary position:

Spoken English versus British Sign Language (BSL).

Constructively, both sides of the debate agree on a number of factors
- Fluent language acquisition is the ultimate goal.
- Fluent language use enables literacy and other cognitive skills
- Attempting to use two languages simultaneously, as in Sign Supported English, results in a poor quality of both BSL and speech and does not benefit long term language acquisition.
- Learning to be fluent in two languages (separately) is beneficial to cognitive and social development.
- Fluent language must be attained, before approximately the age 5, whilst the language centres of the brain have sufficient plasticity.
- The term 'Verbal skills' refers to the use of language in either speech or sign.

Areas that the two sides disagree on:
Oral: there is enough evidence of technology (hearing aids, cochlear implants etc.) successfully enabling deaf babies and children to access sound, that fluent speech and hearing is a realistic aim.

BSL: there are enough examples of deaf children having language deprivation that the attempt and then failure to facilitate their use of speech and hearing, followed by accessing BSL post lingually, is not good enough.

Oral: with the right technology and support, deaf children can successfully integrate with their hearing peers.

BSL: deaf children benefit more from the shared language and culture of BSL, and experience isolation when striving to fit in with others who are not their peer group.

Silo mentality
It is human nature to surround ourselves with those that agree with us, rather than embrace diversity of thinking. Instead of observing and learning from those with different experience, we tend to avoid those whose views differ from us - and evolve blinkered and blaming cultures.

At the 1880 Second International Congress on Education of the Deaf, in Milan, it was agreed that signed education be entirely replaced by oral education. Educators banning signing in schools passionately believed they were helping. Deaf people who were consequently punished for signing at school described this as unhelpful. Of the 164 delegates at the Milan Conference, only one was deaf. Perhaps outcomes would have differed had the conference been more diverse.

When cochlear implants were first being trialed in the UK, some deaf people protested against what they viewed as unnecessary physical risks for what they saw as the implementation of a eugenic like audiological improvements in children who were unable to consent for themselves. Many deaf people were happy to place themselves as boycotters and protesters, but few were invited or offered themselves as deaf consultants (voluntary or paid).

Where passionate, hard-working people remain in opposing silos and resist amalgamating, we do not get the best from either side - and the client misses out on the benefits of their joint curiosity and study.

Marschark et al. (2016), summarised it perfectly:
'The insistence of many in the field that 'the one true path' is before us does not change the fact that both history and the existing literature tell us that many paths are needed, even if our goal of optimizing education opportunities and outcomes for all DHH learners is the same'.

References
Marschark M., Lampropoulou, V., & Skordilis E.K. (Eds) (2016). Diversity in Deaf Education, 2016. Oxford University Press: New York

C6 Deaf education: past, present and future
Dr Kate Rowley and Dr Sally Austen

When describing their schooling, your deaf client may use names and concepts that are specific to the deaf experience. This chapter aims to provide a frame of reference for the history that your client may provide.

Deaf specialist boarding schools

Those born prior to 1960s are most likely to have been educated in specialist deaf boarding schools. The choice offered to their parents would have been either a Deaf boarding school or local (hearing) primary school.

Costs and benefits

Assuming that their parents couldn't sign, and the local school had no specialist deaf provision, the Deaf boarding schools took children from the age of 3. At the time this was understood to give children access to language from a young age, although we now know that 3 is far too late for a child to start to receive good language input. Often, when the child left home, they had no idea where they were going or whether they would ever return. Many clients describe leaving for boarding school as traumatic.

Children would be taken to and from school in taxis at the beginning and end of term. Many describe abuse from other children they shared the taxi with, and occasionally from the taxi driver.

The benefits of these schools were the strong sense of identity and allegiance that children developed, so much so that some sign language features are specific to particular schools. Many deaf people's first question to each other is which school they went to. The psychosocial value of a peer group of cognitive and linguistic equals is immense. However, prevalence of abuse was high in some Deaf boarding schools, usually starting with abuse by a teacher and continuing with abuse by older or stronger peers (see Chapter F2).

Children being abused had no way of phoning home, as this was prior to the invention of video or visual technology; and even if there had been their call home would have been monitored by staff. Many never shared a full language with their parents so could not even explain what was happening to them when they went home for holidays.

Some children took exams at 16, few stayed on to 18. Deaf people in this period were more likely to carry out vocational training due to the inaccessibility of further and/or higher education.

Communication
Throughout the years of deaf education, and within each type of school, the 'oral-manual' debate will have influenced whether children were taught using a strict oral policy (not allowing deaf children to learn sign language and/or to be taught in sign language) (see Chapter C5).

Most schools insisted on oral communication. Thus, the levels of educational (and pastoral) access varied amongst individuals depending on their ability to lipread and use residual hearing. However, in most oral schools children used sign language outside of the classroom. They would usually learn sign from the minority of deaf children who had deaf parents and mostly had to sign secretly to avoid punishment.

Some boarding schools adopted a total communication policy, where teachers would use British Sign Language (BSL) signs along with spoken English. Signs would follow English word order. Levels of access varied across individuals, as total communication is often quite taxing and most teachers were not able to sign fluently. Thus, for many deaf people, the language of instruction remained inaccessible. The small number of schools that purported to use sign language in the classroom, rarely employed fluent signers. Thus, for the most part, deaf individuals rarely received a good education.

Those deaf adults who are well educated may well have attended one of the few selective schools for deaf children. To get into such schools, deaf children had to take an exam (similar to the 11+ exams for hearing children) and then be interviewed. Such schools were mostly oral and most deaf people left with relatively good educational qualifications - often because they arrived at the school with age-appropriate language and cognitive skills, or because they had greater abilities in lipreading and use of residual hearing.

Hearing Impaired Resource Bases (HIRBs)
Formally known as PHUs (Partial Hearing Unit), HIRBs were also known as:
- A deaf specialist unit, usually attached to a mainstream school
- Deaf unit

Those born in the 1960s, 1970s and part of 1980s were increasingly likely to have received their primary education in local mainstreams schools with a resource base providing specialist input. However, many still attended secondary schools for the deaf.

HIRBs allowed deaf children to be educated in a deaf environment when necessary and to gradually be integrated in the hearing school as they became more skilled or confident. HIRBs allow deaf children to be educated closer to home (travelling mostly by taxi) rather than go to a boarding school many hours away.

For some children this was, (and is) a positive experience of being supported in both the deaf and hearing world. However, HIRBs are generally quite small and deaf groups are generally very heterogeneous. So, although there may have been 10 deaf children, the range of ages and abilities could mean that the deaf child still had no real peer group.

Mainstreamed or integrated education
Over time, especially those born in the 1990s or later are most likely to have been educated in mainstream schools for the majority of their education.

Most boarding schools closed and mainstreaming increased. This was promoted so that children could be taught in their own home community. However, it appears that local authorities will often favour local provisions with minimal support over sending deaf children out of borough to specialist provisions that better meet their needs, because it is cheaper.

Mainstream or Integrated schooling is often promoted as an opportunity for deaf children to experience equality. However, in order for mainstreaming to work two things are crucial:

1. That the child has a peer group
Integration is nothing more than tokenism if that child has no one with whom they can relate, communicate and play. Many deaf children remain isolated in hearing schools. Those that use interpreters or communication support workers often build more of a relationship, and spend more time, with that adult than they do with the other children.

2. That the placement is appropriately resourced
In order for oral education to work, deaf related knowledge and resources are crucial. Deaf children need loop systems, FM systems, Teachers for the Deaf, whole schools that had deaf awareness training, SENCO support, teachers that will talk to them face to face – not talk while facing the board, staff that know how to replace hearing aid batteries, staff that are willing and able to stop two people talking at once to allow the deaf child to follow what is being said.

Where sign language is used in the classroom and/or playground, the deaf child needs peers, teachers and Teachers of the Deaf who can sign. While some schools provide CSWs/TAs that will translate from English to BSL in the classroom, the majority are not able to sign fluently and are not qualified to interpret. This gives the 'illusion of inclusion', as people around the child believe their needs are being met and that they are following all that goes on in the classroom.

Further specialist resources, both internal and external are required for children who present with additional disabilities (language delay or deprivation; concurrent medical conditions; Autistic Spectrum Disorder; challenging behaviour; see Chapters B1, H1, E4 & F12 respectively).

Special schools
In the context of asking a deaf person about their past education, a 'Special School' refers to a school for children with complex, multiple needs including significant learning disability and limited daily living skills.

However, if you are talking with independent deaf adults of middle age and above, it is highly likely that professionals without experience of deaf people had assumed that deafness equated with learning disability and had wrongly placed the child in a school that neither met their needs as a deaf person, nor made best use of their higher cognitive abilities.

If the adult that you are interviewing has good functional ability and lives fairly independently, then the fact that they tell you they went to a 'Special school' may not be an indication of them having complex cognitive needs.

Special schools, past and present, tend to diagnostically overshadow the child's deafness (see Chapter E1). They do not see the communication difficulty as a function of deafness, but as a factor of a (oft times invented) learning disability. They do not use fluent sign language, so are not able to role model good language and, at best, the child learns some functional skills but ends up with preventable language deprivation.

Remaining deaf schools
Few deaf specialist schools remain. Those that do remain tend only to accept children who have significant learning disabilities. As with many changes in resources (cuts!) this leaves mainstream schools to deal with children with lesser needs or behaviour problems; and parents desperately fighting to get their children a diagnosis so that appropriate extra resources can be provided.

The consequence of poor educational access
As with hearing clients, your deaf clients' cognitive abilities will vary (see Chapter E2 & H1). However, even well educated, intelligent deaf clients may experience difficulties with empathy and executive functioning as a result of language deprivation (see Chapter B1) and from different attachment relationships associated with being the only deaf person in a hearing family. Other deaf people experience difficulties with literacy (see Chapter B3) and gaps in knowledge (see Chapter B4). Although the numbers of deaf people completing degrees and doctorates is steadily rising, deaf people are generally underemployed compared to their hearing peers (see Chapter F1).

Deaf education: the future
Throughout history deaf learners of equal intelligence to hearing learners, have not reached equal levels of educational achievement.

Deaf education has been well documented since the Milan Conference of 1880 (see Chapter C5) but there has been little improvement in deaf children's attainment and the trends it has followed have not always been evidence based. Educational policies in relation to deaf children have very much reflected society's attitudes towards deafness and sign languages.

To improve language, cognition and attainment in the deaf population, proponents of all styles of education need to come together, with an open mind, to review the evidence. Deaf professionals should be involved at every stage, bringing their lived experience to research (see Chapter G6), development, teaching and regulatory roles (such as Ofsted and CQC).

Ensuring the deaf child has access to deaf peers and deaf adult role models throughout their lives promotes psychosocial, linguistic and educational success.

To prevent language deprivation and poor attainment, professionals need to be involved with deaf children and their families, providing them with ways to communicate and access learning environments from birth. Starting specialist provision in Reception class, aged 4, is FAR too late. We have the shared knowledge to work preventatively with deaf children and to ensure that they never have anything less than full access to communication and education.

C7 Bi- and multi-lingualism: how it can aid cochlear implantation
Dr Kate Rowley

Hearing children in bilingual families
When hearing children from immigrant bilingual/multi-lingual families arrive at school, they may not have fully acquired the language that is spoken at school. However, these children will likely have picked up their home language age appropriately. This language platform enables them to acquire a second or even a third language once they start school. Compared to children who already speak the language of the school, they may be slow to start and will need support to develop the language used at school but are most likely to catch up.

Deaf children in hearing families
For deaf children, the situation is usually quite different in that deaf children are rarely born into environments where they can fully access the language that surrounds them (see Chapter C2 & B1). Those that experience language deprivation will have age inappropriate language and cognitive skills upon arriving at school and will lag quite far behind their hearing peers. Throughout the school years, they often struggle to catch up and are often still in environments (at school) where the language used is not accessible to them.

Deaf children in bilingual hearing families
Some deaf children will be born into bilingual/multilingual families. If the child's home language differs to the language used at school, and the child was already struggling to access the home language, they almost certainly will struggle to learn a second language. If a child does not acquire a fluent first language, they typically never achieve fluency in any language and such deaf children will struggle even more at school.

Deaf children in deaf families
Deaf children born into deaf families, where fluent sign language is accessible, are not likely to struggle in this way. Their language skills follow a similar timetable to hearing children learning spoken language. Being exposed to an accessible language from birth, promotes the development

of age appropriate cognitive skills that will support their learning upon arriving at school.

It is important to note that although deaf children from deaf families will have good sign language skills, they will not have had the same opportunities as hearing children to develop spoken language skills (whether in its printed or spoken forms) and will require support to catch up once arriving at school – similar to hearing bilingual/multilingual children whose home language differs to the school language. In addition, although deaf children from deaf families will already be fluent in one or more sign languages, many people working in deaf education are not. This will impact communication and deaf children's learning.

Bimodal-bilingual education to support language development in children with cochlear implants

Although neo-natal hearing screening allows for early diagnosis of deafness (see Chapter C3), and the age of cochlear implantation is rapidly reducing, babies and children are still missing a large proportion of the critical brain development phase to develop language fluency. Any emphasis solely on speech development detracts from the knowledge that proficiency in one language promotes proficiency in the other and that simultaneous development of two languages allows transfer between the two. Humphries et al. (2014) propose that implanted children should be given the opportunity to develop both signed and a spoken language in order to achieve fluency in both.

Their recommendation is that deaf babies and their families are taught to use sign language before, during and after implantation. Language during the critical first six months plays a crucial role in the development of auditory processing. Thus, if a deaf child acquires a sign language (compared with no language) prior and during implantation, they will be in a better position to acquire a spoken language. An added advantage is that pre-implant exposure to visual languages harnesses the child's natural desire to communicate through gesture.

It is impossible to predict which children will gain from a cochlear implant and which will not. Some children gain no linguistic benefit while others will become fully integrated into a hearing environment. If parents and educators only introduce sign language once a deaf child has failed to attain useful speech, then the next critical period, up to 5 or 6 years will be missed, increasing the risk of significant impairments of Theory of Mind (see Chapter B5), executive functioning and academic ability.

Bimodal bilingual education means children acquire proficiency in both sign and spoken language. Some deaf children will demonstrate verbal language fluency via speech, others will be better able to demonstrate it through the printed form.

Language development begins before speech development and sign can be learnt from when a baby is first born. The bimodal bilingual model helps parents focus on language development rather than just speech development and brings with it a number of advantages:

- strengthening sensory motor pathways to the brain
- facilitating early development of spatial awareness
- ensuring the brains of deaf children follow normal language development pathways so when the time comes for implantation, they are primed to acquire spoken language

Reference
Humphries, T., Kushalnagar, P., Mathur, G., Napoli, D.J., Padden, C., Rathmann, C., & Smith, S. (2014). Bilingualism: a pearl to overcome certain perils of cochlear implants. *Journal of Medical Speech Language Pathology, 21(2)*, 107-125

C8 British Sign Language
Herbert Klein and Dr Sally Austen

British Sign Language (BSL) is a beautiful language that should be protected and promoted.

It is a cultural identification.

It prevents language deprivation.

BSL is a unique language

British Sign Language is a native language of Deaf people in Britain and the UK. It fulfils all of the design features of a language, and a 'fully fledged indigenous language' (Hockett, 1960; Leeson, 2006). It is not a sign system, a code for English, or a manual pidgin.

Like the different sign languages of other countries, it has evolved and will continue to evolve naturally amongst the members of the Deaf Community for as long as Deaf people communicate together.

The rich lexicon of sign is made up from more than just handshapes:
- locations and movements of manual sign components
- it includes 'spoken' and 'oral' components (mouth-patterns that do and do not represent English words respectively)
- facial expression
- eye gaze
- head nods and shakes

Language forms that are created (e.g. Paget Gorman, Makaton or Esperanto) cannot evolve in the same way as native spoken or native signed languages. To the untrained eye, gesture systems appear to be providing a linguistic complexity that they are not. A collection of words or signs is not a language.

How is BSL different from Signed English?

BSL has its own grammar and vocabulary, distinct from English. Therefore, like any two distinct languages, there is no direct word-for-sign correspondence between English and BSL.

Signed English
There are forms of English supported with signs. The language is English. It is being represented (with varying degrees of success) with hand shapes:
- Sign-Supported English - simplified BSL vocabulary within an English grammatical structure, akin to 'Franglais'.
- Cued Speech - a phoneme-based system of hand shapes that assists lip-reading.
- Makaton - a program integrating speech, signs and symbols to aid communication in people with significant learning difficulties.
- Paget Gorman - Developed in the 1930s, it is a sign system that reflects normal patterns of English. Originally used with deaf children, it is now used mostly in speech and language therapy.

BSL as a preventer of language deprivation (see Chapter B1)
Incorrectly, there is a long-standing belief that sign language interferes with spoken language development in deaf children. On the contrary, the fully accessible nature of BSL allows healthy early language development. Relying only on augmented hearing technology and speech therapies, can leave children with language deprivation, which negatively affects cognitive development, literacy, mental health, empathy and behaviour control.

Deaf activist, model and actor, Nyle DiMarco provides an excellent video to explain the role of sign language in the prevention of language deprivation: https://www.youtube.com/watch?v=cUTymzn5FEc.

Dialects and differences in BSL
Just as with spoken languages, BSL has many regional dialects. Signs may differ from the north to the south of the UK, or even from town to town. Some signs or signing may go in or out of fashion or evolve over time, meaning that older and younger Deaf people may use different signs.

Families, friendship groups or Deaf schools may have signs unique to them. The BSL Corpus Project, based at Deafness Cognition and Language Research Centre, University College London, explores and records this: https://bslcorpusproject.org/

Sign language internationally
Each Deaf community around the world evolves its own language, just as with spoken languages. Increased travel, video contact and increasing

numbers of Deaf refugees and immigrants, enables the sharing of language features, however there is no such things as a standardised international sign language.

What is currently referral to as International Sign (IS) is a pidgin sign language, with features of many indigenous sign languages. It is used in contexts such as international conferences and sporting events – and informally when travelling and socialising. The iconic nature of some signs means that deaf people mixing internationally with other deaf people, will generally fare better than hearing people mixing internationally with other hearing people.

BSL is all around
Within health care, you will come across Deaf professionals - nurses, clinical psychologists, social workers, occupational therapists etc. Deaf professionals usually work alongside interpreters who are largely funded by governmental Access to Work (ATW) facility.

Within academia Deaf people take roles from undergraduates through to professors. Deaf people are present in politics, engineering, IT, journalism, art, astrophysics and education – to name but a few.

As well as within mainstream sport, Deaf amateur and professional sports people flourish in Deaf sport (e.g. Deaf rugby, golf, Deaflympics).

There are numerous Deaf led charities such as National Deaf Children's Society (NDCS), British Deaf Association (BDA) and Deaf Hope (for survivors of domestic abuse).

Within the arts there are Deaf theatre companies (e.g. Deafinitely Theatre), TV companies (e.g. BSLBT) and deaf TV programs (e.g. Magic Hands on CBeebies). The number of Deaf film companies increases each year.

You will find deaf professionals, with or without interpreters, in guided tours in art galleries and museums, interpreters in mainstream theatre, music festivals and literary festivals. BSL interpreters are commonly placed in re-runs of childrens' and adults' TV shows. And deaf presenters lead the whole of the TV Channel, BSL Zone. Deaf rappers, Deaf Raves and Deaf poetry are also expanding rapidly.

Deaf multicultural and faith groups are growing, with places and means of worship being provided by and for Deaf people (e.g. www.muslimdeaf.org; deafchurch.co.uk).

New Video Relay Service technology (see Chapter D7) is being used now by most banks, mobile phone companies and public service (e.g. Department of Work and Pensions).

Deaf people are also visible as teachers of BSL and language consultants. It is crucial that Deaf people lead in these roles in order to maintain the authenticity of the language.

BSL is missing
However, there are also shocking gaps in the visibility of BSL.

Given that BSL was officially recognised as a native UK language in 2003, and there are approximately 120,000 UK users, it is still shockingly absent at times. During the Covid-19 information and news summaries, the Welsh and Scottish parliaments had live BSL interpretation from the very start. The English government, for its parliament briefing, shown live daily on the BBC, was extremely reticent to provide an interpreter, despite pressure from Twitter's '#WhereIsTheInterpreter?' and a legal challenge.

Although the Equality Act (2010) requires 'reasonable adjustment' it is still common for the hearing majority to fail to reliably provide BSL interpreters in vital situations (e.g. surgical consent discussions, school parents' evenings, psychiatric assessment, court proceedings).

Children are regularly refused qualified BSL interpreters or signing teachers in schools. The closure of numerous deaf schools in the last two decades was justified on the basis that integrated schooling would be sufficiently resourced to give deaf children equity of education (both academically and socially). This has not been the case. Most Teachers of the Deaf (ToD) and most speech and language therapists (SALT) are not fluent in sign language.

Worryingly, it appears that still within the fields that most require equality of information and choice (i.e. audiology and education) BSL language, information and role modelling is often poor. A lone deaf child in a mainstream school is unlikely to have an older deaf role model. Parents making choices about cochlear implants and educational pathways for their child are unlikely to meet a successful deaf professional or advocate from whom to gather information. Deaf Ex Mainstreamers (DEX) campaign on this topic: https://dex.org.uk/.

Increasingly film and TV are including Deaf characters in roles but the emphasis is often with the Deaf person in the 'victim' role. As diversity is encouraged in mainstream media there is still a paucity of deaf role models who could enable the linguistic and social development of deaf children. And there still seems to be a naive acceptability among the hearing world that it is acceptable for hearing people to take deaf roles, even if they are non-fluent (or incompetent) signers.

Language extinction
There are concerns that BSL, as any other minority language, may deliberately or inadvertently wither.

Oppression
#Deaflivesmatter draws similarities with other oppressed minority communities. In such scenarios, it is common for political movements or invading forces to ban the use of the native languages of their enemies or by their newly acquired 'subjects'. As language embodies a community's history, culture and solidarity, it is often this the oppressor wants rid of.

Ignorance
BSL is often considered by those who do not know it, to be less eloquent or functional than spoken English. This is not the case and, as a recognised native language of the UK, there are no valid linguistic arguments as to why deaf children should be preferentially taught in English over British Sign Language.

Arguments are often made from a societal position – most commonly in the form of "these deaf children will have to function in the hearing world". But this is often fuelled by an ignorance about the difference between language and speech. Speech has great value in a predominantly hearing world, but language is crucial for cognitive development.

This can be an emotionally evocative argument but the hearing majority, who have a first-language-English bias, is likely to affect the outcome of decisions about the needs of deaf adults or children.

The counter argument is that BSL contributes to language development in deaf children and can prevent language deprivation (see Chapters B1 & C2). Unfortunately, parents in many countries are not provided with clear information about what it means to be deaf, the value and accessibility of sign language or what it means to deprive a child of that accessible language. Significant misinformation is passed to parents at a time when they are often traumatised by their child's diagnosis and struggling to weigh up the facts (see Chapter C3).

Ironically, 'baby-sign' is being happily introduced to hearing newborns, but BSL for deaf babies is not!

Diminishing populations
BSL is used by both deaf and hearing people, although it is likely that, if there were no deaf people, BSL would cease to be a regularly used British language.

Despite increasing medical and technological knowledge there is not a reduction in overall prevalence of deafness in the UK, although the demographics of the deaf populations are changing. For example, there are reductions in deafness associated with conditions such as Rubella due to vaccination; but increases in deafness associated with premature birth due to increased survival rates in pre-term babies. Such changes, alongside other factors could see BSL being used by proportionally different demographic groups in future.

Conclusion
BSL is a valuable linguistic and cultural asset, which has a massive part to play in preventing language deprivation. It must be treasured.

References
Hockett, C. F. (1960). The Origin of Speech. *Scientific American, 203*, 88-111

Leeson, L. (2006). *Signed Languages in Education in Europe - a preliminary exploration.* Strasbourg: Language Policy Division

C9 BSL alphabet

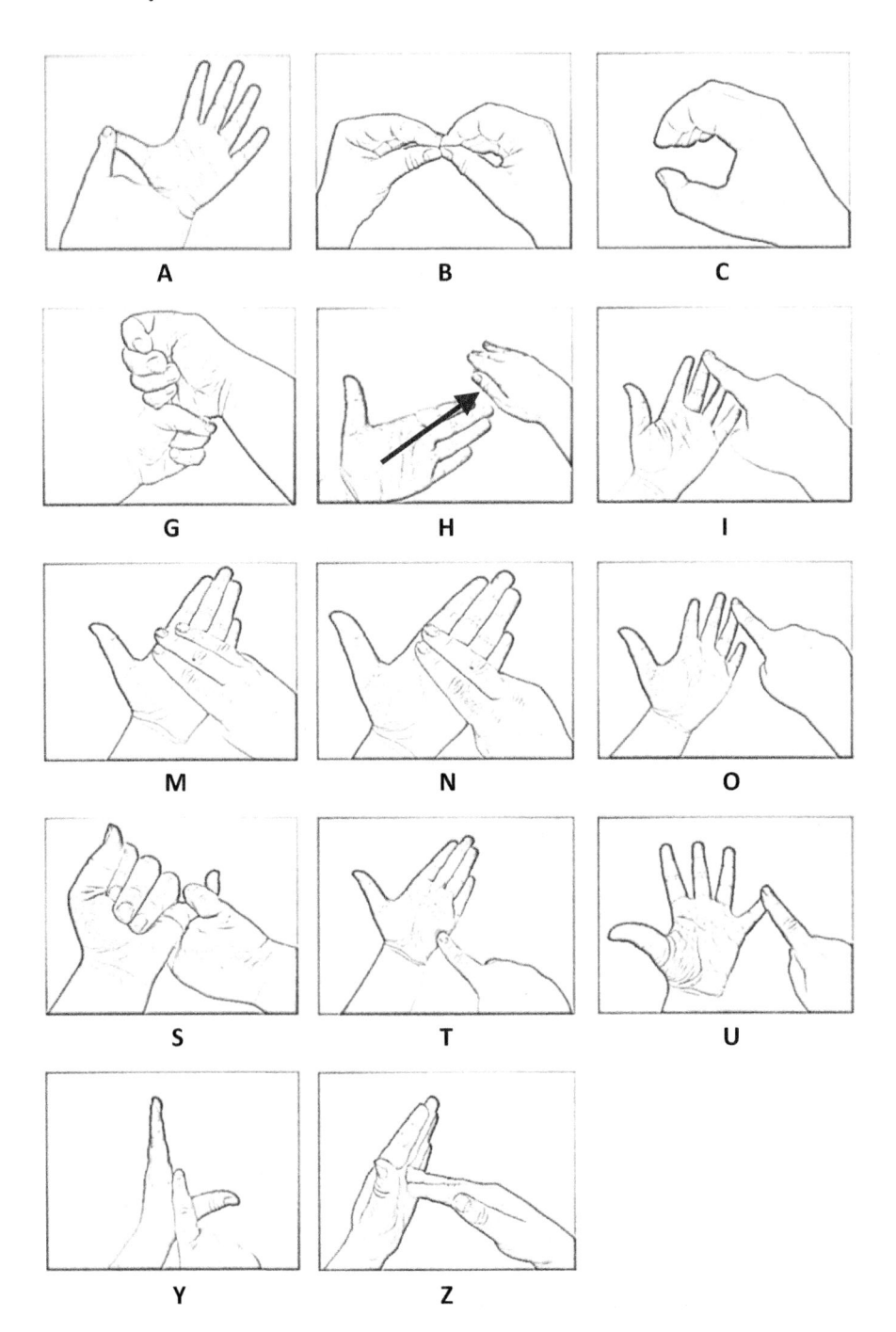

D	E	F
J	K	L
P	Q	R
V	W	X

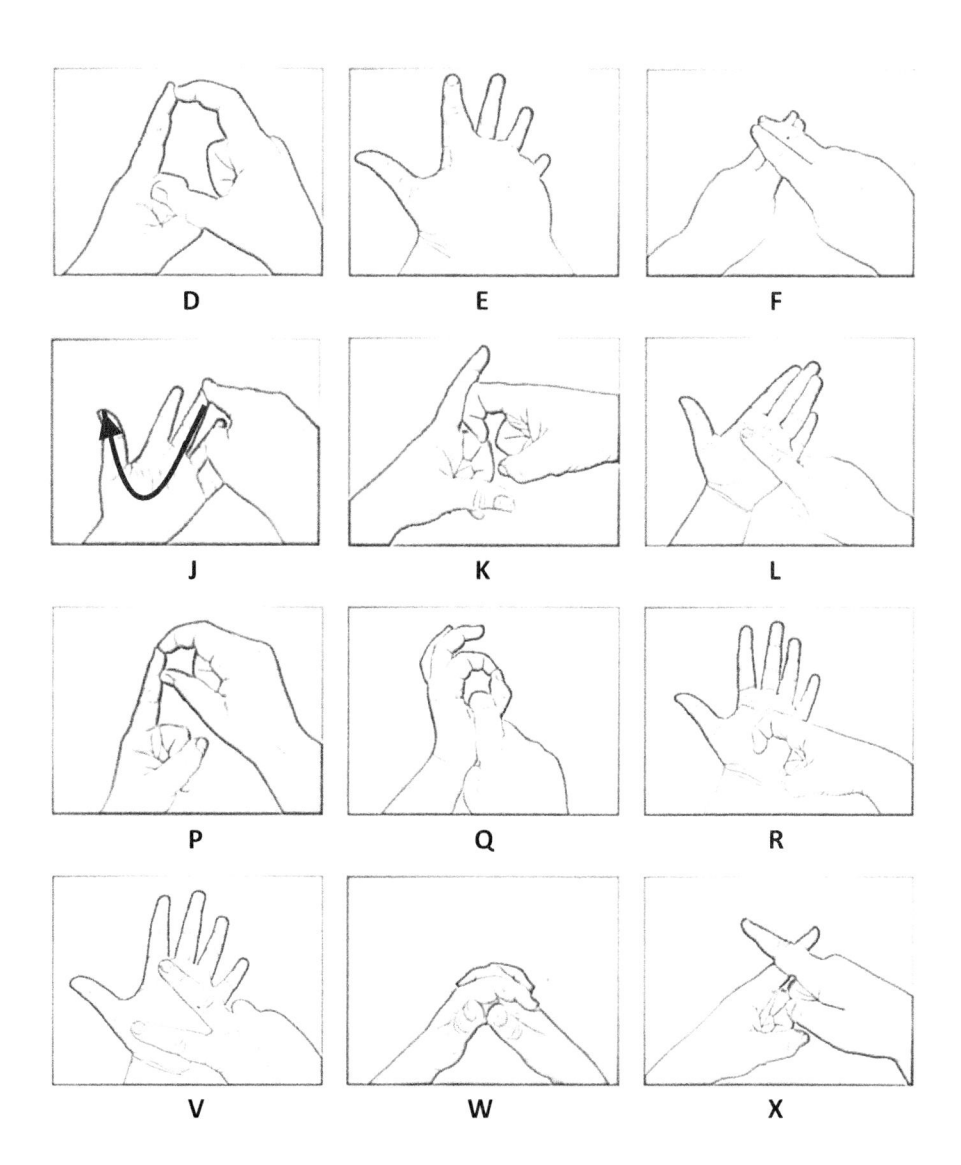

C10 Being hearing, cultural naiveté and some audist assumptions
Neil S. Glickman PhD

Chances are that if you are learning about deaf people for the first time, you are hearing. Notice that I didn't say, "You can hear". I said, "You are hearing". That's because from a culturally Deaf point of view, being "hearing" is primarily about identity, not the ability to hear.

This has direct parallels to other minority vs. majority group dynamics. Whether you agree with it or not, many minority group members think in terms of in-group vs. out-group.

To African Americans, being African-American or White refers to identity. To GLBTQ people, there are varying terms for the in-group that have changed over time such as "gay," "lesbian", "queer", etc. and there are varying terms for the outgroup, such as "straight" referring to sexual orientation or "cis-gender" referring to people who identify with their biological identity.

Religious groups often have terms for "our group" vs. "everyone else". For example, Jews may refer to all Christians as "goyim". As a Jewish child growing up in New York, I frequently heard my family, especially my grandparents, refer to the goyim as if all Christians were the same.

Thus "Deaf" with a capital D, "hearing", usually, but not always, with a lower case h, or "hard-of-hearing," or "hearing-impaired" are all terms that connote identity more than degree of hearing loss. People from the dominant group usually don't feel the need to make these distinctions. They are more inclined to believe that people are people.

A great deal of political struggle focuses on this. Thus, in the US, many African-Americans have felt the need to argue that "Black lives matter" in response to systemic racism and oppression, such as the dangers that African-American men often face with police. In response, many White Americans respond that "all lives matter" because they don't appreciate the ways that society disadvantages racial minorities.

Audism
The same dynamics plays out between Deaf and hearing people. If you can hear, most likely Deaf people will see you as "hearing", and they will

expect you to show, unless you demonstrate otherwise, attitudes that hearing people typically show. From a culturally Deaf point of view, these hearing attitudes may be seen as insensitive or, at their extreme, oppressive.

The name often given to identify oppressive attitudes towards deaf people is "audism". Obviously, this is the analogue of racism, sexism, anti-Semitism, homophobia, etc.

As a professional working with deaf people, your grasping this idea, and working with it non-defensively, may make the difference between you establishing rapport with a culturally Deaf person or not.

A few Audist assumptions
1. Deafness refers to hearing loss or a kind of sensory deprivation
With no reference to Deaf culture, language and community, this attitude can get you into trouble. It can predispose you to assume that all deaf people view deafness as a problem. It is easy to assume that nobody would choose to be deaf. Generations of Deaf families however, say otherwise.

The word "deafness" itself has cultural connotations. "Deafness" typically refers to severe hearing loss. The term is embedded in what has been called the "medical-pathological" model of Deaf people. Many culturally Deaf people prefer to talk about Deaf people, Deaf culture, Deaf community, Deaf history, Deaf schools, etc., using "Deaf" with its' more "culturally-affirmative" connotations.

Thus, you may think that discussing "deafness" is neutral or objective, but be aware that, from a culturally Deaf perspective, the term is loaded. To give an analogy, GLTBG people would likely not hear discussions of homosexuality or even, masculinity and femininity, as neutral and objective. For them, these terms are laden with cultural baggage and it is for this reason that minority groups often promote new terms or new ways of using language. The same dynamics occur within the Deaf/hearing context.

2. Deafness is a medical problem and inevitably associated with psychological problems like depression, anxiety, anger, even personality disorders

The assumption that being deaf is inevitably a problem with great psychological significance can be a source of diagnostic error if you are not culturally sensitive. It sometimes is but often isn't. It is very easy for hearing clinicians to project their own feelings and beliefs about what it is like to be deaf onto deaf people.

By starting from the perspective that deafness is a medical problem, rather than a language and cultural difference, they can then make easy leaps to see connections between deafness and personality disorders or even deafness and psychosis.

The idea that deaf people must be paranoid is a long-established trope. Indeed, the history of hearing people working with deaf people in mental health settings is largely a story of diagnostic and treatment errors based on a failure to empathically see the world the way deaf people do.

3. Speech is superior to signing as a form of communication; deaf people should use their voices and lipread

Speech may be the dominant medium for language in our world but even a cursory exploration of sign languages can lead one to discover how eloquently one can express oneself in sign and how captivatingly beautiful sign languages can be. From a culturally Deaf perspective, signing is at least as good, if not better, as a medium for language as speech.

Many people who are born deaf do not have clear speech and may be reluctant to use their voices. They may have a lifetime of experience of being judged for their speaking skills, and some may resent the expectation that they speak to accommodate the hearing person as opposed to having the hearing person try to accommodate them. Indeed, some may receive comments about how well they speak as patronising. It is somewhat equivalent to telling a light skinned African American that they don't look Black, as if that were a good thing.

In addition, spoken and sign languages have very different grammars so that it is nearly impossible to sign well in ASL or BSL while simultaneously speaking. There are lots of good reasons why Deaf people may not use their voices, and it can be culturally insensitive to assume that their inability or unwillingness to speak is a bigger problem than your inability or unwillingness to sign.

If you are working with a signing Deaf person, the right questions to ask are how they prefer to communicate and how you can best accommodate those preferences. It is helpful to be mindful of one's assumptions.

Conclusion
There are many other cultural differences between Deaf and hearing people. So, if you are new to working with Deaf people, welcome to a new perspective. You are not just someone who can hear. You are hearing.

Recommended readings
Glickman, N.S. (Ed.) (2013). *Deaf mental health care.* New York City: Routledge

Leigh, I. W. (2009). *A lens on Deaf identities.* Oxford, England: Oxford University Press

Section D

D1 Interpreters and communication professionals
Dr Ben Holmes

Interpreting is a specialist occupation that requires a high level of proficiency in two fundamentally different languages or modes of communication. An interpreter's role is to facilitate communication between and within languages. In the case of a British Sign Language (BSL)/English interpreter this means translating spoken English into BSL and BSL into spoken English (the latter may be referred to as a 'voice over').

The interpreter you work with, is a fellow professional; someone with whom you can plan, discuss and evaluate communication, in order to provide the best experience for all involved. This chapter outlines some of the different types of interpreters and communication professionals you might encounter in your work with deaf clients, colleagues or professionals. For more specific information about how to work with interpreters please also refer to chapters D2, D3, D4, D7, D9 & D11.

Registered Sign Language Interpreters (RSLI)
Qualification
In the UK, working as a registered BSL interpreter requires significant training and qualification that is not always required in spoken language interpreting roles. Qualified, registered, BSL interpreters will have:
- A degree level qualification (or level 6 diploma) from a recognised course in sign language interpreting
- DBS check
- Professional indemnity insurance
- Annual Continued Professional Development

UK regulation
Registration with a regulatory body is not required for qualification. However, as most employing organisations require registration, it is the norm. The UK registration bodies are:

National Registers of Communication Professionals working with Deaf and Deafblind people (NRCPD) - https://www.nrcpd.org.uk

Regulatory Body for Sign Language Interpreters and Translators (RBSLI) - https://rbsli.org

In Scotland there is also the Scottish Association of Sign Language Interpreters (SASLI) - http://www.sasli.org.uk

Identification

Qualified, registered interpreters will have a 'yellow card' as proof of their status. It will also be possible to find their details on their respective regulatory body database online.

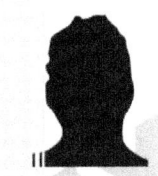

NRCPD | REGISTERED

A N Other

Sign Language Interpreter

ID: 1234567 Valid until: 31 January 2021
NRCPD | The National Registers of Communication Professionals working with Deaf and Deafblind People | www.nrcpd.org.uk

Printed with permission from NRCPD

Trainee Sign Language Interpreters' ID cards are purple. Other registered interpreting and communication professionals (e.g. lipspeakers) have badges of different colours.

Trainee Sign Language Interpreters (TSLI)

Trainee Sign Language Interpreters can also register with the professional bodies above and can work under supervision in certain settings. However, they should not practice in legal, mental health work or child protection interpreting. This requires further post-qualification experience.

Deaf Relay Interpreter (DRI) or Sign Language Interpreter (Relay-Intralingual) (see Chapter D4 for more information)

Where a deaf person has an additional language need due to disability, language dysfluency or not being a native BSL user, an additional Deaf Relay Interpreter (DRI) will need to co-work with the BSL interpreter. A DRI is a deaf professional that adapts information from the BSL interpreter into a form of BSL that is more accessible to the deaf person you are working with. The DRI then relays the deaf person's response back to the BSL interpreter who will translate this into spoken English.

Although previously the role of a DRI had a diverse range of routes to becoming registered, this is now being overseen by NRCPD with a specific training and registration route to attain the qualification of Sign Language Interpreter (Relay-Intralingual).

Lipspeaker (see Chapter D9 for more information)
A hearing person trained to clearly reproduce the words of another person, in order to maximise a lipreader's understanding.

Deafblind interpreters
Qualified interpreters who specialise in communicating with Deafblind people and may use a variety of different communication methods (see Chapter D11 for more information).

Other communication professionals
Other communication professionals that you might work with include:

Note takers
Record notes of what is said, either in writing or electronically. Deaf people may require this when they need a written record for later reference but cannot write at the same time as watching what is being interpreted.

Speech to Text operator (also known as a Palantypist)
Trained to produce a written English record of everything that is said between deaf and/or hearing people. The text is shown on a screen and includes spoken words as well as information about surroundings (e.g. laughter or applause).

Code of conduct
Interpreters and communication professionals have a strict code of conduct that they are expected to follow. This includes:

Confidentiality for the client
The interpreter cannot tell you about what was discussed in previous meetings or appointments even if the same interpreter happened to be involved. You must ask the deaf person or other people that were involved in the meeting.

Interpreting everything that is said
Interpreters will interpret everything that is said or signed. They are not able to omit information at the request of either party.

Working within the bounds of own competence
Interpreters are only allowed to work in fields where they believe themselves sufficiently competent. In order to gain competence, qualified interpreters may work with supervision before operating fully independently in newer specialisms (e.g. mental health, courts).

This means that it is important to provide a brief explanation about the aim of the meeting when requesting an interpreter to help them know whether they are able to accept the booking (see Chapter D2 & D5)

Professional membership associations
Support networks exist to encourage good practice, promote training and represent the interests and views of sign language interpreters and the interpreting profession in the UK.

For more information see:
ASLI (Association of Sign Language Interpreters) www.asli.org.uk
IOCN (Interpreters of Colour Network) www.interpretersofcolour.net
VLP (Visual Language Professionals) www.vlp.org.uk

D2 Working with Sign Language Interpreters (SLIs)
Dr Ben Holmes and Jackie Dennis

Sign Language Interpreters (SLI) are employed for the benefit of both the hearing and deaf person or people. Optimum work using a SLI therefore requires investment and preparation by:
- The hearing person
- The interpreter
- The deaf person

Eye contact
The interpreter is facilitating a primary relationship between the hearing and deaf people present. Thus, the hearing person must keep eye contact with the deaf person. Even if the hearing person has no sign language skills, they will gain a lot from observing the deaf person's facial expression and body language. It is also a sign of respect to maintain eye contact.

The deaf person will look back and forth between the interpreter and the hearing person thus also monitoring their facial expression and body language.

Physical positioning
Positioning will depend on the number of people and type of meeting. The BSL interpreter should always be visible to all the deaf people. Positioning within the room should be negotiated primarily with the deaf person and then with other people present. Light should fall on the face of the interpreter but not dazzle them. No one should sit with a window behind them.

Positioning should include consideration of:
- Personal space
- Visual abilities
- Equipment (projector screens)
- Lighting
- Safety

It is typical for the interpreter to sit to the side of the person speaking, as indicated below (D=Deaf person, I=Interpreter, H=Hearing person):

```
    D         I
              H
```

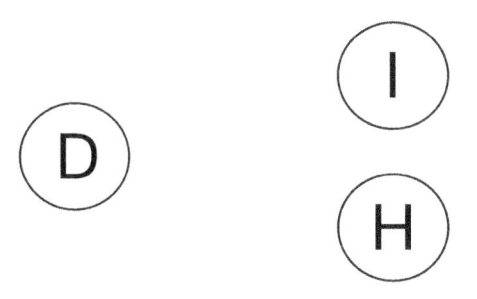

It is also worth considering how the positioning of the interpreter can affect the relationship dynamics in the room. For example, if the deaf person and interpreter already know each other, but are unknown to the hearing person, then starting with a triangular seating pattern may imply equality, welcome and sharing of information. In contrast, in therapy, where the primary relationship is between the therapist and patient, the interpreter may sit slightly behind the hearing person. This positioning works equally well for a deaf therapist and hearing client.

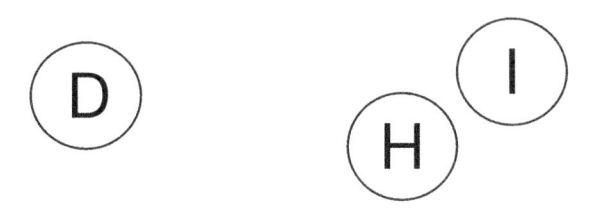

```
    D              I
              H
```

Providing background information ('Feeding the interpreter')
The greater the available information about the content to be interpreted, the greater the ease and accuracy of interpretation.

Briefing prior to meeting
The more information you give the interpreter the better, including:
- The purpose of the meeting
- Any paperwork or presentations that will be used
- Information about the client's communication and other needs
- Relevant background information such as family dynamics/members or anything particularly pertinent

On meeting
- Share updated information (e.g. how is the client today)
- Discuss timings, seating, questions from either party
- The interpreter may be able to advise on how to present information to ensure maximum accessibility

Debriefing
Clarify points about communication and meaning. Interpreters are not allowed to offer opinions beyond their communication role. For example:
- They can advise on improving future accessibility of information for the purpose of mental health assessment
- They can comment on change in communication or language style that they have noticed but not offer an opinion on why this may be
- They cannot comment on whether the client has a mental illness

Debriefing should also be used to prepare for future meetings.

Pacing
In contrast to spoken language interpreters, BSL interpreters sign at the same time as the speaker. There may, however, be a slight lag because of differences in grammar between BSL and English or because context is needed before a concept can be explained:
- Speak at a steady pace so that the interpreter can follow
- Do not stop mid-sentence as the interpreter may be waiting for a key piece of information to enable them to continue
- Pauses in between sentences are sometimes necessary to enable the interpreter to catch up
- Regular pauses are crucial to allow the deaf person a chance to respond to what is said

Considering the needs of your interpreter
Interpreters needing to tune in
Interpreters need time to get used to clients' communication (in speech or sign): their accents, dialects (see Chapter C8) and their language fluency (see Chapter B1). Some repetition or additional time may therefore be required, especially at the beginning of the appointment.

Interpreting specialist subjects
Interpreting is not a matter of word for word translation. Working with two distinct languages, the interpreter must understand the concepts and the language they are being asked to convey.

Interpreting for clients with dysfluent language requires a great deal more training, time and adaptation (see Chapter D3).

The interpreter Code of Conduct requires interpreters to work within their areas of competence. Interpreters working in health, mental health settings or the criminal justice system are expected to have specific training and experience. However, often the descriptions of the tasks put out by interpreting agencies or the employer are vague and the interpreter can find themselves in unfamiliar situations.

Example
An interpreter is called to a team meeting. However, when they arrive the deaf person is expecting to present their adaptations to complex computer software, to demonstrate how this improves the efficiency of car engines.

There are multiple responsibilities here:
- the interpreting agency must advertise their bookings accurately
- the interpreter must be clear about their competencies in this area
- the deaf professional should express if they have a preference for an interpreter and this person should be booked if possible
- the professionals leading the meetings must check the overall success of the communication and provide additional information and explanation to the interpreter, where this can be effective
- If accurate communication is not possible the meeting should be brought to a halt

Jargon, acronyms and names
Professionals should avoid jargon or provide explanation to ensure clarity. Acronyms and complex names should be spelt and explained.

Cognitive demand
Breaks are required to cope with the fatiguing, cognitive demands of prolonged or complex interactions. The more demanding the information or communication, the more frequent the breaks. Ask your interpreter.

In some complex situations, having a break is not always convenient or appropriate and so a second interpreter may be needed. The extreme cognitive overload of the interpreting process means that at times interpreters need to work alongside a colleague in order to share the active function of the process.

If only one interpreter is used, someone must take responsibility for ensuring breaks happen at certain points. It is best for the interpreter to remove themselves from the room to allow a proper break otherwise informal conversation often happens, requiring interpretation, meaning the only person that has not had a break is the interpreter.

Considering the safety and wellbeing of your Interpreter
Vicarious trauma
Interpreting in stressful situations (e.g. restraint, child protection, medical diagnosis) or for traumatic information (e.g. in mental health assessment or sexual abuse debrief) can impact on emotional wellbeing. Allowing time to prepare and debrief with interpreters is crucial.

When booking interpreters, they should be given sufficient information about potentially distressing topics, such that they are able to choose not to take certain jobs before arriving.

Physical safety
The safety of the interpreter should be considered in situations where there is challenging behaviour, lone working, travel, or sharing personal identifying material.

Interpreting for groups (see also Chapter F8)
To ensure that information is not missed, groups must be well chaired. The interpreter must be aware of who is talking/signing at all times and gaps must be provided between speakers.

Simultaneous speaking or signing cannot be interpreted - everyone must agree to a turn-taking system (e.g. raising a hand before speaking or standing when talking). This will also ensure the deaf person, or persons, will have an equal opportunity to contribute. Without fair turn-taking deaf people are often left out due to the slight time lag with interpretation.

Use of spoken and sign language interpreters
Sometimes, deaf people come from a family where there are one or more family members that are hearing and are non-English speakers or have English as a second language. In this situation you may need to book both spoken and signed language interpreters (e.g. an Urdu interpreter and a BSL interpreter). Such appointments take approximately twice as long as the same meeting with no interpreters. The person leading the meeting will also need to check with all parties that there has been adequate opportunity to understand what each person has been saying.

D3 Using interpreters with non-fluent or language deprived sign language users
Dr Ben Holmes and Maria Kilbride

Identifying language dysfluency

As with any language, in sign language there is a spectrum of ability. Not all sign language users are fluent. Among those who appear fluent, some will have experienced a degree of language deprivation (see Chapter B1) or experienced limitations to information access in early life (see Chapter B4), which can affect their communication.

A deaf client may have enough functional language to seem initially articulate but not enough to successfully engage in more complex conversations. Initial conversations with clients tend to spotlight social niceties (about the weather or their journey to the meeting) or their history (clinical, legal, family etc.) – all of which utilise factual, linear and rehearsed material. Be mindful that these initial interactions are not necessarily a gauge of language competence or understanding of more complex concepts.

Hearing professionals who do not sign will not be able to judge a sign language users' level of fluency and may therefore be unaware of the need for additional interpreting strategies. Hence the importance of working closely with interpreters and Deaf Relay Interpreters (see Chapters D2 & D4).

Trusting the interpreter

All interpreting work requires a degree of cultural and linguistic mediation. For example, certain collective terms, such as 'substance misuse' or 'weapons' in English do not directly translate in BSL. In such cases, the interpreter will often need to negotiate with the hearing professional a way to present information in the most accessible and explicit way possible (see Chapter D2).

When working with dysfluent sign language the need for more extensive language adaptation may only become apparent during the interpreted situation – and the interpreter will need to make this apparent to the hearing professional. These adaptations may affect the way in which information is provided and the responses that are subsequently received.

Co-working between professionals and interpreters should not just occur during preparation and debrief meetings, but throughout the whole meeting. The interpreter needs to be given time and flexibility to stop, go back, try various approaches. This is at its hardest when both the hearing professional and the interpreter are unfamiliar with the deaf client.

The hearing professional may feel discomfort with the level of necessary adaptation and that it impacts rapport between them and the deaf client. Whilst the interpreter's efforts can feel intrusive, it is important to remember that they are not trying to commandeer the relationship with the client. They wish to facilitate the aims of the professional by way of achieving understanding, good communication and rapport between the professional and the client.

When working with clients with dysfluent language it is even more important, where possible, to retain continuity of interpreter. Once the interpreter has found ways to unpack certain concepts or use certain imagery, it is less efficient to have to start this anew with a different interpreter, should subsequent meetings be necessary.

Example of some mediations that might be used include:

Characterisations
Sometimes interpreters will make language adjustments that may include characterisations or physical descriptions. This can be extremely useful and necessary but can feel extreme or uncomfortable to an inexperienced hearing professional.

Example
Professional: How are you getting on with Mrs Doyle?
Interpreter in BSL: Mrs Doyle. You like her? Good relationship with her?
Client: Who?
Interpreter in BSL with characterisation: Me. I am the new teacher. I am a Lady, big with round glasses. Do you like me?

Characterisation is not limited to humans. At various times the second author has characterised the HIV virus, a computer algorithm and a bumblebee!

The degree of characterisation and role play can impact on the well-being of both interpreter and client depending on the sensitivity of the subjects being characterised. For example, 'becoming' the character who is the perpetrator or victim of a sexual assault could be traumatising. This should be discussed in the brief/de-brief. (This is an example of why interpreters' own supervision is extremely valuable too).

Role play
Alongside willing hearing professionals, role play can be extremely useful in facilitating 'meta' reflection. For example, in therapy: by acting out a known scenario from a client's past, with him as the audience, it may then be possible to elicit what older client Bob now thinks of younger Bob's behaviour.

Conditional clauses are notoriously difficult for people with language deprivation to understand. Role play is invaluable in replicating 'what if' discussions (e.g. Client is at risk of financial scammers). Role play could include receiving an email from a friend asking from money, thinking this is normal and transferring money or thinking this is suspicious and refusing. At each stage, the deaf person's reaction can be observed to judge whether they are able to understand and make an informed decision.

Comprehension of concepts ('Unpacking')
Some clients will struggle to understand complex or abstract concepts (see Chapters B1 & B7). Some may also have gaps in knowledge (see Chapter B4). Additional information may therefore be needed to aid understanding – this is sometimes referred to as 'unpacking the concept'. If you are unsure whether the client has understood, check with them by asking them to repeat back what they think was said.

Example of unpacking an information gap
Hearing professional: *Did you get into debt because of the interest payments?*
Interpreter in BSL: *When you borrowed money you had to pay back firstly the money you borrowed, and second the extra money called 'interest'. Did paying back the extra money cause you to go into debt?*

Example of unpacking a concept
A deaf person with highly complex communication needs is ready to leave hospital after a prolonged stay. They have a little functional BSL, mostly idiosyncratic signing, little lipreading and no written English. They have been brought on a planned orientation visit to a supported living environment closer to family, accompanied by staff and an interpreter who are well-known to them. An informal chat with the Manager takes place, by way of introduction.

Manager to deaf person: Do you know what this place is and why you are here today?

The question is interpreted in this way, with no response from the deaf person. The interpreter asks the Manager for time to get to the question in a different way.

Interpreter: This morning you woke up in your room. Staff woke you up, right?
Deaf client: yes, Dave woke me, I was asleep!
Interpreter: Oh dear, Dave woke you early! Then you shower? Breakfast?
Deaf person: yes, shower and toast.
Interpreter: Yes, you, Dave and me ate toast. Then we got into the big silver van, yes?
Deaf client: Yes, long way!
Interpreter: Yes, a long time in that van! So, you arrived at this new building. Never seen before.
Deaf client: Different place, new place.
Interpreter: Yes, this place different, new! You've come here today, a visit here, what for?
Deaf Client: See bedroom. Go shopping with sister. Cup of tea, relax.

In this example the client does not know the sign for 'supported living accommodation' and lacks expressive language. But with the interpreter's extensive adaptation to engage the Deaf person and provide context, a working hypothesis is agreed that the client has understood enough to know that they are visiting a place where people sleep, see family and enjoy recreational activity.

Closing down questions
Some deaf people with non-fluent language may have difficulty responding to open questions. Interpreters therefore sometimes provide a list of options to help them respond.

Example
Hearing professional: How have you been feeling this week?
Interpreter in BSL: This week have you been happy, sad, angry or worried?

However, in closing the question off in this way the Deaf person may only respond to the options provided. This may give the hearing professional the perception of a completed answer when further questioning and clarification may be needed.

Example
Hearing professional: How have you been feeling this week?
Interpreter in BSL: This week have you been happy, sad, angry or scared?
Client: No, fine.

The interpreter should explain to the hearing professional the form of their interpretation, as well as the deaf person's reply. If the interpreter has given options, the professional needs to know what they were and whether further enquiry is needed.

Hearing professional: I was told that you had been a bit worried about going out.
Interpreter in BSL: This week, were you worried about going out?
Client: Yes, I was worried about going to the shop because a new person has started working there that I do not know.

In these situations, it is useful for the interpreter and professional to work together to check how best to repeat or reframe the question.

In certain clinical or legal situations, a question may need to be left open (e.g. to avoid 'leading' a witness in a legal procedure). If there is a need to ask questions in a specific way, it is advisable to meet with the interpreter beforehand to discuss and plan.

That said, the level of language adjustment that will be required to assess understanding for a non-standard signer will not change just because the setting is more formal, leaving a situation where open questions are asked but an unreliable or unhelpful answer is given. In these circumstances the (legal) team should employ a Deaf Intermediary (see Chapter 18).

Mixed language and communication
Where clients are non-fluent signers, reliance on mixed communication may be the best, imperfect, solution. A mixture of sign language, role play, lip-reading and even writing/drawing may be needed.

Interpreting from sign to spoken English
In an ideal situation, the hearing interpreter (with or without a relay interpreter) would be able to deliver a clear, simultaneous first-person rendition into spoken language. However, some of the linguistic features that make for fully comprehensible language may be missing in the signing of a dysfluent Deaf person. The absence of role shift, directional verbs,

times lines or placement, and the inclusion of idiosyncratic signs all impact the interpretation into spoken English.

Where meaning is not clear, the interpreter must be circumspect, and their rendition may need to be narrative or reported.

Deaf Client: 'America brother must '

Without the additional linguistic information this could mean 'I must go to America to see my brother' or 'My brother must go to America' or 'My American brother is a bully' etc. The interpreter cannot assign meaning that is not apparent, instead saying only what they can see.

Research shows that psychosis is under-diagnosed in foreign language clients being assessed with a spoken language interpreter, because interpreters feel pressured to make sense of what the client is saying, even when the meaning in unclear. It takes confidence to relay something meaningless to a professional - and the interpreter should be supported in this.

Communication: a working hypothesis or fact?

When working with clients who have non-fluent sign language there will be situations where communication about certain topics is difficult or even impossible. It is vital that this uncertainty is acknowledged and recorded, so that it is both referred to in subsequent meetings, and so that ongoing attempts are made to gain greater clarity. Otherwise, this tentative communication becomes fact, which then gets passed on as such, and can end up in legal documentation.

Summary

In working with deaf people with dysfluent language, the relationship between the hearing professional and the interpreter(s) is vital. Additional time must be allowed for their co-working.

In a mental health setting, if it is believed that a client may have non-fluent language a referral to specialist mental health services is recommended (see Chapters G3 & G4). In a legal setting a Deaf Intermediary (see Chapter I8) should be engaged.

D4 Deaf Relay Interpreters (Relay-Intralingual Interpreters)
Lenka Novakova

What is a Deaf Relay Interpreter (DRI)?
Whereas a British Sign Language (BSL)/English Sign Language Interpreter (SLI) provides interpretation between spoken English and sign language, a DRI is a deaf communication professional who provides additional interpretation between the deaf sign language user and the SLI.

DRIs need to have an extensive knowledge and understanding of deaf related issues, deaf culture and the Deaf community – and have excellent communication skills to adapt to the client's communication needs.

As of 2021 a new name, Relay-Intralingual interpreter, is being introduced to formalise the registration of DRIs as a distinct category of interpreters.

Why might a DRI be needed?
SLIs work with clients who have varying degrees of language fluency and within a multitude of complex contexts (see Chapters D1 & D3).

A DRI may work alongside the SLI to maximise overall translation in situations where the client has severe language deprivation (Chapter B1), mental health problems (Chapter F4), cognitive difficulties (Chapter E3) or poor Theory of Mind (Chapter B5).

A DRI may also be effective when communication between BSL and other signed language is not fully mutual intelligible (Chapter D13).

Interpreting process with DRI and SLI
As the hearing professional's words are translated into sign (by the SLI), the DRI then modifies the message linguistically and culturally in a way that is most understandable to the deaf client. Essentially, it becomes one deaf person interpreting for another deaf person.

As the deaf client replies in sign, the DRI will modify the client's (perhaps idiosyncratic) sign in such a way that the SLI can then provide the spoken English voice over to the hearing professional. This works the same whether the deaf person is the professional or the client (see Figure 1).

Figure 1

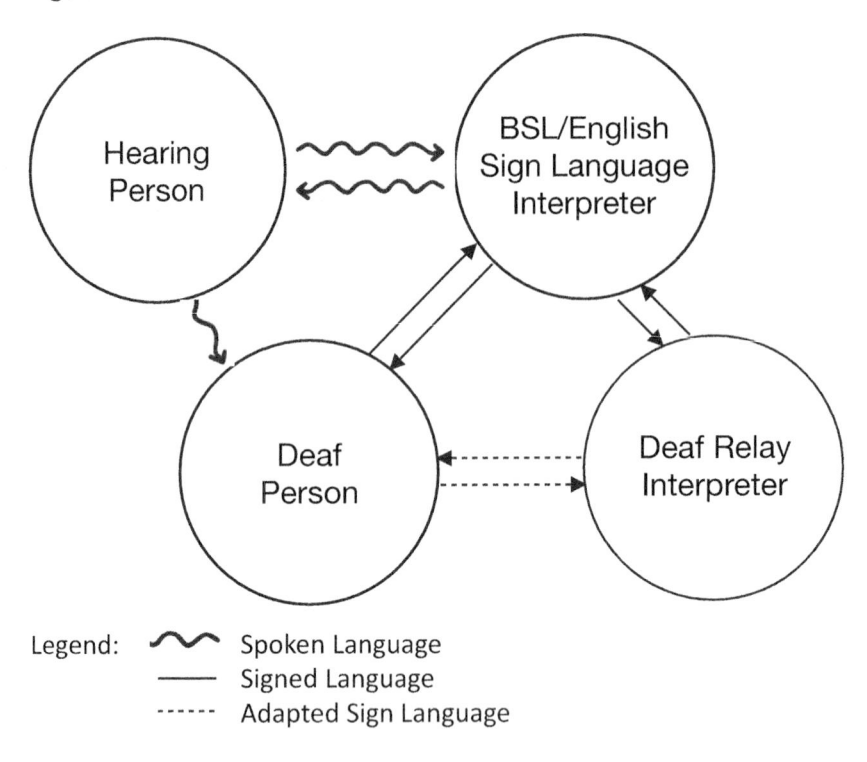

Legend:
- ～ Spoken Language
- — Signed Language
- ------ Adapted Sign Language

Trusting the DRI, and giving them the latitude to make language adjustments, is important. For example, a DRI may choose to use role play in order to augment their communication.

In a less linear mode, the DRI's role is also to check, monitor and clarify dialogue to maximise the client's understanding. Thus, it is not always necessary for all dialogue to be translated by both SLI and DRI. Often the DRI will observe and contribute where they think they would be most useful.

The hearing professional should endeavour to be explicit, so the interpreter has less to infer. In some situations (e.g. cognitive assessments, legal settings), it may be important that certain information is not provided to the person being assessed so as to not give an inaccurate impression of their knowledge. Where this is the case, it is essential to have a pre-assessment meeting with communication professionals involved to discuss how questions might be interpreted most effectively.

DRI training
Being Deaf and a native signer is not a qualification in itself. Until 2021, there was no one formal route to qualifying as a DRI. Up to this time, DRIs gained their experience through a combination of different qualifications that enabled them to do this role effectively (e.g. BSL level 6, BSL translation, BSL tutoring, deaf awareness).

However, as of 2021 DRIs will be required to have a level 6 diploma in sign language interpreting and translation or completed the NRCPD practice assessment for DRIs. Registered DRIs, or Registered Sign Language Interpreter (Relay-Intralingual) as the new registration process will call them, will have a yellow badge to prove their registered status, as with other SLIs. Trainees will have a purple badge (see Chapter D1 for more information).

Lack of training for DRIs in mental health/healthcare settings
Despite this formalisation of the registration process, there remains no specialist training in mental or physical health for DRIs. Instead, this is gained through supervised practice.

Similar to SLIs, DRIs should not undertake any assignment that is not within their capacity. There are not many DRIs in practice currently, fewer still with experience in mental health settings. The introduction of this specialism should hopefully swell their numbers.

How to book a DRI
A DRI can be booked in the same way as an SLI (see Chapter D5).

If the client is from a specific ethnic background, consider the value of the DRI's cultural capital. Where the client and interpreter (SLI or DRI) are from the same ethnic background, a shared understanding of language and culture may improve overall interpretation.

The responsibility of the lead professional (e.g. clinician, solicitor etc.)
For hearing professionals, the experience of working with a deaf client and (various) interpreters can be unnerving and deskilling. While the professional should be willing to accept communication advice from the SLI, DRI and the deaf client, the onus of responsibility is on the lead

professional to establish whether they consider the interpretation arrangements sufficient for the task being undertaken and, if not, to make decisions accordingly.

Where possible, advice should be sought from deaf services and deaf professionals. However, in some scenarios there is no opportunity to postpone action. For example, if the client is clearly suicidal, is reporting chest pains or is threatening assault with a weapon. However, there are opportunities to consider how a diagnosis or legal decision will be downgraded to a 'working hypothesis' until further information can be collated.

In situations where a DRI is required, a linguistic conversation may not be sufficient in itself to enable to the person to access all information being discussed. In these situations, further adaptation may be required. For example:

1. Consider the role of observation in collating information (e.g. rather than discussing whether the client can manage their finances, take them to the bank and observe them paying their bills).

2. Offer a repeat meeting, allowing each person involved more time to hone their communication. Invite additional, or different interpreters, use more visual props and gather more background information to facilitate discussion (e.g. names or photos of specific people that might be discussed).

D5 Booking a sign language interpreter
Dr Ben Holmes

Right to an interpreter
Deaf people have a right under the Equality Act (2010) and the Accessible Information Standard (2016) to interpreters for meeting with professionals (see Chapter 19). This includes all health care, education and legal settings.

It is the service provider's responsibility to book and pay for the interpreter, not the deaf client's. Deaf professionals may be able to reclaim the cost of their interpreters through UK government funded 'Access to Work' (ATW).

Family and friends as interpreters
It is always preferable to book a professional interpreter.

A client may say that they prefer a family member or friend to interpret for them, but they may also be saying this if it seems easier or because that is what they have always done (see also Chapter C4).

Family and friends are unlikely to have the level of expertise and their presence can shift the dynamics of the meeting. For example, the client may withhold information that they would otherwise have disclosed. Furthermore, the family/friend interpreter may withhold information from the deaf client because they consider it too upsetting for them or they think they are protecting the deaf person from difficult issues.

Using children to interpret in a professional context is wholly inappropriate and may be considered a Safeguarding issue.

Booking an Interpreter
Interpreters can be booked via interpreting agencies or as freelance professionals. Details can be found via online search engines – or your organisation may already have a contract with an agency.

To provide the most appropriate interpreter:
- be as specific as possible about the communication needs of the deaf and hearing people who require the interpreter (e.g. hearing psychiatrist with no sign language, fluent signing deaf teenager)
- the aim, length and whereabouts of the meeting
- other preferences, such as gender, dialect, experience in particular fields

Interpreters are in high demand and may need to be booked several weeks in advance of an appointment. In emergency situations, interpreting agencies will try their best to provide an interpreter faster. Freelance interpreters are likely to charge for travel and to have a minimum fee.

Where it is not possible to get a face to face interpreter, an online interpreting service might also be suitable. These require either connecting to a website or downloading an App (see Chapter D7).

Privacy and boundaries
The Deaf world is small. There is therefore a high chance that your interpreter may have met the deaf person prior to the appointment. This can be an advantage, as the interpreter will quickly tune in to the deaf person's communication. However, it could also negatively affect engagement, the client's sense of confidentiality or the dynamics of the interaction. Depending on the context, it may be appropriate to choose an alternative interpreter (e.g. if engaging in psychotherapy).

Evolving working relationships with interpreters
The more often you work with a particular interpreter, the more able they are to tune into the style and language of the professional and the preferences and language of the client. By ensuring a debrief session, you can build an understanding of the goals of the sessions and develop a collaborative style of working. It is worth keeping the contact details of these interpreters to continue working together in future bookings. Shared CPD events are extremely useful, to increase the fund of knowledge for all, and thus shared language.

For further information see Chapters D1, D2, D3, D4, D6, D7 and:
https://nubsli.com/guidance/interpreter-awareness-guide/

D6 NUBSLI: checklist for booking a BSL/English interpreter

Checklist for booking a BSL/English interpreter

Before you book a BSL/English interpreter:

- ☑ What is the date, start time and location of the booking?
- ☑ What is the nature of the booking? (e.g. an interview, a meeting, a conference etc).
- ☑ How many interpreters will you need?
- ☑ Have you set a realistic budget for access costs?
- ☑ Are there any specific Language requirements? (e.g. BSL/SSE/Deafblind/Visual frame)
- ☑ How many participants will there be? (is it a 1:1 or a group? How many Deaf BSL users will be present?)

Details for on the day of the booking:

- ☑ How long will the assignment last (and have you allowed extra time for the event running over)?
- ☑ Have you accounted for breaks? (It's not only the interpreters that require breaks - Deaf people using interpreting services will need regular eye breaks, as focusing for long periods is very tiring)
- ☑ Will there be multiple rooms or break out groups at the event?
- ☑ Who is the point of contact for the event?
- ☑ Are there any access issues to be aware of (e.g. you need to arrive 30 minutes ahead of time to get through security/parking etc)

Preparation to provide interpreter/s at least one week before the booking:

- ☑ Is there an agenda, previous minutes or a presentation that can be shared with the interpreter/s?
- ☑ Will you be using video or sound clips during the event? Are these subtitled or can transcripts be made available?
- ☑ Will handouts be used? Can a copy of these be sent to the interpreter ahead of the assignment?

Original checklist developed by NUBSLI and included with their permission
www.nubsli.com

D7 Video interpreting
Herbert Klein and Dr Sally Austen

Online interpreting services have existed for many years but have massively expanded due to Covid-19 related social distancing and remote working.

Booking and prepping remote interpreters
There is no dispute that most social interactions are better done face to face. However, there are times when this is not possible. This may be due to issues with safety (e.g. during the Covid-19 pandemic) distance (e.g. when the therapist is in Oxford and the client is on the Hebrides) or time (e.g. attending remotely fits one's diary, attending in person would not).

Just as face to face interpreters can be booked via agencies or as freelancers (see Chapter D5), some also provide remote interpreting services. Online interpreting is arguably made harder than face to face, in that some aspects of verbal and nonverbal communication are lost, wifi and technological difficulties such as 'freezing' abound and deaf accessible protocols are harder to maintain (e.g. people forget to pause to allow the deaf person equal chance to contribute; screen sharing without considering that this obliterates the view of the interpreter etc).

All regular aspects of working with interpreters should be followed: allowing time for the client and interpreter to attune to each other's communication style; preparatory information; discussion to ensure the right interpreter is booked for the job; debriefing to maximise future working and to consider the wellbeing of the interpreter.

The debrief should include discussion of whether the online working was of sufficient standard to ensure governance.

Video Relay Services (VRS) and Video Remote Interpreting (VRI)
VRS and VRI were established before the Covid-19 pandemic, as an alternative to face to face interpreting.

Video Remote Interpreting (VRI) refers to services provided as and when needed for situations where all participants are in the same location. The remote interpreter is introduced to the conversation via a web-based video link for events such as school parent's evening or a staff meeting.

Services in the UK are mostly provided by independent interpreting service providers and are therefore not evenly distributed across the country. As the service is provided online, distance is not a problem in that the interpreter could be booked from anywhere in the country. However, dialectical differences should be considered.

Currently, video interpreting services are provided through contracts and individual agreements.

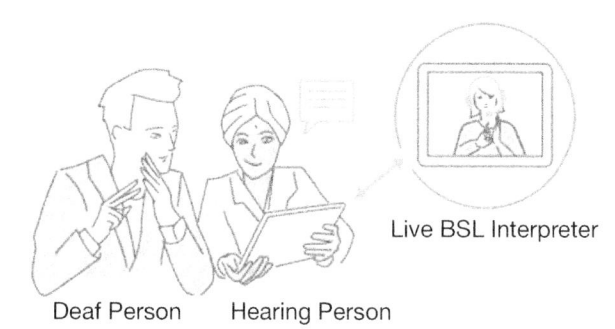

Deaf Person   Hearing Person   Live BSL Interpreter

Video Remote Interpreting
Image Courtesy of SignVideo

Video Relay Service (VRS) differs from VRI in that it connects two people in separate locations: the hearing party using a standard telephone, and the deaf party using internet video link (on their smart phones, tablet or laptop). A small time-lag should be expected, to allow the interpretation between speech and sign.

A deaf person might use VRS to call their GP to make an appointment; a hearing person might use it to contact a deaf colleague.

Many banking, utility companies, councils and NHS facilities have VRS contracts to enable customers to contact their call centres, and which are free for the deaf caller.

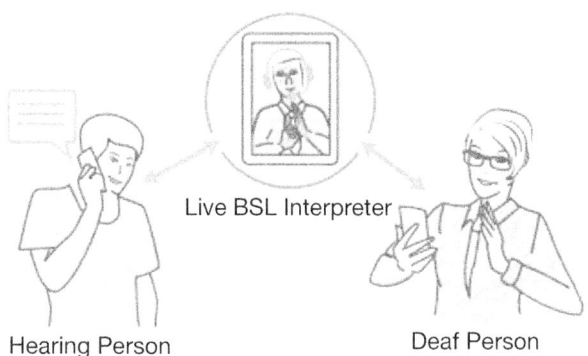

Hearing Person   Live BSL Interpreter   Deaf Person

Video Relay Service
Image Courtesy of SignVideo

VRS services, available 24/7/365 and accessed from anywhere, are the ideal means by which deaf people can contact 999 emergency services and NHS 111. The service is accessed via an App., which provides a service that is equitable to that of hearing people. In Scotland this service is provided by the government combined with their health service; whereas in the rest of the UK this is still in a consultation phase.

Limitations of VRS and VRI
VRS and VRI are a great development and promote more rapid communication equality and access. However, the interpreters used are generally not known to the participants and do not have any preparation for the specific job. This means that the topics that they are interpreting may not be within their specialist skills, they have not had opportunity to get to know the individual's communication style and they have no contextual or background history.

Thus, interpreting tasks that require specialist skills such as physical or mental health or legal matters should be restricted, where possible, to face to face interpreting or booking and prepping online interpreters. Likewise, working with idiosyncratic signers (such as refugees, those who use family signs or old-fashioned signs, or those with disabilities) can require more time, space and specialist skills than the VRS or VRI service can provide.

VRS calls should be considered as gateway calls, to consider what future communication support the client may need. For example, a VRS to a mental health service may be sufficient to make the referral but the decision is then made that the more in-depth mental health assessment will require a face to face (or booked and prepped remote) appointment with an interpreter who has mental health experience and perhaps a Deaf Relay interpreter.

Summary
Booking and prepping a remote BSL interpreter or using VRS or VRI services have great benefits. However, it is the professionals' responsibility to consider if this meets the needs of each particular client, for each particular task.

D8 Oral communication: lip reading
Dr Sally Austen and Hellen McDonald

Oral communication combines lipreading with the use of any (residual) hearing the deaf person has. Natural gesture is also important for receptive and expressive oral communication.

Lip reading is incredibly difficult. Estimates typically report up to around 30-40% effectiveness but there is evidence that at a sentence level people accurately identify as little as 12% of what they see (Altieri, 2011).

It is often assumed that deaf people will be well-practiced at lipreading and therefore better at it. However, there is evidence to show that deaf, hard of hearing (HOH)and hearing people are equally inaccurate. A good knowledge of the spoken language supports lipreading skill, with those who have been deafened gradually being more accurate than those deafened suddenly.

In order to maximise effectiveness of lipreading various factors should be considered:
- The language used
- Who the speaker is
- The behaviour of the speaker
- The positioning of the speaker
- The environment of the speaker
- The emotional and cognitive wellbeing of the lipreader
- Clear context

The language
Some sounds have identical lip-patterns (e.g. in English T and D differ according to the position of the tongue behind the teeth, which cannot be seen). So, if someone is struggling to lipread you, try choosing different words to recreate the same meaning.

Speakers
Some people are easier to lipread than others. Those with expressive faces are easier. Those with facial hair are harder (e.g. beards, moustaches, long hair over face or eyes). Accents other than our own are harder to lipread.

Your speech
Speak as normally as possible but at a slightly slower pace, making lip movements clear:
- Do not exaggerate lip movements as this will change how words appear
- Do not shout
- Be prepared to repeat things, rephrase things or write/draw them down.
- Check the lip-reader has understood you

If you are meeting remotely, via video conferencing, use platforms that offer closed captioning.

Deepness of the speaker's voice, relative to the listener's frequencies of hearing loss can also impact on understanding.

Your position
Make sure you can be seen by the person you are communicating with and you are not too far away. Do not cover your lips or turn your head whilst talking. Lip reading is best when face to face. The side of a face limits accuracy. The back of the head is impossible!

Example (Clinical psychologist working on an Expert Witness Court assessment): Client was charged with deliberately ignoring police request to leave his upstairs flat. The police knew the client was profoundly deaf. The police informed him that he should leave the flat – by shouting through the ground floor letterbox!

If you can't stay face to face (e.g. needing to use a flipchart, look down at your notes, consult another person), then the lipreader will not understand you. If looking away is inevitable, you will either need to repeat yourself when you can look directly at the lipreader or employ a lip-speaker (see Chapter D9). Employing a lip-speaker will improve the lipreader's effectiveness.

Group situations make lip-reading extremely difficult. Only one person should speak at a time and all in the group should be visible (i.e. in a circle or a staggered line). A competent chairperson should indicate when the next person is about to speak.

The environment
- Use a room that is well lit
- Make sure the face of the speaker is well lit and that the lipreader is not dazzled by light
- Do not stand with your back to the window, as the light will cast a shadow on your face
- Where possible reduce auditory distraction (e.g. background music, other conversations, fish tanks bubbling, builders outside)
- Where possible reduce visual distractions (e.g. lots of posters on a wall behind you, flickering lights, people moving about)

The emotional and cognitive wellbeing of the lipreader
The speaker should not expect consistency of lipreading. Lipreading skills diminish when concentration is impaired (e.g. due to tiredness, anxiety or distraction). Ability to hear or lipread, can vary through the day for no apparent reason. Time needs to be given to process verbal information as some words may need to be mentally added to fill the gaps of what has not been heard or lipread.

Example: Client K identifies as deaf and works in an office. He can communicate orally much of the time and, in the right circumstances (familiar person and confident context), use a telephone. However, when his mental health deteriorates and he needs a psychiatric community visit or inpatient stay, he requires a BSL interpreter for all meetings with hearing professionals. Hearing professionals have been known to be dismissive 'Oh he can lipread when he wants to!' However, the crucial point is not about 'wanting to', but about available energy, confidence, and cognition to devote to the lipreading, in that particular situation and time.

Example: Client B is highly intelligent, is hard of hearing and has Autistic Spectrum Disorder. In the early stages of a social encounter she is unable to maintain eye contact. As she becomes more at ease, and can make use of eye contact, her ability to lipread improves.

Clear context
Start with the topic of conversation and then move into the details. Avoid quick changes into other topics without making sure the listener is following.

Professional lipreaders

Often referred to as Expert Lipreaders, due to their occasional instruction as expert witnesses in court, professional lipreaders use their skills to provide information where a visual, but not audio, record of the speaker exists. For example, lipreaders were employed by the media to comment on whether Jeremy Corbyn in the House of Commons (2018) had said 'stupid people' or 'stupid woman' in response to PM Theresa May's speech.

In court, lipreaders may be asked to view CCTV footage of alleged criminals talking. Given the imprecision of lipreading, and the lack of recognised lipreading qualifications, the reports provided by Expert Lipreaders should be used cautiously.

Professional Lipspeakers (see Chapter D9)

A 'Lipspeaker' is a registered qualified hearing communication expert, trained to be easy to lipread; and employed to maximise the effective relaying of information to lipreaders.

Communicating via video conferencing meetings

Since Covid-19, many more remote meetings are taking place and communication styles need to be adapted. To maximise access:
- Allow time for adjusting volume and headphones
- Ensure that additional background noises are kept to a minimum and mute yourself when possible
- Where possible, use platforms that have live captions
- Of those that do have live captions, the availability of the captions can vary according to whether you are the purchased account user or whether you are the joining 'guest'
- If your guest is using captions, make sure to put captions on for yourself so that you can monitor the accuracy and correct words where necessary. This will save stress and misunderstandings
- If multiple people are in the call, use platforms that enable a user to 'Pin' a person, to fix on specific speakers and increase the size of their picture
- Check your lighting. The light should come from in front of you and fall onto your face. Lighting from behind creates darkness around the face and lips, which interferes with lip reading
- Try to eradicate reflections on people's glasses

- Check your seating position. Ensure that your face is in the middle of the screen and not too far away
- If you will also be using sign or gesture, ensure that both your face and your hands can be seen
- Try not to turn away from the camera whilst talking as the guest may not be able to follow the conversation
- If there are more than 2 people in the meeting, ensure that some etiquette is agreed by all so that only one person talks at a time
- Encourage attenders to allow pauses between speakers: it can take a moment to orient to the next talker
- Remember that any delays or freezes due to connection issues can cause lip read words or captions to be missed
- Avoid using distracting or busy 'backgrounds'

Conclusion

Lipreading is an exhausting and imprecise form of communication. To maximise the success of the interaction, the hearing person must commit to considering their own communication and the environment in which their meeting with the deaf person will take place.

References

Altieri, N. A. A. (2011). Some normative data on lip-reading skills. *The Journal of the Acoustical Society of America, 130(1)*, 1-4

D9 What is a Lipspeaker?
Lesley Weatherspoon and Dr Sally Austen

A 'Lipspeaker' is a hearing person trained to be easy to lipread. They will clearly reproduce the shapes of the words and the natural rhythm and stress used by the speaker using facial expression and gesture. They will use additional finger spelling if requested. Some will use additional sign if requested.

A lipspeaker may be asked to lipspeak with 'voice off' or with 'voice on'. Clients who benefit from any residual hearing may request the lipspeaker to use their voice.

If requested, lipspeakers can relay a deaf person's voice.

As with sign language interpreters (see Chapter D1), lipspeakers are required to undertake specific and tailored legal training before being able to accept work and support deaf people in the legal domain.

Lipspeakers should be qualified and registered with The National Registers of Communication Professionals working with Deaf and Deafblind People (NRCPD). They follow a Code of Conduct and should have an up-to-date Disclosure and Barring Service (DBS) check.

Booking a Lipspeaker
Currently the only UK agency for lipspeakers is www.lipspeaker.co.uk.

Provide the lipspeaker with as much information as possible, in advance of the booking. For example:
- Meeting notes/slides/background history
- Agenda/aim of the meeting
- Attendees and their roles
- Name of the Chair/responsible clinician

Working with a Lipspeaker
- The lipspeaker must be clearly visible to the lipreader.
- The lipspeaker should have a solid dark colour background behind them. This prevents 'visual noise' as sustained lipreading is tiring.

- The upper body and face of the lipspeaker should be well lit, without the presence of shadows.
- Allow time for the deaf person to receive the conveyed message and allow time for them to interject/question.
- Check with the client regularly that they are understanding.
- Check with the Lipreader regularly to see if anything needs to be adapted to improve communication.
- Meetings over an hour will need breaks.
- Complex meetings or those over two hours may require a second Lipspeaker. The agency will discuss with you and advise.

D10 Oral communication: improving the effectiveness of communication using residual hearing
Dr Sally Austen and Nikki Stephens

One in five of the UK population has some kind of hearing loss (RNID, 2020). That equates to about 12 million people and includes 900,000 with severe to profound deafness. It is therefore safe to assume that you will come across many clients whose hearing deficit may hamper their ability to hear and understand what is being said.

Hidden disability
Hearing loss is a 'hidden disability': either because hearing people are unaware of it and/or because many people with hearing loss attempt to keep it hidden. On average a person with an acquired loss takes about ten years to seek help and address their difficulties with hearing.

Some people experience their hearing loss as stigmatising, worrying that others may regard it is a sign of ageing, of stupidity or of 'being a nuisance' (see Chapter F3). Whilst it is understandable that in these circumstances someone might not want to disclose their hearing loss, failure to do so prevents others from taking their share of responsibility for the mutual communication.

A universal responsibility
Hearing loss is described as mild, moderate, severe, or profound, depending on how loud a noise needs to be for the person to hear it (see Chapter A3). Each person has a unique hearing threshold, that can vary across frequencies and volume. However, whether a person can hear a noise, and whether there is sufficient acoustic quality for them to comprehend the noise are not the same thing. Both depend on the environment in which the noise is being made.

Thus, there are three ways to improve the effectiveness of a person's residual hearing.
- Adjust the way we all communicate
- Improve the quality of the acoustic environment
- Boost residual hearing through technology

Adjusting our communication

Many of the adjustments promoted in chapter D8, to enable more effective lip reading, also apply to the use of residual hearing.

In the current COVID-19 pandemic, a major barrier to communication has been the wearing of masks. Lipreading is impossible and the facial expressions that are crucial to BSL are significantly reduced. Clear masks and visors are now being used in some areas, but there is still debate between their availability, their cost and safety.

- Ask if the individual needs any support with their hearing. You can simply ask, "Can you hear me OK or shall I try to speak a bit louder? Would you like me to type or write what I am saying?"

- Be prepared to use a Speech to Text App on your smart phone. By holding the phone still and in front of you the App transcribes your words in real time. No such App can be 100% accurate, so watch what is written and correct where necessary. This website has a very comprehensive list of speech to text apps.
  https://www.hearinglink.org/?s=speech+to+text

- If communicating remotely, by video call, ensure you use a platform that has a live captioning facility. Information can be found on the new RNID website: https://rnid.org.uk/coronavirus-response/working-from-home-during-the-coronavirus-covid-19-outbreak/

- For people who have Single Sided Deafness (SSD), position yourself such that their 'good side' is optimised.

- Be aware that some people's hearing loss fluctuates, meaning that they will be able to hear more on some days than others.

- As described in Chapter D8, various factors can affect comprehension at a specific time: fatigue, availability of background and contextual information, the accent of the speaker etc.

- For people using certain Assistive Listening Devices (see below), be prepared to wear or hold a microphone that may come with their device.

- Lipreaders typically need to be no more than 1.5 meters away from the speaker, and those with hearing aids or cochlear implants may need to be even closer. This close proximity can be uncomfortable for both parties.

- Allow 'eye breaks' as often as required, and certainly after thirty minutes.

- Be willing to learn how you make helpful changes, without feeling defensive.

As we may not be able to tell who has a hearing loss or not, we should provide services in a way that is accessible to those who would identify as Deaf, deaf or Hard of Hearing (HOH). From jurors in court rooms to patients awaiting test results and college students attempting to follow lectures, difficulty following what is being said is detrimental to all parties involved. Missing information may be simply frustrating but, in situations such as listening to advice about a crucial health condition or the safety instructions on an aeroplane, it could be life threatening.

Acoustic environment
As mentioned in chapter D8, lighting is important to maximise the visual aspect of receptive communication. Good acoustics are just as important. Acoustic environment, in this context, refers to the quality of the received sound and what might promote or distort it.

Clearly, a conversation held in a room near a building site is going to be difficult. However, other, more subtle noises can overpower the reception of speech (e.g. air conditioning, a bubbling fish tank, a background radio). Other, occasional noises can be distracting or even painful (e.g. a rustling crisp packet, someone clicking their biro). These noises are mostly filtered out by hearing people or easily solved: move to a different room, close a window, switch off the radio, ask someone to stop clicking their pen. For someone who is trying to avoid drawing attention to their hearing loss, asking for help or asserting their need, can be very difficult. Thus, negotiating the communication environment must be a shared event.

In the absence of competing noise, the design of the space, can have massive effects on quality of sound. The crucial factor is whether there is sound absorption or sound echo. An echo distorts the sound being heard;

sound absorption improves the quality of the sound and makes it easier to hear and comprehend.

The larger the space and the fewer sound absorbing features, the harder it will be for any of us to hear clearly. Acoustics can be improved by adding acoustic panels, or more simply by the inclusion of soft furnishings (e.g. carpets, curtains, table clothes). Even adding pictures to the walls can help with acoustics, although 'busy' backgrounds can make lipreading and watching sign language more difficult.

Fashion trends are often the enemy of accessibility for people with hearing loss. The evolution of open plan restaurants with minimal soft furnishings are a nightmare for people trying to use residual hearing. Decisions made without thought for people who are deaf or Hard of Hearing, can ruin lives and careers. Open plan and minimalist offices, created to save money or bring teams together, create audiological warzones of competing noises.

Boosting residual hearing through technology
Hearing aids, cochlear implants, BAHAs have all evolved into very sophisticated devices.

Hearing aids amplify sound and can be directional. Some can compress sound and cut down on some background noise. They can offer access to room or personal loop systems if the Telecoil feature is activated.

NHS aids use digital technology, but they do not restore hearing in the way that putting on a pair of spectacles may correct a person's vision - and they never will. Nor do they offer access to all the technology that private hearing aids do. NHS aids may be compatible with some of the Assistive Listening Devices described below that give better access to speech.

Cochlear Implants (CIs) are surgically implanted devices with an external component called a 'speech processor'. They are offered to certain patients whose hearing aids no longer give them access to the sound they need to hear and understand speech. Having a cochlear implant can be life changing for a person with an acquired or sudden hearing loss. The outcomes for pre-lingually deaf people are less dramatic but some people find the sensation of sound reassuring in different surroundings and that it aids lipreading. Cochlear implants do not amplify sound but present it electronically to the brain via the nerves in the cochlea rather than normal hearing which stimulates the hair cells in the cochlea. For more information visit: www.bcig.org.uk

Bone Anchored Hearing Aids (BAHAs) are also surgically implanted and are based on bone conduction. They are used for patients whose conductive hearing loss or other loss means they are unable to benefit from or tolerate the in the ear or behind the ear hearing aids.

Functional use of hearing technology

Even with the best device some people may struggle to put it in, replace batteries or make full use of it. People with dementia may not always be compliant with wearing their recommended device. Support is available from local Audiology Departments, RNID and HearingLink:
https://rnid.org.uk
https://www.hearinglink.org

Assistive Listening Devices (ALDs) and other aids

At their most basic, ALDs are amplifiers with microphones that bring the sound you want to hear closer to the ears. Some may filter out background noise. The more sophisticated Bluetooth or wireless radio devices deliver the sound direct into the hearing aid or CI speech processor.

These devices are designed to help people with a mild/moderate to severe hearing loss communicate better particularly in 1:1 conversation. Some ALDs can also be used to access sound direct from the TV or mobile telephone.

Personal Listeners

These can be used with a hearing aid through the personal neck-loop provided with the hearing aid on the telecoil setting, or without a hearing aid through a headset or earbuds.

Sarabec Crescendo

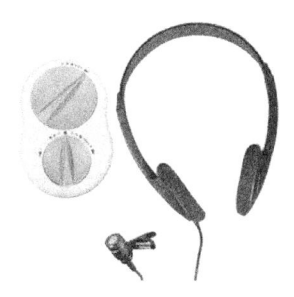

Communicator

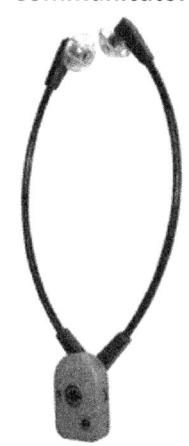

Bellman personal amplifier

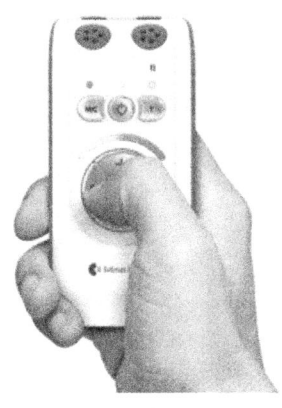

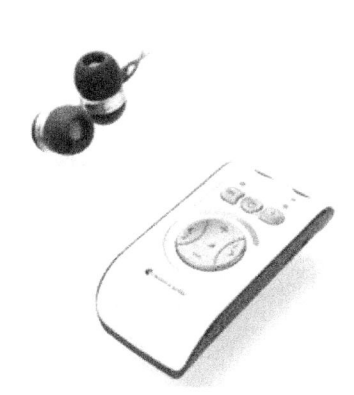

Images courtesy of Connevans

Bluetooth/wireless technology
Hearing aid and cochlear implant users are able to access devices such as the Compilot and Roger Pen using Bluetooth and other wireless technology. These devices are not provided on the NHS, but funding may be available through Access to Work (see below). It may help if the practitioner wears the microphone so that what is said is delivered direct to the hearing aid or speech processor. If there is more than one hearing person, the microphone will have to be passed between them.

Compilot   **Roger Pen system**

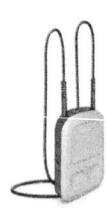

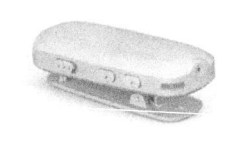

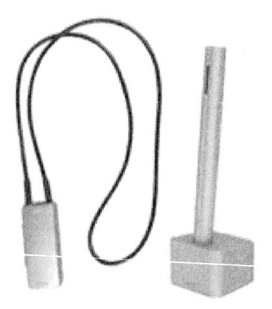

Images courtesy of Connevans

The Roger Pen and MyLink
The Roger Pen and Roger Select are microphones that automatically pick up sound that is transmitted to hearing aids/sound processor. This is done through a receiver and the microphone settings automatically adjust to noise levels around the user.

Loop systems
You may see the sign that indicates that a loop system is available for a hearing aid user with the Telecoil facility activated on their aid.

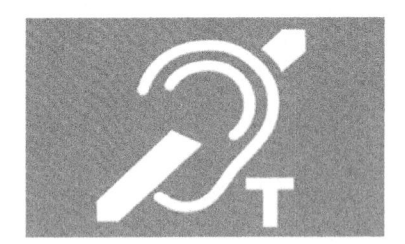

Loop systems are used variably in churches, banks, and shops. Theatres and cinemas tend to use more sophisticated systems. Seeing the symbol is no guarantee that the loop system is switched on, or even working. They are being used less, as other technologies improve.

Other access support
Environmental equipment can come in the form of alerting devices, mainly for use in the home. Some local authority Social Services departments will still do a home visit and after assessment will provide: Flashing doorbells, flashing phone alert, room loop systems for use with TV, vibrating under pillow smoke alarms, or vibrating alarm clocks.

Equipment for use in the workplace may be available from Access to Work, a government scheme where the employer shares the cost of the equipment recommended to enable the deaf/HOH person to do their job. More information can be found at: https://www.gov.uk/access-to-work

Assistance dogs
Assistance dogs can be trained to alert deaf/HOH people to noises such as fire alarms and doorbells. There are almost 1,000 working partnerships in the UK between Hearing Dogs for deaf People and those they are supporting. When the dogs are working, they are not allowed to be petted. In an appointment or consultation, they will just settle down and wait at their owner's feet until they are needed again.

Conclusion
Each of us - as individuals, workplace managers, or governments establishing policies on equality and accessibility – must consider our role in communicating with people who are Deaf, deaf, HOH. For those who have access to it, technological developments play a huge part in improving noises that can be heard and understood. However, it can only improve communication, it does not eradicate hearing loss. Practicing good communication tactics and strategies, and being aware of the difficulties that others may be experiencing, is essential to deliver and understand information quickly and accurately.

D11 Communication with deafblind people
Dr Ben Holmes and Jayne Oakes

For all of us vision and hearing vary along a continuum. For deafblind people it is also true that there are variations in the degree of vision and hearing a person has. This can result in a broad range of different communication systems that are preferred by deafblind individuals.

Depending on sensory ability, individual deafblind people may prefer to use any combination of:
- Clear speech
- Lip reading
- Adapted BSL systems (e.g. Visual frame, or Hands on sign language)
- Makaton, gesture or other sign-based communication systems
- Manual communication systems such as Deafblind manual, Block, tracking or hand to hand contact.
- Objects of reference
- Written English
- Braille or Moon

Some people may be able to use these systems with minimal adaptation or technological enhancement (e.g. enlarging text). Others may require significant adaptations or need to learn new communication systems.

Age of onset and pre-existing language
Deafblindness may be congenital (from birth) or acquired (the result of loss in later life). Preference for a communication system is typically influenced by the individual's:
- degree of vision and hearing
- age of onset that deafness and blindness commenced

Pre-existing language fluency levels will influence later communication style. For example, someone born deaf may be a fluent sign language user whereas someone born blind may prefer spoken English.

Preparation for later sensory loss
Most commonly, the two senses of vision and hearing are affected at different times and at different rates. When progressive sensory loss can be anticipated, people can prepare for their changing needs. Although,

generally people prefer to adapt existing communication methods rather than learn new ones, it is crucial that professionals are aware of the potential loss trajectory and that appropriate services are provided in a timely manner.

Common causes of deafblindness
- Medical complications during pregnancy or birth (e.g. cerebral palsy)
- Genetic conditions (e.g. CHARGE syndrome, congenital rubella syndrome, Down Syndrome or Usher Syndrome; see Chapter H1)
- Illness (such as cancer and its treatments) and accidents
- Ageing

Communication systems
The following summary provides a brief description of some of the main communication systems that are used by deafblind people where some level of adaptation is required. It should be recognised that more time will be required to communicate with Deafblind people.

In addition to using any of these specific communication systems, it is essential that the communication environment is set up well (see Chapters D8 & D10 for more information):
- Speak clearly
- Make sure the room is lit to that individual's preference
- Reduce background noise and visual clutter
- If the person has hearing aids or cochlear implants, check they are working and switched on
- Make sure the physical environment enables the person to access any interpreters present (e.g. adequate space and lines of sight)

Visual frame signing
When someone has residual vision but with a restricted visual field, they may use visual frame signing. This is where the communication partner provides adapted signs but within a smaller area so that all the signs stay within the visual field of the person receiving information.

For example, the sign for bath - two hands holding a towel is adapted to an alternative sign - a rubbing chest sign to show wash; moving signs such as fire are signed slowly to enable the deafblind person to see these;

fingerspelling is altered (e.g. "y" is produced as deafblind manual "y") so that the person may see this (see Chapter D12).

Tracking
Tracking also relies on some residual vision. The person receiving information places their hands on the wrists or forearms of their communication partner. This contact allows them to ensure that signs remain within their field of vision whilst making use of information from other sensory inputs (e.g. touch and proprioception) to follow or 'track' the conversation.

Hands on Sign
Hands on signing is similar to tracking but tends to be used when the person has less residual vision. The person receiving information places their hands on the hands of their communication partner. They then feel arm, hand and body movements to understand what is being said. This method of communication can also be called co-active signing.

Deafblind manual (See Chapter D12 for deafblind manual alphabet)
Deafblind manual communication is very similar to the BSL alphabet but with all letters spelt out on the palm and fingers of the person receiving information. This means that some letters (e.g. vowels) are essentially the same, whereas other letters have to be modified (e.g. for 'P' the finger is pinched to distinguish it from 'E').

Abbreviations are also used in this method of communication (e.g. pp = people) depending on the skills/knowledge and preferences of the deafblind person. Tracking is used, to reference speakers or objects within the situation and hand taps or rubs are used to provide positive or negative affirmation and confirm understanding.

Block communication
Block is a system that is more likely to be used by people who have a preference, for written and spoken English - or whose family and friends are unwilling or unable to learn other communication methods. Communication occurs through 'drawing' the capital form of different letters on the hand of the person receiving information using one finger.

Braille
Letters and words in Braille are represented by a series of raised dots in recognisable patterns that can be felt by the fingertips. Whilst perhaps

more commonly associated with blind people, deafblind people can also use Braille.

Moon
This is similar to Braille but uses raised patterns that are similar to the shapes of English letters, rather than dots. Meaning is determined through feeling the shape of the letters.

Tadoma
This method of communication requires the individual to place their hand on the throat, lips or cheeks of their communication partner. They then determine what is being said by feeling the movements and vibrations created by speech.

Haptic communication
Pre-agreed signs are made on the body to provide information that could be gained visually or aurally (e.g. about the environment or emotional responses). The signs can be on any part of the body that the deafblind person is comfortable with and that does not interfere with other aspects of communication; this is typically the back or upper arms.

Objects of reference and other methods of communication
Some deafblind people will use idiosyncratic communication systems that they develop in collaboration with partners, family, friends and carers to 'short-cut' to a shared understanding of meaning. For example, using number systems (e.g. 3 = dinner is ready) or using objects of reference (e.g. being given a coat means we are going out).

An alternative means of communication is the use of tactile prompts. For example, when acting as a guide touching the person's arm or hand to indicate readiness to start walking. For congenitally deafblind people – objects of reference and other bespoke communication systems may be the only communication accessible to them.

Gaining the attention of someone who is deafblind
Different deafblind people will have different preferences about how to notify them of your presence or intention to communicate. Some may be able to see or hear sufficiently well to notice you stand in front of them or speak their name. Others may have sufficient vision to notice changes in shadow and light – here, switching a light off and on may be best.

Some deafblind people can feel disturbances in the air or vibrations from movement and prefer you to bang a nearby surface or stamp the ground. When none of these are possible being gently touched on the shoulder can also be used. However, for someone not expecting an interaction this might be quite alarming and may not be preferred. If communicating regularly with a deafblind person the communicating partner may wear a specific item (e.g. a bracelet) that allows them to know who is there.

Challenges with communication
As might be expected, when adaptations are made to language or communication systems there is the possibility that miscommunications may occur either expressively or receptively. For example, in BSL some signs appear the same but are differentiated by head nods/shakes, eye gaze, lip patterns and facial expression. As this information may not be accessible alternative ways of clarifying meaning may be required (e.g. showing negation of a concept).

Many deafblind people will have Communicator Guides to help them with access, to aid their safety and to help with communication. Some people also rely on friends or carers for communication support. As the formality, or importance, of the communication setting increases the greater the likelihood that specialist interpreters will need to be involved. Given the potential for miscommunication and mis-diagnosis to occur, it is also important that understanding of information is regularly checked. In some settings, such as healthcare or legal settings, specialist interpreters should always be used.

Non-verbal communication and mental health
Deafblind people are more likely to experience conditions that increase their risk of mental health problems:
- Vulnerability - deafblind people are at greater risk of exploitation and abuse
- Loss - acquired sensory loss may bring with it other losses, such as to mobility, independence and control, role, and fear of the future
- Isolation and sensory deprivation - isolation is a known catalyst for new mental health conditions and to worsen pre-existing conditions, such as anxiety, depression, and psychosis (see Chapter F4)

With changes to mental health there may also be changes in behaviour that are indicative of emotional distress. These behavioural changes can be considered as non-verbal communications and may indicate the need for help from statutory or specialist mental health services (see Chapters G3 & G4).

Links
For further information and resources please see:
Deafblind UK https://deafblind.org.uk
Sense https://www.sense.org.uk
Department of Health (1997) Think Dual Sensory – www.deafblind.com/thinkold.html

D12 BSL deafblind alphabet

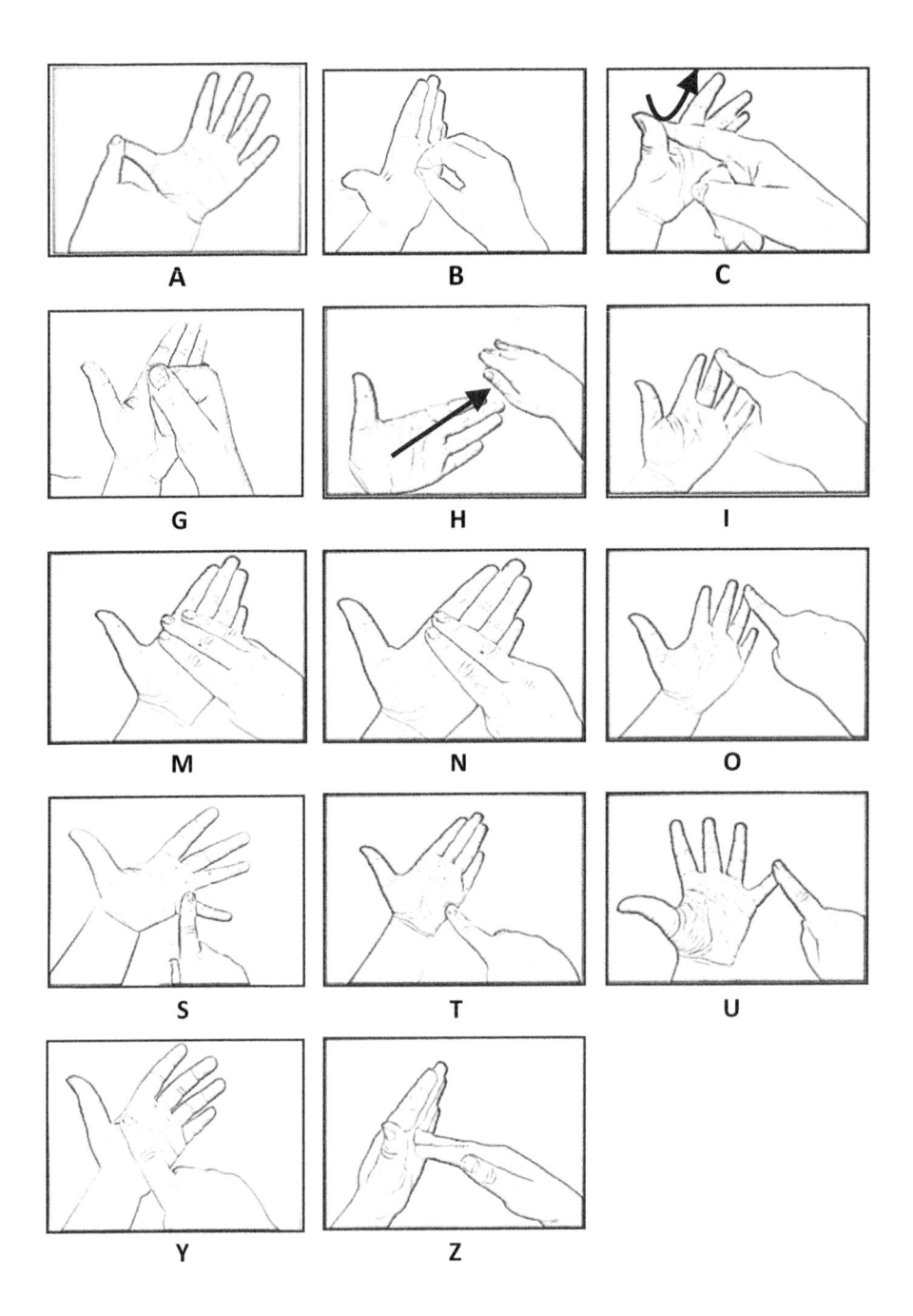

D	E	F
J	K	L
P	Q	R
V	W	X

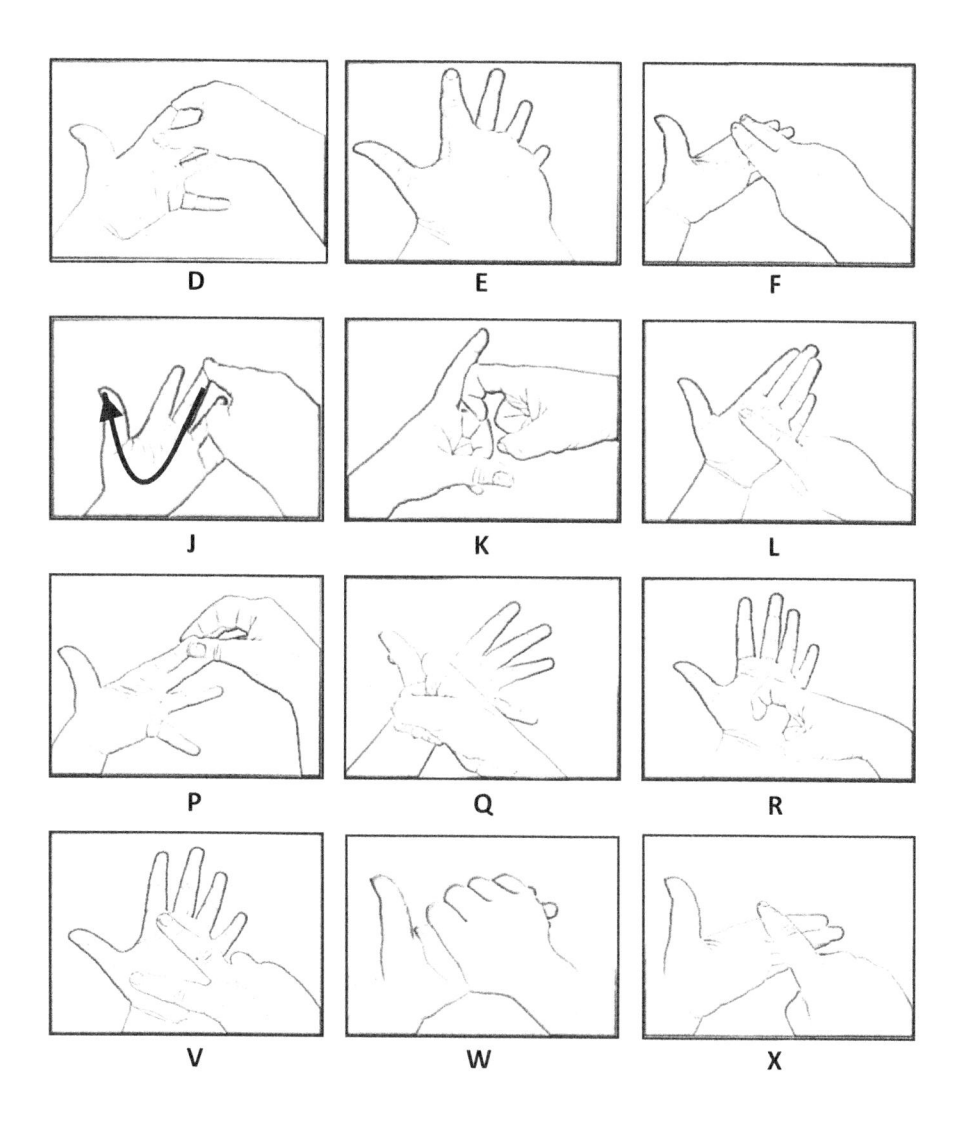

Note: The left hand represents that of the deafblind person receiving information and the right hand represents the person communicating with them.

D13 Non-native BSL users
Lenka Novakova

Whether you work in health, education or legal settings meeting the cultural and linguistic needs of your client will ensure efficiency and efficacy in your work: ensuring a positive experience for them and minimising the chance of misdiagnosis or inadequate interventions.

If your deaf client uses sign language as their first or preferred language this should be respected and adhered to. There is often a misconception that sign language is the same across the world, but this is not the case. Other countries have their own sign languages and deaf immigrants to Britain will need to learn British Sign Language (BSL) as a new language.

As with the difference between BSL and spoken English, each country's native sign language has its own unique syntax, structure and grammar, that differs from their country's spoken and written language form.

The Deaf community in the UK is diverse with nationalities and languages used. As with UK citizens, non-UK citizens also require accessible and informed services.

Deaf people around the world will have very different experiences in terms of:
- access to sign language or audiological technologies
- access to education and the work place
- stigma around being deaf
- and even religious beliefs that being deaf has been a punishment from a higher power.

These differing experiences will impact on any assessment or intervention.

Booking interpreters for non-native BSL signers
It is crucial to ask your deaf client how they wish to communicate and in which language. The National Register for Communication Professionals working with Deaf and Deafblind People (NRCPD) identifies a small number of interpreters across the country who can work in Irish Sign Language (ISL), American Sign Language (ASL), Australian Sign Language

(AUSLAN), New Zealand Sign Language (NZSL), French Sign Language (LSF) and BSL to spoken Welsh.

Interpreters who can work in other languages may not be formally qualified to do so in the UK and finding them would require the professional to phone around various sign language interpreting agencies.

This puts the professional leading the work with the deaf client in a difficult situation as it is always recommended that only fully qualified, NRCPD registered Sign Language Interpreters (SLIs) are booked (Chapter D1). Likewise, trainee sign language interpreters, communication support workers or family members should not be requested to interpret.

Deaf Relay Interpreters (DRI) or Relay-Intralingual (see Chapter D4)
In the likely situation that you cannot find a qualified, registered hearing SLI with the appropriate foreign sign language skills, you may need to book a deaf relay (or Relay-Intralingual) interpreter (DRI) alongside a BSL interpreter. This is also the case where the deaf client has language dysfluency or cognitive difficulties (see Chapters B1 & E2).

Spoken language translators for family members
Only about 5% of deaf people are born into deaf families. Thus, it is very likely that if your deaf client is a non-native BSL signer, they will have hearing family members who will need a spoken language interpreter at appointments. Whereas BSL interpreters simultaneously interpret as you speak, the spoken language interpreter will pause you regularly to speak in their language to the hearing family member. All parties will wait for translation back to English, and this can then be conveyed to the deaf client in sign.

Difficulties
Additional time
A clinician should lead and facilitate the session as they usually would with an SLI (see Chapter D2), allowing enough time for the DRI to further interpret what is being communicated. Working in such settings requires significant preparation beforehand and can take twice as long as a meeting without interpreters. Multiple meetings might be needed to ensure that this person grasps the context and content of the meeting,

particularly if the client has additional cognitive or linguistic difficulties or is particularly traumatised.

Potential conflict of interest

If it is a possibility to find a DRI who is competent in the same language as the client, this will work better for all parties involved. However, it may come with a burden of conflict of interest. The professional should ask the DRI if they know the client in a personal manner before the booking is made. Likewise, the client should be asked (preferably away from the DRI) whether they are comfortable to work with this DRI.

Sign language evolves geographically rather than politically. Thus, it is common for two people to use the same sign language but to be on opposing political or warring sides. For those non-native BSL signing clients who have fled unrest, it is particularly important to ensure they feel safe with their SLI and DRI and that they trust in the impartiality and confidentiality of the conversations.

Both DRIs and SLIs should declare any conflict of interest, as per their code of conduct.

International Sign (IS)

International Sign is not a language per se: it consists of borrowing signs from different sign languages.

If a deaf person from a different country is fluent in their native sign language, and not yet learnt BSL, they might choose to use International Sign. However, for those who are not aware of their own language limitations this may not be the most effective solution, so an SLI working closely with DRI should determine the best method of interpretation.

D14 Checklist of your client's communication needs
Lindsey Gagan

Client Name: Date:

Completed by: Role:

Sign language?
Does this person use fluent sign language with family and/or friends?
  ☐ Yes   ☐ No

Does this person prefer to have a sign language interpreter in conversations with hearing people?
  ☐ Yes   ☐ No

Does this person require a deafblind interpreter?
  ☐ Yes   ☐ No

If the person answers yes to any of these questions, an interpreter must be sought to support the conversation, provided that the delay incurred does not compromise the person's wellbeing.

An interpreter must be booked in advance of further arranged appointments in accordance with the Accessible Information Standard (2016) and Equality Act (2010)

Does the person have a preference around interpreter support?
☐ Yes – a familiar individual / agency (specify:..)
☐ Yes – a male / female interpreter
☐ Other (specify: ....)

Using the deaf or hard of hearing person's friend or relative as an unqualified interpreter is not advised. They may not be accurate or impartial. Consider also the impact on the confidentiality of the conversation. Seek the preference of your client and weigh up the need to proceed immediately against postponing until an interpreter is available (see Chapter D5 for how to book an interpreter).

For immediate interaction with the person, consider points overleaf...

Level of functional hearing

Does the person use hearing aids or a cochlear implant?
- ☐ Cochlear implant
- ☐ Hearing aid left side
- ☐ Hearing aid right side
- ☐ Hearing aids both sides

Is the person wearing these today and are they in working order?
- ☐ Worn today and working well
- ☐ Prefers to use but aids/implant not working well (detail..)
- ☐ The person chooses not to use aids/implant (why? ....)

Do aids/implant support communication usefully?
- ☐ Yes - the person can follow telephone conversations
- ☐ Yes – the person can follow some speech face to face (with need for clarification)
- ☐ The person does not follow what is said but can hear some sounds with aids/implants
- ☐ No

Is hearing better in one ear?
- ☐ The left side   ☐ The right side   ☐ No

What does the person hear without hearing aids/implant?
- ☐ Some speech
- ☐ Environmental sound only
- ☐ Nothing. Sound is perceived as vibration

Do you need to think about the maintenance of the hearing aids or implant?
- ☐ Not applicable to the conversation today
- ☐ Plans are in place for the person to maintain their aid (supply of batteries, audiology review appointments etc.)
- ☐ A need has been identified and will be followed up by ....[name]

Vision
Does the person have good vision? (Date of last eye test:)
- ☐ Yes
- ☐ Yes, with glasses (have today / do not have today)
- ☐ No (Specify ....)

Does the person make eye contact with you while you are talking?
- ☐ Yes
- ☐ Needs some prompts to look
- ☐ Responds very little

Speech
Does the person use speech?
- ☐ Yes and it is clearly intelligible enough to most people
- ☐ Speech is intelligible to familiar people
- ☐ The person uses speech/voice but this can be difficult to understand
- ☐ Some lipreading is used (be aware that this is often very inadequate for deaf and hard of hearing people)
- ☐ Responds very little

Which spoken language does the person use?...

Is a spoken language interpreter needed for this conversation?
- ☐ Yes   ☐ No

If the person has adequate hearing, available amplification and speech to engage in a spoken conversation, think about the following:
- Does the person prefer you to speak on their better side or face?
- What is a comfortable face to face distance for the person to see you speak?
- Sit with good light on your face (not behind you as your face will be in shadow
- Reduce noise - close windows, turn off tv, be aware of echo.
- Speak clearly so the person can see your mouth but do not exaggerate words

If the person is a sign language user, it will not be appropriate to attempt any detailed conversation that can be safely revisited later when an interpreter is available

---

Consider whether writing may support your conversation…..

Reading and writing
What does the person report about reading?
- ☐ No difficulty reading written information on any topic which is designed to be accessible to a lay person
- ☐ Reads newspapers, letters and follows TV subtitles, with just occasional unfamiliar words
- ☐ Reads some everyday short messages but not lengthier or more in depth information
- ☐ Does not find written information helpful

What does the person report about writing/typing?
- ☐ Writes or types a letter confidently
- ☐ Prefers to write or type short, routine messages
- ☐ Writing is not a useful way to communicate

Does the person use any of the following?
- ☐ Mobile phone text messaging
- ☐ Email or Social Media (which?..)
- ☐ Typetalk
- ☐ Fax or other (....)

Does this person have any additional disabilities which may impact the conversation?
☐ No   ☐ Yes (Specify ....)

Reviewing your conversation – was it successful?
Was the person able to repeat back the information?   ☐ Yes   ☐ No
Did the person ask relevant questions?   ☐ Yes   ☐ No
Did the person let you know if something was not clear? ☐ Yes   ☐ No
Did the person repeat or clarify information when you needed?
                                                        ☐ Yes   ☐ No

Make note of helpful strategies:-
- ☐ breaking information down into small, key points
- ☐ using plainer, more familiar language (e.g................................
  ....)
- ☐ drawing
- ☐ writing key words / short sentences

Section E

E1 Diagnostic overshadowing
Dr Sally Austen

Categorisation is implicit in diagnostic frameworks. But it is important also to avoid blanket assumptions.

Diagnostic overshadowing refers to the attribution of a person's symptoms to their primary presentation, when their symptoms may actually suggest a comorbid condition.

The term first came about as a result of physical illness being missed in people with Intellectual Disabilities (ID). Symptoms of the physical illness (new behaviours or demonstrations of emotions) were being blamed on the ID, resulting in misdiagnosis and delay in treatment.

Diagnostic overshadowing in deaf people is more likely to result in missed opportunity: to treat or provide services. Something that is compounded by already poor access (see Chapter G1).

For example, autism is missed in a deaf child with early language delay and seen as an inevitable feature of deafness, rather than a difficulty that will respond to additional resources and intervention (see Chapter E4).

Similarly, challenging behaviour (including criminal behaviour) in deaf adults is often attributed to a person's deafness resulting in lack of rehabilitative interventions or punitive consequences (see Chapters F12, I1& I2).

There are multiple causes of deafness (see Chapter H1) that may have been associated with concurrent health or cognitive conditions. Deaf people are just as liable to have any of the other conditions and experiences that hearing people present with (e.g. asthma, appendicitis, cancer, dementia, bereavement).

Thus, it is the professional's responsibility to review their work in case of diagnostic overshadowing. Contact can be made with specialist deaf services if in doubt (see Chapters G3 & G4).

E2 Cognitive assessment
Dr Ben Holmes

A cognitive assessment aims to understand how an individual processes information, makes sense of their world and responds to problems they face.

Theoretically, different aspects of cognition are considered as separate 'domains'; for example, memory, attention, executive functioning, processing speed. However, understanding cognition in the context of day to day functioning is far more complex than this.

Cognitive assessments are useful tools in many settings, including health care, education and in court proceedings. They can be used to diagnose difficulties, inform decisions about support needs and highlight areas of skill that might be developed. Accuracy is therefore key.

Cognitive assessments for deaf people
Any assessment makes certain assumptions about the person being assessed. There are currently few standardised assessments designed or normed for deaf people - the assumptions of most being based on experiences typical to hearing people.

Lack of awareness of the interaction between the differing experiences of deaf people (culturally, linguistically and in terms of opportunity and access to information) and assessments can therefore risk drawing inaccurate conclusions.

Use deaf specialists
Making assessments accessible to deaf people is not as simple as **just** employing an interpreter. It also requires an in depth understanding of the theory behind assessments being used.

When completing cognitive assessments for deaf people, clinicians specialising in this area of work should be contacted to lead, consult or co-work (see Chapters G3 & G4). In court settings, it is crucial that deaf specialists are employed (see Chapter I6).

Standardised tasks
Often, cognitive assessments include the completion of standardised tasks. Developed through years of rigorous research these tests offer reliable points of comparison from which to determine an individual's relative ability.

Tasks are administered verbally, by pen and paper or by computer. Generally, they are completed face to face, but some can also be completed remotely – which has been of particular relevance during Covid-19 (see Chapter E8).

The need for caution
Whilst standardised tasks are often a core component of a cognitive assessment, their use has limitations:
- Task performance represents only a measurable 'snapshot' of ability
- Performance on tasks, and in day to day life, is affected by many factors beyond 'pure' cognition
- Domains are not discreet, they consist of a combination of functions that are hard to separate

Frequently, when assessing deaf people, assessments cannot be delivered in the standardised ways intended. This increases the risk of error associated with their use and the potential for inaccurate conclusions.

A full cognitive assessment relies on far more than just performance data from standardised tasks, for example:
- Contextual information, gathered through clinical interview with the individual, people who know them well and from observation
- Information about early development, psychological wellbeing and history of the presenting difficulty
- Qualitative information about how tasks are completed

It is the combination of these factors, alongside test data, that produce a useful understanding of an individual's cognition.

The importance of normative data
The purpose of cognitive assessment is to determine ability within the context of the broader population. Normative data are therefore an essential part of assessment.

Normative data are collected by administering tasks in a standardised way to a sample of a given population. Without a reference sample to compare to it is not possible to know what typical performance for that population might look like. For example, scoring 4 out of 10 on a task might appear problematic but if the average score is 2 it is actually very good.

Normative data for deaf people
Some measures have been developed that provide test norms for Deaf people (e.g. BSL-CST; Atkinson et al., 2015). However, availability of such data is unfortunately still limited.

The experiences of deaf people vary hugely, causing greater heterogeneity than within the general population. Even where norms do exist, consideration of other factors that might affect performance, and of the question being asked, is still crucial.

Despite the lack of deaf norms, there may be times when understanding functioning in absolute, rather than relative, terms is still necessary. For example, literacy levels in deaf people are, on average, lower (see Chapter B3). Here, deaf norms could indicate an average **relative** ability but miss the client's possible need for support compared to the general population (e.g. linguistic adaptation to access written material).

Deaf gains
Whilst it is important to consider the potential disadvantages deaf people may experience from lack of appropriate norms, it is also important to note where the experience of deaf people might provide advantages; for example, visual attention for peripheral stimuli (Stoll & Dye, 2019).

The use of baselines
In some situations, using a person's performance as a baseline for comparison at repeat assessment is effective. For example, when there is a query about a possible deterioration in function.

Baseline comparisons are a more accurate point of reference than the use of generic norms. Caution is still advised in allowing for the accepted degree of measurement error or practice effect.

Task adaptations
Adaptation will depend upon factors specific to both the individual and the test.

Some tasks work very well with minimal, change (e.g. Raven's Matrices, Colour Trails, Tower of Hanoi). Others are just not appropriate to use (e.g. tests that rely on pronunciation of English words, such as TOPF). The effect of adaptation on which cognitive domain is being assessed, and on the appropriateness of norms being used, must be considered.

For example, number strings are often used to assess working memory. However, other factors (e.g. differing number systems across BSL dialects) may add additional confounds not found with spoken administration. One adaptation might be to assess working memory using a Corsi-type block board instead. However, it is important to note that this changes the task from verbal working memory to visuospatial working memory.

Another example is the assumption of automaticity with written numbers and letters on some tasks of information processing. Depending on the client and their language experiences it may be more appropriate to complete non-verbal information processing tasks, such as those using shape and colour.

Jagged profiles
It is not uncommon for people to have a jagged profile on test batteries. It may therefore happen that the tasks that are accessible represent particular strengths or particular areas of difficulty for that person. This makes it important to consider any results within the context of other information.

Sometimes it is appropriate to omit tasks that have a disproportionate reliance on spoken English or hearing culture. However, that does not mean that scores on remaining subtests can always be generalised to represent overall ability.

Other factors affecting the assessment of deaf people
The effect of opportunity and education
For many deaf people, the opportunities for incidental learning are reduced (see Chapter B4). Historically, education for deaf people has not always provided the same focus on acquisition of knowledge as in

mainstream school (see Chapter C6). Neither reduced opportunity, nor reduced exposure to information, reflects cognitive ability. However, both could impact on the ability to answer questions, even with good communication access.

For example, crystallised intelligence tasks often rely on the ability to recall facts that have been taught or learned. In this instance, simply translating questions does not make them equivalent. A low score may in fact measure 'facts that the client's teacher told them', rather than anything to do with intellect.

Some assessments aim to assess levels of skill proficiency (e.g. functional adaptive behaviour assessment). However, these measures do not always consider whether the person has had adequate opportunity to develop skill mastery (e.g. through overprotection of others - see Chapter B8). Assessments may thus, show level of exposure to a task, rather than cognitive ability to engage with it.

The effect of language
Sign language is not a gestural form of spoken language. Sign languages have their own structure, grammar and syntax that sometimes express concepts in very different ways to spoken language (see Chapter C8). Different dialects in sign language mean that a good match between client and interpreter is important (see Chapter D2).

The translation of task instructions from English to BSL also needs careful consideration as translation may require the use of gesture, demonstration or object function being described in a way that was not intended for the task. To withhold this linguistic information may deprive the deaf person of the opportunity to understand what is expected of them. To include it, may change what the task is assessing.

This makes some tasks or questions inappropriate to use. For example:
- Questions such as "What shape is a ball?" cannot be translated without giving the answer away
- Instructions that give the answer away through the action of signing (e.g. 'Fold the paper in half.')
- Arithmetic tasks assessing working memory where the visual nature of sign language makes the answer very apparent

- Word generation tasks that rely on the use of starting letters (e.g. "name objects beginning with F") - the spelling of a sign is the written English translation and so not a comparable question to ask

Language can particularly affect tasks of executive functioning where instructions are often deliberately vague or abstract, to assess how a person solves the problem. For example, the Key Search task, in the Behavioural Assessment of Dysexecutive Syndrome (BADS) battery, requires you to draw how you would search for a set of keys that has been lost in a field. The instructions in BSL will give some indication of required strategy, thereby defeating the purpose of assessment.

A further consideration is the possible impact of language deprivation (see Chapter B1). This may impact on test performance either directly (because language is the medium of assessment) or indirectly (because linguistic coding of information will aid task completion).

The effect of culture
Difficulty with a task is not always indicative of impairment but can sometimes result from cultural difference. What is 'normal' within one culture may not be in another. It is important that a different set of cultural norms is not pathologised or seen as an 'impairment'.

For example, the BSL adaptation to the Addenbrook's Cognitive Examination (ACE-III) memory task uses biographical information about a man (his age, the school he attended and wife's name), rather than his address, because this is more culturally appropriate (Atkinson et al., 2015). By translating the questions found in ACE-III without this adaptation, there is a risk of disadvantaging the person being assessed because, culturally, obtaining and recalling information of the type in the original version is less typical for deaf people.

The effect of interpreters
Many interpreters will have worked with clinicians that are naive to working with deaf people. In their role of maximising understanding, they often provide additional explanation to their deaf client, that may not have been provided by the hearing professional.

Most interpreters will not have extensive experience of completing cognitive assessments, nor an understanding of the theoretical concepts being assessed. Equally, hearing professionals may not know the best way of explaining a task so as to facilitate interpretation. This creates a risk that gaps may inadvertently be filled in the process of interpretation that means the test then assesses something different.

It is important that, before any assessment, interpreters and clinicians discuss the aims of the appointment so that there can be a collaborative conversation about how certain instructions are best provided (see Chapter D2).

The effect of power
Many deaf people will have experienced situations where hearing people make incorrect assumptions about their ability, and treat them in a patronising or discriminatory way.

Negative experiences such as these could impact on the client's confidence or motivation, which could affect task performance. There is also a risk that a client may want to give the impression of having understood instructions when they have not (See Chapter B2). Thus, it is crucial to allow extra time to engage with a client, helping them to feel at ease before starting formal assessment.

Summary
Completing cognitive assessments with deaf people requires careful consideration of many factors. An understanding is needed of the theory behind assessments, and how individual experiences may impact on engagement, so that appropriate adaptations or test selections can be made. Without this, there is a risk that assessments will be inaccessible and misinterpretation of information will lead to erroneous conclusions.

References
Atkinson, J., Denmark, T., Marshall, J., Mummery, C., & Woll, B. (2015). Detecting cognitive impairment and dementia in deaf people: the British Sign Language cognitive screening test. *Archives of Clinical Neuropsychology, 30(7)*, 694-711

Stoll, C. & Dye, M.W.G. (2019). Sign language experience redistributes attentional resources to the inferior visual field. Cognition, 191, 103957

E3 Deaf and Hard of Hearing people with intellectual disabilities
Dr Sara Rhys Jones and Dr Kevin L. Baker

Introduction
Recognising deafness and hearing loss in people with an intellectual disability (ID) shares similar challenges to identifying ID in people who are deaf or have a hearing loss. However, understanding the overlap between deafness and intellectual disability is vital.

Communication is a common factor but must be contextualised with the recognition that a person with an ID often finds it difficult to adapt to their environment and other people. This means that support staff and professionals have to adapt their communication to the person's.

Recognising deafness/hearing in people with an ID
The prevalence of deafness is *at least* 40 times higher in people with ID than the general population (Carvill, 2001). However, the majority of these people are unknown to Audiology services. In one survey, 97% of people with ID, were found to have a hearing loss of which only 6% of carers were aware. It is quite common for people to assume that the person with ID does not understand them because of their ID, rather than their hearing.

Deaf people with ID are often missed by a range of health professionals, including Audiologists. Assessments are often complicated by communication difficulties associated with both hearing loss and cognitive processing. Unfortunately, when professionals fall back on a medical approach to understand someone they see as 'complex', they then attempt to fix the parts they see as 'broken'. If hearing aids are prescribed, there may be other challenges related to cognitive difficulties which can interfere with the person's acceptance of wearing the aids, keeping them safe, and using them. The British Society of Audiologists have addressed this with national guidance (https://www.thebsa.org.uk).

Many deaf people with an ID rely on staff to understand the reasons for being prescribed hearing aids and their support to get the best from them. McShea et al. (2016) found that many staff significantly underestimated the number of people in their service with a hearing loss and advocated that training is essential. Staff turnover frequently results in important information being lost or degraded. Many service users miss follow up appointments and are subsequently discharged from Audiology.

Diagnosing intellectual disability in people who are deaf or HOH
An ID diagnosis is based on the following three criteria:
- a significant impairment of intellectual functioning
- a significant impairment of adaptive behaviour
- the impairments being present before the age of 18

The assessment of Intellectual disability with a deaf person is not straight forward. There are difficulties in adapting standardised assessments of intellectual functioning and adaptive behaviour (see Chapter E2).

Many deaf children also do not receive an assessment of their cognitive functioning as adolescents, as it is often assumed that the difficulties they experience are due to their deafness and communication difficulties, rather than their cognitive functioning (see Chapter E1), leaving teachers and parents unclear in understanding a deaf child's difficulties.

The diagnosis or categorisation of ID is important as part of a holistic assessment, providing the rationale for support and plans for improved quality of life. Misdiagnosis can mean that a person may not get the opportunities appropriate to their ability to adapt or cope. A holistic assessment of cognitive or intellectual ability would normally include a good assessment of any sensory impairment, including hearing and vision (Carvill, 2001). Additionally, any limitations of adaptive behaviour should be assessed with other conditions in mind such as ASD, ADHD, and a specific language disorder.

Communication is part of adaptive behaviour
Adaptive behaviour refers to the collection of conceptual, social and practical skills that are learned and performed by people in everyday lives. Communication assumes more importance for people who are deaf and have an ID.

A deaf person who is able to communicate well and has good problem solving abilities, will often be able to adapt to a wide range of educational and social situations. They may struggle if others cannot adapt to their individual communication style. However, their adaptive behaviour will allow them to develop coping and support mechanisms, such as meeting other deaf people, developing friendships with both deaf and hearing people, engaging with education, and finding employment.

A deaf person with an ID may experience significant difficulties adapting their communication and problem-solving abilities because of cognitive limitations such as shorter attention span, poor short term memory, difficulties in flexible thinking, limited planning ability and poor imagination. In our experience, if a deaf person experiences difficulty in adapting their communication to others, they frequently have learning and social difficulties, which may suggest a ID.

It is useful to assess a person's ability to communicate with both hearing people and deaf people, to gain a more complete understanding of their abilities. Exploration of a range of communication modes in addition to sign language and speech (writing, gesture, pictures, symbols, drawings) is informative. It also helps to collect information about how an adult has experienced communication in their family home and while at school.

Deaf people with intellectual disability who use sign language
A small number of deaf people who have Deaf parents will have been exposed to BSL from an early age and developed some fluency in their sign language. Others may learn from their hearing parents who made the choice to give them access to BSL. Those who may have only be exposed to sign language at a later age (see Chapter B1) may have language skills significantly poorer than their cognitive ability.

Unfortunately, within mainstream services there is less awareness about sign language. Some perceive signing as useful only after the client 'fails' to use their residual hearing, speech and lipreading. Others may suggest the use of Makaton, without appreciating that it is only a signed system designed to augment and support speech, and not a rich and adaptive or expressive language like BSL (see Chapter C8). Others regard the basic signing of hearing staff as sufficient because this matches that of the client, without understanding that staff require superior language and communication skills to correctly interpret a deaf person with poor communication abilities.

Deaf people with ID and "challenging" behaviours
The majority of referrals for people with ID to specialist services are for behavioural reasons: challenging behaviour; increase in anger outbursts; social isolation and withdrawal; anxiety, low mood and depression; and inappropriate sexual behaviours. Deaf people with ID can find specialist services difficult to access (see Chapter G1).

Frequent miscommunication leading to frustration and fear can understandably result in behaviours that challenge staff and services. Studies have found that there is an association between sensory impairments and challenging behaviour in people with learning disabilities (Timehin & Timehin, 2004). Behaviour management plans without information about the hearing and vision of a service user, may be missing fundamental information that can help make sense of challenging behaviour (McShea et al., 2014).

It is essential to recognise that all behaviours function as communication. For a deaf person with an ID the following are likely to be important when attempting to understand their behaviour when it challenges others:

Communication and attachment: most people born deaf experience delays in language acquisition (see Chapter C2) and development in communication skills and many experience difficulties communicating with their hearing family, who often have little or no experience in communicating with deaf people. This is more so with deaf people with ID. This can lead to maladaptive attachment behaviour patterns in order to seek safety, containment or emotional understanding.

Culture: Some cultures respond to individuals with a disability in a very different way to the individualism promoted in Westernised cultures. It is important to be aware of the cultural background of the family to help make sense of how a deaf person with an ID responds to family and social situations.

Isolation: Many deaf people with ID experience exclusion from their local Deaf community, as well as the hearing-majority culture. This is often because of their difficulties with signed communication and adaptive behaviour, but also due to the Deaf community having few opportunities to understand intellectual disability.

Common difficulties experienced by the support system

Working with deaf clients with ID can be challenging and professionals can feel deskilled.

We asked a range of staff about their thoughts and feelings about the support they provide to deaf people with an ID. Below we have listed some of their responses:

- Some hearing staff with little to no signing skills feel limited and frustrated by their ability to communicate but are unaware of how this impacts on the client - the deaf client having to repeatedly adapt to the staff's limitations (e.g. writing key words, gesturing, pointing)
- Hearing staff can find learning to sign very difficult and time consuming. Some do not get the support from their managers to learn sign language
- Some hearing staff struggle to express themselves visually (e.g. facial expressions, gestures, signs) and report feeling 'silly' or embarrassed. Some don't understand the importance of facial expressions (i.e. facial expressions for deaf people are the equivalent to tones in voices in spoken languages)
- Care staff are frequently influenced by 'normalisation' policies and training, responding to the client as 'hearing and different'. The aim of this approach is to reduce feelings of exclusion and isolation. However, staff tend to use speech with the client regardless of whether the client can lip-read and/or understand their speech
- Some hearing staff think the client's difficulties are to do with cognitive difficulties and not because their communication needs are not being met
- Some Deaf staff assume that their client's communication problems are solely because they have not had enough exposure to fluent BSL and a Deaf environment
- Deaf staff are often excluded from quality training or even basic information about how to understand their client with an ID, ASD, or both
- Deaf staff often experience difficulties working in a hearing-focused environment due to lack of interpreters
- Relay interpreting (see Chapter D4) may be poorly understood, and a lack of supervision and training provided

Recommendations for successful interventions

The deaf person with ID may be supported directly or by working with their support system (i.e. staff, families and commissioners). We suggest that the following guidelines for good practice:

Working directly with client: Adapt communication, assess the level and nature of cognitive functioning difficulties, adapting support to ensure a client can reach their full potential and achieve a good quality of life.

Advise regular health checks as per the White Paper, Valuing People:
(https://www.gov.uk/government/publications/valuing-people-a-new-strategy-for-learning-disability-for-the-21st-century)
and the Sick of It report:
(https://signhealth.org.uk/resources/report-sick-of-it/).

Working with generic (hearing) support staff: Provide training on d/Deafness, Deaf awareness, and BSL. Share information about the person with all involved, including hearing and visual assessment as well as intellectual and adaptive behaviour assessments.

Working with Deaf support staff: Provide training on ID and ensure Deaf support workers can access a range of training courses in BSL (e.g. providing interpreters and time for discussion).

For all professionals and support staff: Personalised training for staff improves care of clients. Regular meetings to review and check information prevents information loss and allows for information to be shared across the support system.

Summary

Deafness is frequently ignored in the field of intellectual disability - and intellectual disability ignored in the Deaf community. The individual should be viewed as having dual diagnoses (i.e. a D/deaf person WITH an ID).

References

Carvill S (2001). Sensory impairments, intellectual disability and psychiatry. J Intellectual Disability Research. Vol 45; 6, Pp 467-83

McShea L, Corkish C, McAnelly S (2014) Audiology services: access, assessment and aftercare. Learning Disability Practice. 17, 2, 20-25

McShea L, Fulton J and Hayes C. (2016). Paid Support Workers for Adults with Intellectual Disabilities; Their Current Knowledge of Hearing Loss and Future Training Needs. Journal of Applied Research in Intellectual Disabilities, 29(5): p. 422-432

Timehin C & Timehin E (2004). Prevalence of hearing impairment in a community population of adults with learning disability: access to audiology and impact on behaviour. Br J of Learning Disabilities 32: 128-32

E4 Autism Spectrum Disorders in deaf children and young people
Dr Hannah George

Autism Spectrum Disorders (ASDs) are pervasive developmental disorders which affect up to 1% of the UK population. Difficulties associated with ASDs can be grouped into three categories:
- Social interaction - Poor/unusual features such as: eye-contact, facial expression, use of gesture, social smiling; problems with peer relationships, social responses and/or empathy; lack of showing and/or sharing interests or pleasure.
- Language and communication - Language delay (without gesture compensation), poor conversational reciprocity, unusual or repetitive language, poor imagination or imaginative play.
- Repetitive behaviours and preoccupations – Preoccupations that are unusual in their intensity or content; compulsions or rituals; physical mannerisms (e.g. spinning, jumping, flapping, unusual hand mannerisms), preoccupation with parts of objects, sensory interests or aversions.

Rates of ASDs in deaf children and young people
The prevalence rates of ASDs in deaf children and young people is reported to be higher than in the general population. However, Wright and Oakes (2012) raise research methodology cautions in that many such prevalence studies have:
- poor representative sampling
- inaccurate diagnoses
- questionable validity of the assessments used to make diagnoses

ASDs are diagnosed later in deaf children than hearing children (Mandell et al., 2005). Research also suggests that children with ASDs are more likely to have a degree of deafness compared to children without ASDs (Rosenhall et al., 1999).

Causes of ASDs in deaf children and young people
There is undoubtedly a common pathway in some of the known causes of deafness that are also associated with the increased prevalence of ASDs (e.g. prematurity, congenital rubella, cytomegalovirus (CMV), CHARGE Syndrome). One explanation is that these affect the neural networking of

the foetus/baby, which then impacts on hearing and potentially behaviour.

However, comorbidities alone would not account for the high prevalence of ASDs in deaf children. Behavioural features of ASDs and deafness significantly overlap and can cause inaccurate diagnoses of ASDs.

The diagnostic challenge
Overlapping difficulties
Problems defining the source of difficulties makes diagnosing ASDs in deaf children challenging. Key features of ASDs overlap with some of the difficulties that many deaf children without ASDs have. Most deaf children grow up in a hearing environment, which impacts on their language development, theory of mind, social development and often their tolerance to change and uncertainty.

Many people diagnosing ASD, for clinical or research purposes, have a poor understanding of the developmental trajectory of deaf children and how this may differ from hearing children.

Misdiagnosis can occur in both directions. Social awkwardness, poor social interaction, poor social and emotional understanding and social isolation are all features associated with ASDs. Therefore, deaf children displaying these features can mistakenly be thought of as potentially being on the autism spectrum. Equally concerning is that where these difficulties do exist, they could be mis-attributed to the child being deaf, when there may be undetected evidence of an ASD (see Chapter E1).

PRACTICAL TIP: *When assessing deaf children or young people, work alongside and seek advice from deaf professionals/deaf specialists (see chapter G3).*

Theory of Mind (also see Chapter B5)
Theory of Mind (ToM) is the ability to see things from another's perspective and make accurate guesses about other's feelings, attitudes and beliefs.

Impaired ToM is a key feature of ASD. Poor ToM is also a common difficulty for deaf children, particularly those born into hearing families. Such delays are not typically seen in deaf children who are native signers born into

British Sign Language (BSL) using deaf families (see Wright & Oakes, 2012). This suggests a relation to language acquisition and other non-linguistic developmental factors.

Language ability and ToM are inextricably linked and therefore late language acquisition is likely to be related to delayed ToM in deaf children (see Chapters B1 & C2)

Distinguishing the cause of poor ToM is important. Evidence suggests that ToM is delayed in younger deaf children but not in older teenagers and that learning programmes for emotional understanding are helpful in the development of ToM in deaf children (Rhys-Jones & Ellis, 2000; Marschark et al., 2000), suggesting that deaf children can "catch up" in their development of ToM. Therefore, poor ToM in a deaf child does not necessarily indicate they also have ASD.

Socio-emotional delay
Poor social and emotional understanding, resulting from poor ToM, is a significant indicator of ASD. Deaf children may also show difficulties in this area. Social and emotional delay is highly linked with language acquisition (Chapter C2) and language deprivation (Chapter B1).

Language delay is a diagnostic feature of ASDs, but also common in deaf children who do not have an ASD. The two differing sources of the delay must not be confused.

If a child is deprived of language then they will be prevented from social communication, unable to access the social world, and will not develop the "emotional language" necessary to understand and express their own emotional world, let alone others'.

Even if the child/young person does develop language, they are often likely to have poor access to social communication and incidental information. Deaf children who are brought up in a 'hearing world' frequently miss out on incidental learning and background comments. They are less likely to be exposed to social and emotional language; instead their learning is needs based and face-to-face.

This type of indirect, unplanned learning is very important in understanding our social world and how to behave within it; also in developing an emotional understanding and vocabulary.

As a result, deaf children and young people may lack developmentally appropriate social skills and can often come across as "socially clumsy", seemingly not knowing how to interact well with others, not following social norms and rules, and (subsequently) struggling with peer relationships.

Being included in two-way conversations is crucial for the development of social knowledge. However, deaf children are often excluded from everyday interactions due to communication barriers or because they lack the social skills. Therefore, the gap in what is seen as "normal" social behaviour increases as the young deaf child develops.

PRACTICAL TIP: Consider how the child/young person's developmental environment may link to their social and emotional understanding. Seek deaf specialist opinion on their language development.

Social isolation

Social isolation can be an indicator of ASDs but it is also relatively common in deaf children and young people who do not have an ASD. In a hearing world they are often isolated from social interaction either intentionally or unintentionally, and lack the skills (social and linguistic) to interact well with their peers and feel truly involved.

Socially unstructured environments are often busier, faster paced, and noisier, leaving deaf people struggling to follow conversation. Thus, they are more socially isolated and more likely to isolate themselves, to avoid these challenges. Deaf children in mainstream education, may be the only deaf child in the school. Even if there is a "base" or resource for deaf children, they may be in the minority and have little or no peer group (see Chapter C6).

In some cases the only communication accessible relationship the deaf child has is with their communication support worker or teaching assistant. This can be misidentified in an ASD assessment as the child preferring relationships with adults, rather than recognising it as their only option.

PRACTICAL TIP: Consider whether limited social engagement in deaf children and young people being assessed for ASD could be the result of poor communication access or lack of a peer group.

Anxiety

Increased levels of anxiety are common in deaf children and young people. A lack of access to incidental information (information gained from the environment rather than directly communicated) as a result of not hearing things around them can lead to their world being unpredictable and confusing. This anxiety can lead to behaviours such as need for routine, rituals, obsessions, poor reaction to change/new people/new places.

These are also common behavioural features in people with ASDs and are often picked up in deaf children as an indicator of possible ASD.

PRACTICAL TIP: Use behavioural analysis to differentiate between behaviours related to ASDs and those related to alternative explanations such as anxiety: for example, use visual calendars; encourage parents/carers/teachers to be explicit about day to day plans and routines.

Sensory issues

Sensory interests and aversion are common features of ASDs, but do not necessarily indicate an ASD in a deaf child.

Deaf children will have a different sensory experience to hearing children to various extents depending on the nature of their hearing loss. This can lead to some sensory aversions or sensory seeking behaviours. For example, children with cochlear implants may be averse to loud and noisy environments due to the tuning of their processors, or some deaf children may make seemingly odd guttural noises or vocalisations because of the sensory stimulation in absence of auditory stimulation and feedback.

PRACTICAL TIP: Consider alternative explanations for sensory aversions/sensory seeking behaviours. Involve an occupational therapist (preferably one experienced in working with deaf children) to develop a sensory profile for a child and a sensory diet, which may help with these behaviours.

Lack of standardised assessment

A major cause of late diagnosis, misdiagnosis, and failing to correctly diagnose ASDs in deaf children relates to problematic assessment methods and processes. This presents significant challenge for clinicians.

Until very recently there were no standardised, validated tools for assessing ASDs in deaf people. Deaf adaptations of the Autism Diagnostic Observation Schedule-2 (ADOS-2), the Autism Diagnostic Interview Revised (ADI-R) and the Social Responsiveness Scale-2 (SRS-2) have recently been developed and validated (Phillips et al., 2021; Wright, Phillips, Algar et al., 2020; Wright, Phillips, Le Couteur., et al., in submission).

Problems that needed to be addressed included:
- assessment of language and linguistics (given that signed language is not directly comparable with spoken language)
- communication during assessment (where the assessor is not able to communicate with the child/young person or family in their native language e.g. BSL)
- ensuring the process is accessible for deaf children and families (e.g. written communication, feedback, reports, care planning)

PRACTICAL TIP:
Deaf Child and Adolescent Mental Health Services (Deaf CAMHS) are situated around the country and provide specialist assessment for deaf children and consultation to generic services (see Chapter G3).

Early intervention
Where there is an early and correct diagnosis of ASD, and the correct support for deaf children and young people is implemented, their outcomes can be greatly improved. This can vastly improve the lives and experiences for them and their families.

Complications for deaf children and young people with ASDs and their families include access to services and appropriate interventions, suitable education placements, peer support, and the additive effects of everyday challenges of being deaf and of having an ASD. As well as specialist consultation and advice from Deaf CAMHS, there are various organisations that exist exclusively to support deaf children, young people and their families (e.g. National Deaf Children's Society).

Conclusion
Identifying and assessing ASDs in deaf children and young people is complex. Even with the best adapted assessment and assessment

protocols, teasing apart what features may be a result of the developmental challenges and impacts of the child being deaf, versus what may be a result of an ASD, can be problematic even for experienced clinicians. Co-working with deaf specialists is crucial.

From referral to assessment, care planning and intervention, working with deaf specialist teams will lead to more valid and reliable assessment and a much better experience for deaf children, young people and families.

References

Wright, B., & Oakes, P. (2012). Does socio-emotional developmental delay masquerade as autism in some deaf children? *International Journal on Mental Health and Deafness, 2(1)*

Mandell, D., Novak, M.,& Zubritsky, C. (2005). Factors associated with age of diagnosis among children with autism spectrum disorders. *Pediatrics, 116*, 1480-1486

Marschark, M., Green, V., Hindmarsh, G., & Walker, S. (2000). Understanding theory of mind in children who are deaf. *Journal of Child Psychology and Psychiatry, 41*, 1067-1073

Phillips, H., Wright, B., Allgar, V., McConnachie, H., Sweetman, J., Hargate, R., Hodkinson, R., Bland, M., George, H., Hughes, A., Hayward, E., Garcia de las Heras, V., & Le Couteur, A. (2021). Adapting and validating the Autism Diagnostic Observation Schedule Version 2 for use with deaf children and young people. *Journal of Autism and Developmental Disorders* https://doi.org/10.1007/s10803-021-04931-y

Rhys-Jones, S.L., & Ellis, H.D. (2000). Theory of Mind. Deaf and hearing children's comprehension of picture stories and judgements of social situations. *Journal of Deaf Studies and Deaf Education, 5*, 248-261

Rosenhall, U., Nordin, V., Sandström, M., Ahlsen, G., & Gillberg, C. (1999). Autism and Hearing Loss. *Journal of Autism and Developmental Disorders, 29*, 349–357

Wright, B., Phillips, H., Allgar, V., Sweetman, J., Hodkinson, R., Hayward, E., Ralph-Lewis, A., Teige, C., & Le Couteur, A. (2021) Adapting and Validating the Autism Diagnostic Interview – Revised for Use with Deaf Children and Young People. *Autism, (in submission)*

Wright, B., Phillips, H., Le Couteur, A., Sweetman, J., Hodkinson, R., Ralph-Lewis, A., Hayward, E., Brenna, A., Mulloy, J., Day, N., Bland, M., & Allgar M. (2020). Modifying and Validating the Social Responsiveness Scale Edition 2 for use with Deaf Children and Young People. *PLOS ONE* https://doi.org/10.1371/journal.pone.0243162

E5 Autistic Spectrum Disorders in deaf adults
Dr Ben Holmes and Dr Sally Austen

Being deaf does not cause Autistic Spectrum Disorders (ASD). However, deaf children and adults do have a higher prevalence of ASD (see Chapter E4). This is because some causes of deafness include neurological difference which can increase the risk of ASD (see Chapter H1). Additionally, deaf people who have been language deprived are more likely to have difficulties that mimic ASD (see Chapter B1).

Although the existence of National Deaf CAMHS (see Chapter G4) has improved services for deaf children, it is not uncommon for a first diagnosis of ASD to be made in deaf people who are well into adulthood or even senior years.

Why would a deaf person reach adulthood before being diagnosed?
Lack of recognition
The current generation of middle aged, and older, deaf adults experienced schooling where diagnoses of ASD were rare. It is only in the last 2-3 decades that ASD has been properly recognised as a spectrum of conditions and identified in mainstream (hearing) schooling. Deaf adults are likely to have experienced poorer access to education (see Chapter C6), often with a very specific focus on speech acquisition. Thus, historically, little thought was given to whether a child may have had additional difficulties, such as ASD.

Another factor affecting recognition of additional needs is the impact of language acquisition (see Chapter C2). So many deaf children are raised in environments where they do not have the language rich environment they require. This has meant that professionals sometimes become habituated to deaf children having linguistic, or social communication difficulties, that these difficulties are misattributed to being deaf (see Chapter E1).

Language acquisition difficulties are in fact preventable for nearly all deaf people, whereas someone with ASD will develop the same difficulties even within a language rich environment. By the time difficulties are recognised as being more significant, the young person may already have left school and missed the opportunity to access assessment clinics through CAMHS.

Adaptation of services to complex needs
More recently, Deaf schools have increasingly accommodated deaf children with additional difficulties. As a result, the schools have become very skilled at adapting their support for, and professionals have become slightly habituated to, working with deaf children with additional needs. Thus, formal diagnoses have not been required or sought in order for appropriate support to be provided.

Whilst school is often a very positive experience with easy access to appropriate support, the lack of a diagnosis on entering adult services means that no additional support is considered necessary. This unfortunately means that the young person often finds themselves without the scaffolding that they are used to and appear to present suddenly with difficulties (such as anxieties, challenging behaviours or cognitive difficulties) that were not apparent at school.

Difficulties being masked by support systems
It is not uncommon for families to find ways of supporting a deaf family member with additional difficulties without the support of services because, historically, services to recognise or support those needs did not exist. This pattern of family coping (e.g. adopting certain routines; providing specific support) can continue into adulthood and give the appearance that there are no difficulties because the system or routine is successful.

It is then not until the adult child's parents die that the additional difficulties start to become apparent, sometimes as late as when the person is in their 60s or 70s. This can create difficulties that affect the assessment process.

Accessing specialist assessment
Ideally the assessor would be both a specialist in assessing ASD and a specialist in working with deaf people.

It is often difficult to facilitate a referral for an ASD assessment when existing services are not aware that a deaf person may have reached adulthood without having had the assessment they need. Services are so stretched that they have difficulty justifying assessments for ASD at a later age when, diagnostically, difficulties should have been observable before. Furthermore, not all areas have specialist adult ASD teams.

This is further complicated as, previously, mental health or learning disability services may not have considered the possibility of ASD because of the individual's age. The client may therefore have various incorrect diagnoses (e.g. psychosis or personality disorder) before reaching an appropriate ASD specialist. By this time, they may already be on medication that can affect presentation.

It is important to remember that misdiagnosis can also occur in both directions. Clients who have been diagnosed with ASD may actually have undiagnosed language deprivation which has either been masked, or misunderstood, as ASD.

How to assess
There are so many potential complicating factors that could affect assessment and diagnosis of a deaf adult with suspected ASD that this should only be done by people that are sufficiently competent to do so. Those without this competence should make contact with specialist deaf services (see Chapters G3 & G4)

Assessment must involve a combination of professionals, that might include: Psychologists, Psychiatrists, Speech and Language Therapists, Interpreters, Occupational Therapists or Nurses.

The assessment must always include someone with the same first language as the client. In the case of a British Sign Language user, this will therefore most likely be a deaf professional.

Standardised, normed and adapted assessments for ASD are not available in a way that is suitable for all deaf adults. Adaptations can be made to standardised assessments such as ADOS-2D. This is created with the intention that there is adjustment based on linguistic and cognitive ability rather than chronological age.

Professionals must accept the need to take significantly more time for assessments, gathering information from a broad range of sources. These might include:
- structured 1:1 observations
- structured group observations with other people with the same first language
- structured tasks
- collateral history from family or significant others
- school reports (where possible)

- neurodevelopment history (where possible)
- unstructured observations with other people with the same first language

Assessment of ASD in deaf adults is particularly difficult when developmental and collateral history from family, school or GP is not available. This may be because of their older age (family members have since died, schools have removed old files, GPs have changed the ways they record client information). It is also partly the result of fewer people in the deaf person's history who were able to communicate fluently with them and thus able to attain useful information.

Despite these difficulties the client's language and communication history is vital to the ASD assessment. Cognitive assessment may also be appropriate to rule out other possible explanations for difficulties or differential diagnoses (see Chapter E2).

Diagnostic overshadowing (see also Chapter E1)
Some behaviours, lifestyle features or experiences for typical deaf people may, to hearing people, appear similar to features of ASD when in fact no ASD is present.

Isolation
It is not uncommon to have little or no peer group and thus spend a lot of time alone. For example, a lone deaf person working in a car factory with entirely hearing colleagues, may spend all their break times on their own because no one else can sign. A deaf person who communicates orally may avoid complex conversations and stick to well rehearsed topics, for fear of being unable to lipread or missing the context.

Routine
Routine can be soothing to those with and without ASD. Aspects of being deaf in a predominantly hearing world can be stressful and routine may provide solace. It also replaces the need for some communication or information gathering. For example, a shop worker who has worked the same shifts for 10 years and becomes anxious when asked to change their shifts. It is not the time per se that is problematic to them, but that to rearrange and relearn their commute, child care and relationship with the new shift supervisor is more complex than for their hearing peers.

Language deprivation (See Chapter B1)
Inadequate access to language, particularly in early life, can significantly impact on communication, cognition and social relationships. This can sometimes present in a way that is similar to ASD. Unfortunately, many deaf people are exposed to language deprivation and this must not be confused with ASD.

Managing ASD in deaf adults
When there are behavioural or emotional regulation difficulties linked to ASD, Deaf CAMHS often seek to transition care to the equivalent adult mental health services because of the crucial support required. However, the different service thresholds mean this is not always possible.

Referral to specialist (tertiary) deaf services (see Chapter G4) requires the deaf client to be care coordinated by the secondary mental health or learning disability team. Care coordination is usually provided to those clients who have severe and complex mental health problems including severe self-harm or acute psychosis. It is often the case that when the client's presentation does not **currently** reach the referral threshold, they are turned down even when services may be able to help.

Thus, a deaf client with ASD, can end up having to deteriorate in terms of mental health or behaviour before they can access specialist services. This is obviously distressing for the client, family and potential service providers.

Deaf CAMHS have initiated some pilot projects extending support for young people with neurodevelopmental conditions until 25. For some clients this allows more time to develop self-management skills. It can also smooth the transition between services for young people and adults, to help establish appropriate support. However, for other deaf adults with ASD their needs will require support beyond 25 and currently services are not set up to provide this. Strong co-working between mental health services, social services and third sectors providers is therefore required.

Conclusion
Assessments for ASD in deaf adults are sometimes required due to historic and systemic factors that prevented appropriate assessment and/or supports earlier in their life. Adapting assessments for deaf adults can be difficult and should be done cautiously. Where there is uncertainty, support should be sought from deaf specialist services.

E6 Attention Deficit Hyperactivity Disorder (ADHD) in deaf children and young people
Dr Rob Walker

This is my clinical opinion developed after more than 25 years of working with deaf young people with ADHD and their families. It is intended as a helpful starting point for discussion and further thinking about this complex topic and it is not intended to provide all of the answers.

Prevalence and cause
As a population, deaf children are at increased risk of ADHD because many of the causes which led to them being deaf (e.g. prematurity, infection etc.) can also impact on neuro development.

ADHD is a developmental disorder, which is present before the age of 6 and is apparent in more than one situation (i.e. at school and at home). Symptoms include poor attention, overactivity and impulsivity. Associated difficulties including social disinhibition, low self-esteem and specific learning difficulties are common.

Impact on communication, learning, and other cognitive skills
For deaf children ADHD is a double jeopardy, as they need to concentrate very hard to communicate and learn - whether they do that by speech and lip reading, sign language or a combination of the two.

Diagnosis
In terms of assessment, standard (hearing) questionnaires for parents and teachers (such as the SDQ, Connors and SNAP-IV) seem to work well with deaf children (unlike autism measures), particularly if the teacher's report is completed by staff who have experience of working with deaf children. However, currently there are no standardised measures for deaf children and therefore the results should be interpreted with caution by an experienced clinician. Observation of the young person in school and clinic by an experienced clinician is equally important.

Cognitive assessment and review by a Speech and Language therapist is helpful in complex cases.

Qb testing is a computer based continuous performance test of the patient's speed and accuracy when responding to geometric shapes appearing on the screen. This is developing rapidly. Whilst it is obviously necessary to ensure that a child understands the requirements of the test it is also true that most deaf children will have experience of similar stimulus-response testing from their experience of audiology assessments and this may be helpful.

Misdiagnosis and Overshadowing (see also Chapter E1)
As with many issues in deaf mental health care, differential diagnosis requires an understanding of deaf norms (see Chapters E2 & G7). A clinician with little experience of working with deaf people may highlight a deaf child's lack of focus on a task as symptomatic of ADHD, when it may be better explained by, for example, poor access to communication.

Conversely, it is also possible that under diagnosis can occur particularly due to 'Diagnostic overshadowing' (i.e. the tendency to attribute difficulties to the young person being deaf rather than to look for other treatable causes; see Chapter E1). This can delay or prevent an appropriate diagnosis of ADHD, which then delays its management.

If a person has both language delay and ADHD it can complicate the process of determining causality. Clinicians in specialist deaf services have observed that language deprivation can lead to delays in a child developing executive functioning, and this might deter clinicians from diagnosing ADHD in favour of attempting to remediate the language issue and improve executive function.

However, more recent clinical experience suggests that focusing on treatment of the ADHD symptoms, including the appropriate use of medication, can lead to greater progress with language learning. This in turn benefits executive functioning, which may reduce the time for which ADHD medication is needed.

Treatment
The treatment of ADHD falls broadly into two categories: 1) behavioural and 2) pharmacological plus behavioural.

i) Behavioural
Much of the behavioural intervention for ADHD focuses on scheduling, planning, and the consideration of cause-effect-consequence. As mentioned in Chapter B1, language delay or language deprivation can restrict a person's ability to learn or practice these strategies.

ii)Pharmacological
In terms of pharmacological treatment prescribers need to be careful regarding the presence of physical health problems particularly any syndrome that might lead to long QT syndrome (see Chapter F10). Some deaf young people have associated complex physical health problems, thus joint management with paediatricians is recommended (see Chapters H1 & H5).

Sleep (see Chapter H8)
Sleep problems are common for people with ADHD. Sleep problems are also common for deaf children - even those who don't have ADHD. The dark may lead to anxiety and behavioural issues in children who can't hear, particularly when they remove hearing aids or cochlear implants at night. Melatonin can be very effective, particularly short courses in order to give parents respite, but sleep hygiene and behavioural approaches should probably be approached more actively in deaf children before turning to medication.

Adult ADHD
Missed diagnosis of childhood ADHD can result in adults presenting with multiple other diagnoses including anxiety, depression and personality disorder. Adults are more able than children to describe the subjective experience of ADHD, particularly symptoms such as restlessness and hyper focus, but this may still be difficult particularly for those with language deprivation or disorder. There are extremely limited specialist services for adult assessment of ADHD in deaf people. Like child assessments, the information gathered should be from multiple views and environments. However, attaining third party information and historical information from families and documents such as school reports, whilst invaluable, can be tricky.

Diagnosis on the basis of just the clients' perspective is particularly unreliable if that client also has cognitive difficulties or language deprivation; or does not want their parents involved.

Conclusion

ADHD is likely to be more common in the deaf population due to neurological risk factors associated with some causes of deafness, yet research and clinical provision is sparse. Under and over diagnosis is reduced, and safe and effective treatment is promoted, when ADHD assessors and clinicians with deaf expertise work together to undertake a careful and comprehensive assessment.

E7 Deaf older adults
Dr Sally Austen and Dr Ben Holmes

It would be an easy but catastrophic mistake to regard all deaf older adults as being the same.

More than ever a thorough history of deafness, language and identity must be taken (see Chapter D14). Although these variables are on a continuum and interact, a simple dichotomous categorisation might help.

Ask yourself, whether your client is:
- Ordinarily a hearing person who, through the process of growing old, has lost some or all of their hearing; or
- A lifelong sign language user, who has now grown old

Age acquired hearing loss (see Chapter D10)
One in five people has some hearing loss and this rises to one in three over the age of 65 and one in two who are over 75.

Presbycusis, or age-related hearing loss, comes on gradually as a person gets older. It may make it hard for a person to tolerate loud noises, as well as hear what others are saying.

As the hearing loss is gradual many people do not realise they have lost some or all of their hearing. The majority will be prescribed hearing aids, but combined with other features of aging, such as finger dexterity or numbness, vision and cognitive issues, some clients may find problems with fitting and using the hearing aids, keeping them in a safe place or letting carers know when batteries need replacing.

Older people can often find themselves isolated as they retire, their mobility reduces and family members move away or die. Hearing loss can significantly add to this sense of isolation (see Chapter D10) even when the person has company.

Many older people try to hide their hearing loss. This is partly due to concerns of stigmatisation and partly that they may not want to draw attention to themselves or burden others with their needs. Unfortunately, the less someone discloses their hearing loss, the less others can help with improved communication strategies.

Whether being supported in the community or in residential care, great thought should go into making the environment and social interactions as accessible as possible to people with a hearing loss (see Chapter D10).

Where communication needs are not met, there are risks not only of isolation but also misdiagnosis and misrepresentation of the client's legal preferences.

Mrs A is in hospital with a suspected broken hip. Her hearing aids were not collected by the ambulance crew and the painkilling medication is slightly blurring her vision. The A&E doctor starts to ask Mrs A about her pain level, whilst looking away to pull the curtains around her bed area. She misses the beginning of the sentence and cannot grasp the context in order to start lipreading. Despite normal intelligence, she gives the doctor an incorrect medical history and signs a consent to surgery form without knowing what she has consented to.

Mr B is visited in his nursing home by a social worker to assess his Capacity to make decisions about his future housing and care needs. The radio is playing in the background and another distressed patient is heard to repeatedly shout out. The social worker has a thick beard, covering much of his mouth, and an accent that is different from Mr B's. The social worker confidently writes that Mr B was unable to answer simple orientation or memory questions and therefore his Capacity is in doubt.

The Covid-19 pandemic has necessitated changes in the way professional consultations take place. Meetings with solicitors, GPs etc. are often conducted over the phone. Unless you are sure that your client is hearing everything you say, this should be replaced by face to face or video consultation.

Face coverings such as masks inhibit lipreading entirely and, where safe and possible, should be replaced by Perspex dividers with microphones to enhance sound, or professional lipspeakers (see Chapter D9) present via video conferencing (see chapter D7).

Sign language users who have grown old

A sign language user who grows old is still a sign language user. It is a common mistake to assume that they have the same needs as elderly people who have been late deafened. Within a care home environment, for example, it is easy for the needs of older sign language users (i.e. for BSL interpreters and the company of others who sign) to be overlooked. Deaf BSL users will generally want to socialise with other Deaf BSL users. There are insufficient care homes that support Deaf BSL users, who may end up in care homes where their physical health needs are prioritised over their social and emotional needs. This results in isolation, communication breakdown and misdiagnosis, which can lead to appropriate frustration/anger/fear being misunderstood as 'challenging behaviour' (see Chapter F12).

Care providers require training to work with deaf residents and employing deaf staff is recommended.

Without the skills to identify the care needs of older deaf people, alongside the relatively small number of clients spread over a wide geographical area, care home providers may claim there is not the critical mass of clients to justify building specialist deaf care homes. However, there is an argument that clients (and their families) would be willing to travel much greater distances for bespoke care.

An example of excellent older age care for sign language users is the De Gelderhorst in Holland (www.gelderhorst.nl). The website can be viewed in English by using the Union Jack icon at the top right.

Many older deaf people whose preferred language is BSL, were in fact raised as first language oral communicators (using speech and lipreading) (see Chapter C5 & C6). A deaf person who is being identified for an assessment of possible dementia, may therefore retain their preference for sign language but actually be more effective at communicating orally.

Age related ailments such as arthritis and neuropathy can affect a person's ability to expressively sign. Worsening eyesight can affect a deaf person's receptive sign language abilities. Changes in language and communication should be noted. This may be an indicator of a need for further investigations.

Assessment of cognitive decline
Assessment for dementia and Capacity are often required when working with older people. Additionally, hearing loss is part of the prodrome of some dementias and concerns about cognitive functioning should be

investigated. However, it is also important to recognise that hearing loss, and being deaf, can have secondary impacts on performance that are not linked to dementia (e.g. isolation or emotional wellbeing).

Whilst individual cognitive screening tests such as the MMSE, ACE-III, MOCA may have been normed on clients in this age group, the adaptations needed to present these tests to people with hearing loss or people who use sign language, have not (see Chapter E2 & G7).

If measures are unreliable this promotes the importance of using (or adapting) cognitive tests to create baseline data, for later comparison to own performance.

People with a hearing loss
Given that the person attending the appointment may not recognise, or may minimise the importance of, any hearing difficulties they have this must be established directly with all older adults (see Chapter D14) and factored into any assessments.

The assessor needs to be completely sure that failure on a particular item is due to the client's inability and not that they just misheard the question. Telephone assessments are particularly at risk of inaccuracies.

Tests of, or via, literacy can be used with people who lost their hearing as adults (see Chapter B3). Many screening tests require an ability to repeat back things that are said, which will be severely affected by hearing loss and the services of a professional lipspeaker may be needed (Chapter D9). Worsening eyesight must also be factored into any analysis of test results or observations of daily life skills.

Sign language users
Cognitive deterioration or assault can affect language and communication. A stroke not only affects the person's dexterity (to form the necessary handshapes and movements) but, as with a hearing person, it affects their fundamental language skills. As with hearing people, strokes in the left hemisphere of the brain, may damage the language centres. However, British Sign Language exists in three dimensions, so some people have more subtle expressive and receptive language difficulties when the stroke is right sided as well (Marshall et al., 2004).

The progression of dementia is often associated with gradual loss of language skills. Acquired language skills appear to be lost via a 'last in, first out' sequence. Thus, a hearing English person who is fluent in a second language French, is likely to experience deterioration firstly in their French and then their English. A deaf person who was raised orally and acquired sign language later in life, is likely to lose their BSL language skills first.

Deaf people often have poorer physical health because of lack of access to information and services (see Chapter G1). This increases their vascular risk factors.

Whilst the use of a sign language interpreter (Chapters D2 & D3) is imperative for communication with your client, a specialist assessment or referral to specialist deaf services is strongly recommended. Referral for dementia assessment associated with severe or complex mental health problems can be made to the adult National Deaf Mental Health Services (see Chapter G4). In the absence of a mental health problem referral can be made to a specialist clinic based in London. See http://research.bmh.manchester.ac.uk/deafwithdementia/clinicinfo/

Some cognitive assessments rely on word reading tasks to predict pre-morbid functioning (see Chapter E2). This is not appropriate for clients who were deaf during their early school years (see Chapter B3) and cannot be translated by an interpreter.

Generational differences in the culture of deaf sign language users
The experiences of deaf people over the last 150 years have varied significantly. The current cohort of deaf older adults experienced significant limits in their access to education and language. Environments that were supposed to be supportive and safe were frequently abusive (see Chapter F2).

History collation
Many older sign language users will have been the only deaf child in their hearing family and been sent to deaf boarding schools at the age of 3 (see Chapter C6). Therefore, their relationship with their birth family may have been less significant than with their deaf friends and peers. Many will have married other deaf people and then had hearing children who are likely to have interpreted and 'brokered' for their deaf parents (see Chapter C4). A small proportion, about 5%, would be part of generations of (genetically) deaf family members.

In education, children of this era were often punished for using sign language, due to an (incorrect) belief that signing would harm their ability to speak (see Chapter C5 & C6). This understandably created a significant mistrust of hearing people (see Chapter C10). It also resulted in impoverished access to language in many cases (see Chapter B1).

Interpreting
The use of a qualified registered interpreter is always recommended (see Chapter D1 & D5) as family members cannot be guaranteed to be sufficiently skilled or impartial. However, there may be times where an older client is unable (due to dementia or distress) to focus on the interpreter. At times like this a family member may need to support communication. Ideally, the decision to do this is made with the involvement of a qualified interpreter.

It should not be assumed that all older profoundly prelingually deaf people are predominantly signers. The ability to access information in written and spoken English held a value that meant that some older deaf people prefer to communicate orally and use lip reading. This must be checked according to the client's preferences. Some deaf older adults may prefer to express themselves through speech but still want to use an interpreter to receive information.

As with all languages, signs and signing in BSL change through the decades. Just as interpreters may need time to adjust to the clients' different dialects, they will also need to adjust to age related differences and may require more time to 'tune in' (see Chapter D2).

Deaf Club
Deaf older adults may talk about the 'Deaf Club', a hub of social fun, support, information, (and sometimes gossip). In the 20th century this was a place where professionals such as social workers for the deaf would offer support. Multiple generations of families would attend. For many who were in schools with oral only communication policy, this is where they learnt to sign. The demise of the Deaf Club (due to improvements in communication technologies, resource cuts in social care and younger deaf people being able, and choosing, to integrate into mainstream society) has been a great loss to many older deaf people.

Summary
Without appropriate care, communication and adapted assessment, older deaf people can be horribly socially isolated, and their needs may be misdiagnosed. Older sign language users and those with late hearing loss have different needs and an early communication assessment is crucial.

Reference
Marshall, J., Atkinson, J., Thacker, A., & Woll, B. (2004). Stroke in users of BSL: investigating sign language impairments *In S. Austen & S. Crocker (Eds.) Deafness in Mind. Pp* 284-302. Whurr Publishers Ltd.

E8 Assessing cognitive functioning remotely
Dr Hannah George and Dr Ben Holmes

Introduction
The Covid-19 pandemic has resulted in many appointments being offered remotely. Whilst the long-term impact of the pandemic is still unknown, the future is likely to hold increased remote working for various reasons.

Remote cognitive assessments for deaf people still carry an unknown degree of error. This limits the conclusions that can be drawn and means they must be considered carefully. However, there is the potential for this to provide a useful function depending on the individual, the circumstance, and the questions being asked.

This chapter aims to provide advice about setting up and adapting cognitive assessments administered remotely to deaf children and adults. Practical considerations, and important caveats, are provided based on clinical experience. The chapter is not intended as a "how to" guide. It must also be read alongside advice in accompanying chapters for full context (see Chapters E2, E3, E4, E5 & E6 respectively).

Existing guidance
Research suggests that some remote cognitive assessments are broadly comparable to face to face (e.g. Brearly et al., 2017). The BPS Division of Neuropsychology provides advice about technology, client and environmental considerations to support successful remote assessment (BPS, 2020a). The use of remote cognitive assessments in expert witness work is also supported in certain circumstances (BPS, 2020b).

Guidance advises clinicians to consider whether remote administration provides a valid substitute for face to face assessment on a case by case basis. However, there are no known studies evaluating remote cognitive assessments in deaf people and many factors that could impact on the validity of this approach for deaf people. Timeliness and accuracy of assessment must therefore always be prioritised over speed or convenience.

Is remote assessment appropriate?
Before undertaking any remote cognitive assessment, consider first:

- What is the purpose of assessment and can it wait?
- Are there any alternative approaches that could be used (e.g. socially distanced assessment)?
- Could other services operating face to face (e.g. social care, educational psychology, SENCo) contribute to an assessment, provide additional information or be supported in their assessments first?
- Assessments that can be offered will be less robust than a full, face to face cognitive assessment. Is a working hypothesis more beneficial to your client than postponing for a more definitive formulation?

Only proceed if the answers to each of these points still indicates that remote assessment is beneficial.

Selecting appropriate assessments
Some assessments are designed to be delivered remotely (e.g. tests on Q-global). However, not all of these are suitable for deaf people and none are known to have deaf norms.

Other tests can easily be adapted for remote administration (e.g. verbally presented tests). However, these are the same tests that are likely to be inaccessible or less appropriate for deaf clients, even if an interpreter is used (see Chapter E2).

Before using any test it is therefore essential to first consider the same factors as for face to face administration, for example: availability of normative data; client language and fluency; and the linguistic and cultural appropriateness of the test (see Chapter E2).

Remote assessment brings additional challenges that particularly affect some cognitive domains. Tests assessing motor speed or response time are unlikely to be suitable. The potential effect of internet connectivity on screens freezing or disrupting displays could affect tests with sequentially presented information. Tests involving manipulables (e.g. Leiter-3) are also not recommended. Resources may also have copyright limitations affecting online use - some are temporarily being relaxed during the Covid-19 pandemic but this should be checked.

For any assessment being considered it is important to remember that service users will not know what they should see and so will not know whether there is a problem (see also Chapter B2). Therefore, as a general rule, if in doubt don't use the assessment and make contact with a Deaf Specialist Service for advice (See Chapters G3 & G4).

Interview measures
Measures that might be particularly suitable for remote assessment include structured or unstructured interviews provided communication has been thoroughly considered and the correct communication support is in place (see below). For example, ADI-R (Autism Diagnostic Schedule Revised) or ADI-RD (Autism Diagnostic Schedule Revised – Deaf version).

Questionnaire measures
Questionnaire measures are also likely to be suitable as they can easily be posted to clients/families and returned for scoring. Alternatively they could be completed during the video appointment. If taking this approach, it is important to ensure the language of the questionnaire is accessible. Direct translation through an interpreter does not always equate to a valid or culturally appropriate assessment.

Jagged profiles
If it is decided that appropriate tests are available to proceed, it is important to be aware that jagged profiles in cognitive assessments are common. Therefore, if only one or two subtests from a battery can be used, assumptions about ability must not be generalised to all domains; - it is possible that the one test selected represents a particular strength or difficulty for that person. To generalise could lead to significant misunderstanding of a person's cognitive profile.

Set-up
Assessment set up is vitally important to ensure the appointment is accessible and any error associated with adapting the approach is minimised. Professional guidance relating to remote assessment should be followed, as should NHS Trust specific guidance regarding remote/video appointments in general. Guidance on remote/video work with deaf people should be sought from specialist Deaf Service professionals. Information can also be found on websites such as https://hearmeoutcc.com/.

A pre-appointment is recommended before assessment to consider: communication needs; risk and consent; access to technology; and whether in-session support will be required. This will also provide an opportunity to check whether materials need to be sent in advance and to discuss how these will be used.

Communication
Ideally, deaf professionals would administer assessments for deaf service users or at least advise hearing professionals during assessment. The reality is that in many situations this may not be possible because there are currently insufficient numbers of qualified deaf professionals.

It is therefore essential that any professional administering cognitive assessments with a deaf person is aware of the importance of communication and the nuances of assessments with deaf people. Professionals must check the client can linguistically engage with tasks (see Chapter D14) and determine whether a BSL or relay interpreter is needed (see Chapters D2, D3, D4 & E2).

During assessment, to maximise good communication:
- Use a good quality camera and microphone. Headphones will improve sound quality but ensure the microphone does not obstruct your mouth.
- Make sure your office space is free from visual clutter and background noise.
- Use a room that will be uninterrupted to maintain confidentiality and minimise distractions, both auditory and visual.

Risk assessment and consent
Risk assessment should inherently be considered as part of any session set-up. When working remotely this is especially important as the clinician has little ability to ensure service user safety should something happen mid-appointment. Risk assessment should consider who to contact during the assessment in case of concern or technological failure.

Service user consent is necessary for any clinical work, including remote work. Agreements about how to gain consent will differ locally (e.g. according to NHS Trusts). Consent to proceed must be gained before the appointment, with additional consent if the session will be recorded.

Technology
In the pre-appointment test call check to make sure:
- The service user has access to the right technology (e.g. a laptop or tablet).

- The service user's screen is sufficiently large to see an interpreter and any resources used; a smartphone may be too small.
- The service user has sufficient knowledge, or support, to access the technology.
- The connection speed is at least 4-5 mbps for visual quality to be sufficient for sign language.
- There is sufficient data allowance.
- You have a webcam with good resolution and no auto-focus. Position this at the top of your screen to make eye contact appear more natural.
- The service user's camera is positioned with them in full view, and face visible, to maximise observation opportunities.
- Listening devices (e.g. Siri, Alexa) are turned off to maintain confidentiality. Advise the service user to do the same.

There are various video call platforms available (e.g. Zoom, Microsoft Teams), each with advantages and disadvantages. Important points to consider prior to the appointment are: security of data transfer; which platform the service user is familiar with; can additional people be invited to the call (e.g. interpreters); is it possible for the service user to 'pin' whoever they want to see if they need to lip read or see an interpreter?

Sending visual "how to" guides for the chosen platform prior to the appointment can be extremely helpful for the service user/parent/carer.

Involving others
Support or supervision may be needed especially for children and young people, or those with additional disabilities. Check who might need to be involved prior to the appointment. It is also important to know who may be present, but not visible on camera, during the appointment.

If someone is supporting the appointment they should be informed about how much support they can provide prior to the assessment so they do not inadvertently influence results. Where possible, the person supporting should not be a family member, because:
- A family member, especially a parent, may be more likely to support the individual, either consciously or unconsciously, if they are struggling.
- An individual may feel more pressured to perform in a certain way, or rely on someone with a 'helper' role. This can increase the risk of the

service user's abilities being under-estimated if help is sought when it is not needed.

If a family member needs to be used, then inform them of the importance of remaining as "neutral" as possible (e.g. sitting away from and out of the eye-line of the individual) so the individual's performance is as reflective of their abilities as possible. It is important to always report who was present during the assessment and details of the set up.

Socially distanced assessments
Remote assessment may be being considered because of infection concern (e.g. Covid-19). If so, an alternative might be a socially distanced assessment (i.e. in the same room but administering items at a distance). One tool currently being explored to facilitate this is the use of visualisers (technology which displays text, objects or images on a screen) to present items at a distance.

Another option is to use computer based platforms (e.g. Q-interactive) whilst in the same room. Both options facilitate collection of additional information that may be missed remotely (e.g. qualitative observations).

If using Personal Protective Equipment (PPE) it is important to consider the affect of face coverings on facial expression and lip pattern, both are crucial aspects of communication for many deaf people (see Chapter D10). Furthermore, PPE could increase client anxiety. Preparing the client for what to expect prior to the assessment is therefore essential.

Summary
There may be good reason to complete a remote cognitive assessment via videocall with deaf clients. However, there are many variables that could impact on the validity of this approach. Accuracy and timeliness of assessments should therefore always be prioritised over speed or convenience. Conclusions should be drawn very cautiously using multiple sources of information to inform decisions. Professionals also need to be sure of their competence in this area, both in terms of remote assessments and assessing deaf people, before attempting assessments.

Remote assessment is likely to be central to future work. Further research into remote assessments with deaf people, and the development of new tests, is therefore needed and welcomed. In the meantime, remote assessment may have a more useful role in informing and developing working hypotheses to help guide action whilst face to face assessment is not possible.

References

Brearly, T. W., Shura, R. D., Martindale, S. L., Lazowski, R. A., Luxton, D. D., Shenal, B. V., & Rowland, J. A. (2017). Neuropsychological test administration by videoconference: A systematic review and meta-analysis. *Neuropsychology review, 27(2)*, 174–186

British Psychological Society (2020a). Division of Neuropsychology Professional Standards Unit Guidelines to colleagues on the use of Tele-neuropsychology. https://www.bps.org.uk/member-microsites/division-neuropsychology/news April 2020

British Psychological Society (2020b). Psychologist expert witnesses undertaking remote psychological assessments. https://www.bps.org.uk/sites/www.bps.org.uk/files/Policy/Policy%20-%20Files/Expert%20witnesses%20undertaking%20remote%20psychological%20assessments.pdf

Roberts, S., Wright, Moore, K., Smith, J., Allgar. V., Tennant, A., Doherty, C., Hughes, E., Collingridge Moore, D., Ogden, R., Phillips, H., Beese, L., & Rogers, K. (2015). Translation in to British Sign Language and validation of the Strengths and Difficulties Questionnaire Health Services and Delivery Research. No 3.2

Acknowledgements

With thanks to the Northern arm of Deaf CAMHS who produced Digital Health Guidance from which some of this chapter draws.

Section F

F1 Depression and anxiety in sign language users
Dr Kevin L. Baker and Paul Redfern

Depression is not the same as feeling tired, sad, or fed-up, but consists of symptoms that can persist for weeks and months. There have been varying opinions about whether it has biological, psychological and social origins. Many accept that it is likely to be due to a combination of causes.

Clinicians usually consider whether a client's presentation is related to a negative life experience and whether their mood could improve if:
- the negative life event improved (e.g. an ill loved one recovered, or bullying ceased)
- the person adapts to the negative event (e.g. thinking about it differently, or making behaviour changes in spite of the event)

Prevalence
In the early days of deaf mental health care (1960's and 70's) research papers tended to show Deaf people as having low rates of depression. There was an assumption that Deaf people would have the same rates of depression as hearing people and that the low numbers were because Deaf people had difficulties accessing mental health services rather than there actually being a lower prevalence of depression. More recent studies show that Deaf people experience depression and anxiety at higher rates and at an earlier age compared to the general population as well as finding it difficult to get help (Kushalnagar et al. 2019).

Research shows that higher levels of stress during childhood and adolescence lead to higher levels of depression, other mental health conditions and poor physical health. This is certainly true for deaf people (Fellinger et al. 2012). Unfortunately, this often leads to a repeating negative cycle, where high levels of stress lead to less effective problem-solving, which lead to feelings of rejection and exclusion that lead to further isolation and less activity.

It has become clear that the additional, multiple disadvantages experienced by some Deaf people in comparison with hearing people, make it difficult to find out where a mental health problem like depression begins and what would be an expected reaction to significant and persistent stressful life events ends.

Symptoms of depression

The symptoms of depression are often enduring, difficult to shift and significantly impact on the person's everyday functioning. They include:

- feeling hopeless and helpless
- having low self-esteem
- feeling tearful, guilty, irritable
- having no motivation or little interest in doing things
- having little interest in sex, eating and being sociable
- finding it difficult to make decisions, remember things, and/or feeling overwhelmed
- lack of energy, not enjoying life
- moving or speaking slowly (or sometimes too fast)
- finding it difficult to sleep, or sleeping too much
- having suicidal thoughts
- somatic symptoms

Each person's depression evolves from their individual history. However, in the context of living in a hearing-majority society many aspects of a deaf person's experiences are shared by a significant proportion of the deaf population.

Stress and depression

Deaf people undoubtedly experience high levels of daily stress due to communication difficulties and exclusion from hearing society. They are more likely to experience poverty, and less likely to be employed or promoted. Deaf people are more likely to have experienced bullying and being called names; and more likely to have been victims of domestic violence, childhood abuse and trauma. Deaf children often do not attain similar levels of education compared to their hearing peers.

When psychological stress becomes repeated and chronic, even at low levels, the body's response involves changes in the level of hormones and neurotransmitters, which after a sustained period of time affects the body's ability to get back into balance. These hormones can affect psychomotor activity meaning that things feel like they take more effort and makes concentration difficult. They also affect sleep patterns (Chapter H8) and make it more difficult to remember things. These changes are reflected in the list of symptoms above. The functioning of the brain and body changes so that clinical depression can be very stubborn.

Repeated exclusion and stress

Regardless of communicate style, deaf people often feel excluded and ignored. Their stress is associated with unequal access to information and services, whether this be the communication failures of hearing people, lack of appropriate technology, the absence of interpreters or subtitles having not been provided. The repeated experiences of exclusion mean that events that are relatively benign to hearing people can become immensely stressful to deaf people (Mousley et al., 2018).

"I am sitting on a train, which suddenly stops. It could be engineering works, signal failure, something on the track, or driver illness etc.. While waiting with other passengers there is an announcement, which I can't hear, but I can see people listening and then using their phones to call people. As a Deaf person I do not know why or exactly what is happening. At this point, I have two choices: to ask someone with a friendly face or do nothing. If I chose to ask, I may learn that there is a new reason why the train has stopped – expanding my knowledge of events in my life. If I don't, I learn nothing. However, to ask someone can also be stressful because communication can be difficult, and I don't know what response I will get."

Deaf people have this kind of dilemma every single day of their lives. There are millions of little bits of knowledge that they may miss because of this kind of information-exclusion. Hearing people rarely experience this.

Exclusion and isolation

When these experiences are part of a person's development and happen daily, they become much more than difficulties in how a deaf person can function in a hearing society. Coming up against linguistic and social barriers create an emotional impact and lead to feelings of rejection and isolation. Stress experiences build from being treated as different and less important than others. This is similar to what is experienced by other minority groups but is arguably more intractable because of the way language and cultural identity is experienced by deaf people.

Consequently, it seems that a protective factor against depression is a Deaf person's identity, which can contribute to improved well-being. Deaf people who perceive themselves as having a marginal identity, that their hearing and language status is due to their "disability" rather than the excluding actions of society, will experience poorer mental health, whereas a Deaf person who perceives themselves as part of a community of like-minded individuals who can share ideas and stories of exclusion between themselves, can feel reassured that the difficulties may not be located within themselves.

Powerlessness, helplessness and low motivation

In some situations, a deaf person may be forced to rely on hearing relatives and friends. Hearing people may try to help, but can easily 'take over', finding it much easier to do things for the deaf person rather than help them to understand and do for themselves. This can contribute to the Deaf person feeling unable to solve problems, or to the feeling that they are not given opportunities to solve their own problems.

We know that depression is often described and talked about differently in different languages and cultures. Whereas hearing-speaking people tend to describe depression using a single set of phrases and words that they may reliably group together as symptoms of "depression", for many Deaf BSL users, there appears to be two main aspects of depression which seem most salient:
- feeling hopeless and bad about yourself
- having poor motivation to do things (Rogers et al., 2013)

Motivation is likely to be moderated by context. For example, a deaf person may be motivated to attend a Deaf event (e.g. going to deaf club, or a deaf comedy performance), but may not feel the same level of enthusiasm to go to a mainstream social event (e.g. going to a cinema) where communication access and cultural affinity may be limited.

Seligman has used the term 'Learned Helplessness' to describe responses to stress that explain depression behaviours, such as poor motivation and perceived lack of control, in animals and humans. It explains to some extent why, even when offered mental health support, Deaf people often do not access it. Repeated absence of health and social care services create an expectation of failure such that help is not sought or engaged with.

"I've never really had much help in the past, why should I expect help to be useful now?"

Negative thinking

Finding out how a person thinks, feels, and behaves is obviously a first step to help them recognise and understand how they can address their 'depression'. It is often difficult for many hearing people who might understand deafness through a lens of 'disability' to recognise the implication of these negative constructs about 'needing help' or 'not being as good as a hearing person'. For the clinician, it can help to reframe these from a cultural perspective.

People with depression often struggle to get help if they do not feel like talking to others or leaving their home. Often their thoughts have a negative bias influenced by their feelings of hopelessness, such as *"No one will be able to help me"*, *"I can't do anything now, I'll do it tomorrow"*, or *"I don't deserve any help"*. Sometimes the person may have a mix of feelings that are difficult to make sense of, they may be anxious or find it difficult to trust others and even be quite paranoid about other people.

Taking a culturally informed approach to these thoughts can contribute to a formulation of the systemic factors that have influenced a client's individual experience of hopelessness. Such a formulation can often suggest ways to reduce the impact of those experiences by finding out more about how a deaf person uses resources within the deaf community for their well-being and resilience. Some deaf people develop and protect their resilience through strong links with other deaf people and culture, in similar ways to other minority cultural groups. Within Deaf culture interdependence is valued more than independence (Ladd, 2003).

Further research

There is some discussion as to whether deaf people are more likely to have somatic representations of depression, than hearing people. It is possible that poor access to primary care information about mental health, delayed diagnosis and a lack of specialist deaf mental health services prevent many deaf people to identify the emotional and cognitive elements of their mental health problem and instead focus on their physical symptoms. It may also be that the visual nature of sign language lends itself to focus on more concrete and physical descriptions of distress than the abstractions often used in spoken languages. We know that people from different cultural traditions can explain their emotional distress in more physical ways.

Conclusion

Deaf people experience numerous and persistent life stresses, which appear to increase the likelihood of higher levels of mental health problems compared to the hearing majority. As a result of inequality in day to day life, and fewer accessible support services, deaf people are often diagnosed later than hearing people, and end up with more chronic and complex problems. This in turn results in a much poorer quality of life, and with less benefit from preventative interventions or personal resilience. Framing a deaf person's difficulties within a systemic and cultural context can add more detail to their understanding of their symptoms of depression and suggest ways that their well-being and resilience can be strengthened.

References

Fellinger, J., Holzinger, D., & Pollard, R. (2012). Mental Health of Deaf People. T*he Lancet, 379(9820)*, 1037-1044

Kushalnagar, P., Reesman, J., Holcomb, T., Ryan, C. (2019). Prevalence of Anxiety or Depression Diagnosis in Deaf Adults, *The Journal of Deaf Studies and Deaf Education, 24(4)*, 378–385

Ladd, P. (2003). *Understanding Deaf Culture: In search of Deafhood.* Multilingual Matters: Clevedon

Mousley, V.L., & Chaudoir, S.R. (2018). Deaf Stigma: Links Between Stigma and Well-Being Among Deaf Emerging Adults, *The Journal of Deaf Studies and Deaf Education*, *23(4)*, 341–350

Rogers, K.D., Young, A., Lovell, K., Campbell, M., Scott, P.R. & Kendal, S. (2013). The British Sign Language Versions of the Patient Health Questionnaire, the Generalized Anxiety Disorder 7-Item Scale, and the Work and Social Adjustment Scale. *The Journal of Deaf Studies and Deaf Education*, *18(1)*, 110–122

F2 Deaf people and trauma
Dr Mary Griggs

Prevalence and prevention
Trauma disproportionally affects people from marginalised populations and is inextricably linked to systems of power and oppression.

Deaf children and adults are more vulnerable to all types of abuse, compared to hearing peers.

Several studies demonstrate higher rates of developmental or childhood trauma in deaf people. Specific factors that increase deaf children's vulnerability particularly to inter-personal trauma include:
- a lack of knowledge about sexual behaviour and boundaries
- for children in residential care, reduced contact with parents/carers for relatively long periods of time
- inadequate language and communication skills to report abuse
- inaccessible professional support
- the increased use of touch as a cultural norm for deaf and deafblind people
- higher concurrence of intellectual disability which can impact on understanding of abuse and seeking help

Effect of trauma
The effects of early or developmental trauma for deaf people, as with hearing people, can be profound. There is some evidence, however, that deaf people are more likely to experience dissociation (a 'disconnection' in a person's thoughts or feelings from their surroundings) than hearing people in response to trauma or reminders of traumatic experiences. One suggestion for this is that deaf people, particularly children, have fewer internal resources with which to deal with trauma.

The literature around trauma within the deaf community has also started to explore the concept of Information Deprivation Trauma (IDT). This idea builds on what we know about late language acquisition for deaf people born into hearing families (see Chapter B1) and the gaps in information (see Chapter B4) and understanding associated with this. IDT can include simply not understanding a traumatic event.

Example: Client Y is deaf. As a child she was not told of the death of a close relative. The impact on the child of not understanding what has happened can be profound. The focus of the deaf person's distress (as a child, or later as an adult) can be as much on 'not being told' as on the death itself.

IDT also looks at the role of information in helping a person protect themselves from future threat, contextualise risk and prepare for similar events in the future.

PTSD
Post Traumatic Stress Disorder (PTSD) can result from a single traumatic event at any time in life or from an accumulation of traumatic events over the life span. Clinical guidance on the treatment of PTSD does not make any specific suggestions for deaf people but states the benefits of specific trauma-facing therapies described later.

Trauma therapies typically converge on the idea that when faced with intense threat for example of assault or abuse, any normal sense-making 'freezes'. Although the traumatic event at some point ends, the trauma memory remains in the person's mind in a raw and 'unprocessed' form, in many ways feeling as intense as it was at the time of the trauma. Reminders of the trauma can then trigger what is known as re-experiencing of trauma. This is one of the key features of PTSD.

Trauma affects people in different ways and the degree to which this happens depends on factors such as prior trauma, a person's internal coping strategies and resources they have to make sense of the trauma. The aim of trauma therapy is essentially to help the brain understand that the trauma is in the past. This necessary updating can help 'process' raw and very real trauma memories. This updating process however relies on things which many deaf people struggle with such as piecing together information about an event or an abuser.

Example: Client X, a deaf, child was sexually abused by a priest. She was told that she 'is lucky' to be in a relationship with him and that she should keep this relationship secret to avoid making other children envious. The abuse was frightening and confusing, but even as an adult it took Client X a long time to start to understand the role of this misinformation, among other things, in facilitating this abuse.

In the case of Client X, the internal ability to make sense of what had happened was compromised. In order to talk about such abuse, the client needs:
- information and understanding that this is abuse
- adequate language skill
- the opportunity to access caring and skilled professionals, who know how to work with deaf people

For some deaf people the ability to process the experience in a more conscious and accessible state is more difficult.

Trauma therapy
Deaf people who have experienced trauma can benefit greatly from specialist psychotherapy and counselling. Access to suitably trained therapists can be problematic because of limited number of therapists or difficulty accessing funding (see Chapter G4).

There is wide agreement that support from a deaf therapist is often the best fit, although sometimes a deaf person may prefer to talk to a hearing therapist, if necessary, via an interpreter.

Adaptations to trauma therapy follow guidance on working with deaf people more generally in mental health settings and highlight, for example: the need to meet and match language and communication skill; pay attention to a person's information 'deficits'; consider storytelling, visual metaphors and role play and use examples to illustrate a concept.

Clearly talking about details of trauma in therapy involves building a trusting relationship between the client and therapist. The use of a chaperone may support some clients.

The developmental environment for deaf people raised in hearing environments differs to the experience of children who share a language with their parents/caregivers. It is particularly important therefore to be open to potential issues of attachment, identity and complex relationship dynamics.

The therapist should be familiar with factors common to both deaf and hearing people, such as shame, fear and feelings of responsibility. They need also to be aware of factors that affect deaf people disproportionately, such as lack of information about sexual relationships, particularly in the context of language deprivation (Chapter B1).

Distress within the Deaf community has resulted from significant barriers to reporting abuse, and at times, disappointing responses to reporting childhood abuse, as an adult. These factors can all help understand vulnerability to trauma and help frame conversations about protective factors and resilience.

> Several investigations have proven significant sexual abuse within Deaf boarding schools in the UK and around the world (St John's Catholic School, Boston Spa School, 2005; St Joseph's National School, Dublin 2012; Provolo Institute for Deaf and Hearing Impaired Children, Argentina, 2019). Other investigations have been hampered by the length of time between alleged offences and attempted prosecution (Woodford School, London, 1999). Refusal by Criminal Justice professionals to prosecute is strongly challenged, as many of the complainants have only been able to attain the necessary knowledge, support and psychological resources later in life.

Trauma-focused CBT (TF-CBT)
TF-CBT is based on the idea that PTSD can result when a traumatic event is processed by the person in a way that leads to a sense of serious and current threat.

Like other trauma therapies, TF-CBT emphasises the need for Psycho-education to understand how trauma effects the brain. It also includes a skills-based component to reduce the more distressing symptoms of PTSD, with 'stabilisation' techniques. These might include relaxation and breathing exercises, which are highly accessible to deaf people.

The trauma-facing component of TF-CBT involves re-visiting details of traumatic events in order to update trauma memories. Therapists may use diagrams to illustrate patterns of thinking and behaviour (e.g. the role of avoidance in maintaining unhelpful thoughts).

Some deaf people struggle to work in the abstract, to think/reflect on their thinking patterns (Chapter B1). The stabilisation phase of TF-CBT is therefore essential. Working at a body level, for example through relaxation techniques, can allow deaf people to see change in the 'here and now'. Experiencing themselves in highly emotional states and then calming their body, can help access calmer and more rational thoughts.

Eye Movement Desensitisation and Re-processing (EMDR)
EMDR is a therapy in which traumatic memories are processed and updated by asking the client to simultaneously:
- complete a task, such as tracking eye movements AND
- think about a certain aspect of a traumatic memory

While a good relationship with the therapist is important, a reduction in PTSD symptoms is primarily due to internal processing/updating within the memory system.

Some components of EMDR require reflection around how a traumatic event from the past is being understood now. Communicating this quite complex concept requires good language and communication skills between client and therapist.

The 'processing' of trauma, using eye movements or other tactile stimuli is fundamentally a visual process and works very well with deaf people. In some circumstances (e.g. if a client has dual sensory impairment), eye movements can be replaced by other bilateral (left-right) stimulation such as tapping on a client's hands or by holding electronic buzzers.

In theory, EMDR can be done with an interpreter. To minimise the visual distraction of any third party during processing, it helps to seat the interpreter slightly behind the therapist and away from the focus of the client's attention. This can also work for a chaperone.

Generally, once all parties are familiar with the technique, therapist and client can agree on certain signs to indicate when to follow eye movements, give feedback etc. The most important thing is that therapists maintain eye contact with the client rather than switching attention back and forth to the interpreter.

Narrative Exposure Therapy (NET)
NET can also be used to good effect with deaf children and adults. This therapy involves constructing a Lifeline (or time-line), using objects to represent positive and negative or traumatic events. Therapy sessions then guide the person to develop a story or narrative of their life which can help them to process and make sense of traumatic events.

Essentially a very visual therapy, NET can work well with deaf people. Key events are laid out in a simple, concrete way and the deaf person is encouraged to choose language and concepts that are both understood and are meaningful to them.

Trauma-informed care

Trauma impacts both the individual and the system around them (e.g. within a ward or team). Mental health services generally are being encouraged to work towards more trauma-informed environments. This is understood as:
- encouraging a culture of listening
- responding in a meaningful way to each person's story
- avoiding re-traumatisation
- creating conditions that can reduce harm and promote healing

Services supporting deaf people are often aware of the negative impact of factors such as isolation, discrimination, communication barriers and inequality. Yet, professionals are often less aware of their own role in potentially re-traumatising survivors of trauma and abuse.

For example, sitting in a meeting with hearing professionals in which some conversations are not interpreted not only prevents a deaf person from equal involvement but can be reminiscent of abusive experiences in which power and control was maintained by this kind of exclusion. These situations can trigger intense distress and anger.

References

Schild, S., Dalenberg, C.J. (2011). Trauma exposure and traumatic symptoms in deaf adults. *Psychologyical Trauma: theory, research, practice and policy, 4(1),* 117-127

Schild, S., Dalenberg, C.J. (2012). Psychoform and somatoform dissociation in deaf adults. *Journal of Trauma and Dissociation, 13(3)*, 361-376

Schild, S. Dalenburg C.J. (2015). Consequences of child and adult sexual and physical trauma among deaf adults. *Journal of Aggression, Maltreatment & Trauma, 24*, 237-256

Schild, S., Dalenberg, C.J. (2016). Information deprivation trauma: definition, assessment and interventions. *Journal of Aggression, Maltreatment and Trauma, 25(8)*, 873-889

F3 Adjustment to hearing loss
Dr Sally Austen and Cath Booth

Introduction
Whilst it is common for British Sign Language (BSL) users to express pride in their deafness, people who have had hearing and then lost it are much more likely to experience it as just that — a loss — something they would wish to reverse.

Deafness varies by degree and type. Each person will also have a unique cohort of strengths and weakness, physical, cognitive and emotional. Whilst each deaf and Hard of Hearing (HOH) person's experiences will be different, there do appear to be some difficulties that collectively span a number of categories. Examples include:

Practical difficulties
The absence of hearing can make a variety of activities harder or impossible depending on degree and type of hearing loss: hearing oncoming traffic, listening to the radio, playing the guitar, correcting your children's reading, hearing a coin drop. Whilst technological or human assistance can help compensate for some such difficulties, the absence of hearing can have a real impact.

Communication and isolation
In a predominantly hearing world being deaf or HOH is associated with communication difficulties, which can have detrimental effects on personal and professional lives. Communication on an individual level can often be difficult and at a group level can be impossible. Background noise, distracting visual environments, and speakers who do not take their share of the responsibility for successful communication can make being deaf or HOH a frustrating and lonely experience.

Isolation and reduced contact with people can have practical and emotional repercussions. Even in the absence of any psychological adjustment difficulties, effective communication will still need to be a significant consideration.

Loss or restriction of role
We each have a number of broad roles: friend, parent, child, employee and other more subtle roles: the helper, the listener, the fixer, the joker,

the organiser etc. For those with acquired hearing loss they may lose roles that they were previously comfortable with. For example, a woman who regards her listening ability when friends have problems as fundamental to her identity feels less of a 'friend'. Likewise, a man who regards his ability to be the breadwinner as paramount and who retires early because of hearing loss can feel 'less of a man'.

In her book Sound, Bella Bathurst describes her own experience of losing her hearing and that of those she interviewed. For those whose income derives from music or the military, they are at great risk of noise induced hearing loss (and tinnitus - see Chapter H2) which then risks the guarantee of their jobs.

Identity
Many people with hearing loss describe difficulties with identity. They may learn about those people who identify as Deaf, with a capital D (see Chapter A3) who share a cultural and linguistic pride, but they do not feel a part of this and yet they no longer feel part of the hearing world either. As such, it is often felt that they 'don't fit in to either world'.

Discrimination and inequity of opportunity
Like restriction of role, discrimination can occur on a broad or more subtle level. Research has shown that deaf and hard of hearing people experience under-employment, financial inequality and restricted access to educational facilities. Advancement in the workplace may also be blocked because of discriminatory attitudes. On a day-to-day basis many deaf and hard of hearing people experience stigmatisation and ill treatment as a result of their deafness (RNID, 2020).

Painful and life threatening conditions
The causes of deafness and hearing loss are numerous (see Chapter H1 & H5). Some are associated with other medical conditions (e.g. acoustic neuroma), or the result of treatment for painful and life threatening conditions (e.g. certain drug treatments for cancer, infection or HIV/Aids).

Whilst some in the Deaf community consider being deaf a lifestyle choice (see Chapter C10), deafness in the context of painful or life threatening conditions is not. Meningitis, which can cause deafness, is still meningitis; a life-threatening condition, with the potential to cause lasting physical, cognitive and sensory damage, and is terrifying for the patient and their loved ones.

Associated disabilities
Many conditions that cause deafness are have associated disabilities and health challenges (e.g. problems with thyroid, kidneys, heart, diabetes, vision, dexterity, and cognition).

For some deaf people this may include cosmetic challenges associated with structural differences to their face or body. Thus, the deaf person will also have thoughts and feelings about any other difficulties they have, whether they are physical, neurological or associated with a specific or global learning disability. It may be that a deaf or hard of hearing person has no negative perception of their deafness, but experiences distress in relation to an associated disability.

Associated audiological difficulties
For many people who are deaf or HOH, other audiological difficulties trouble them. Tinnitus (see Chapter H2) and balance problems (see Chapter H3) affect many. Other audiological conditions such as recurrent ear infections, allergic or painful reactions to the ear moulds of hearing aids, hyperacusis (where noise is perceived as painfully loud) are also common.

Mental well-being
Acquired hearing loss is associated with high levels of depression, social anxiety and isolation – and therefore risk of suicide. Co-work between mental health services and audiology services is crucial (although not always recognised by funding bodies).

Referral to audiology services to maximise use of residual hearing (see Chapter D10) and learning practical coping strategies, such as lip-reading (see Chapter D8) and relaxation strategies for tinnitus management, can help.

Depending on the individual, mental health intervention may be required in terms of:
- Antidepressant or anxiolytic medication
- Therapy (e.g. Cognitive Behavioural Therapy)

Cognitive Behavioural model
The cognitive behavioural model provides a way of understanding an individual's unique experience (of their deafness, being employed, being

tall etc.) and how it contributes to distress. It does this by adopting a scientific approach to measuring and making predictions. However, rather than measuring the event itself, the individual's *perception* of the event is considered.

Example: Two fifty year old women lose their hearing as a result of having an acoustic tumour removed. Person A is devastated. They become depressed. They describe their sadness at not being able to hear their grandchildren laughing. Person B is elated. They thrive. They describe their happiness that they have survived a potentially life-threatening event and will live to watch their grandchildren grow up.

The cognitive behavioural model does not deny that some situations in life are more difficult than others, indeed that some are horrific. However, it purports that negative thoughts and negatively biased perceptions (about oneself, the world or the future) result in depressed or anxious affect - whereas positive appraisal of situations can be psychologically protective.

The impact of deafness is dependent on self-cognition: how one *thinks* about one's deafness will determine how one *feels* about one's deafness. Furthermore, how one *feels* about one's deafness may differ from how one feels about an issue that is *associated* with the deafness.

Behavioural challenges
With therapeutic support, the client is encouraged to test their negative hypotheses about being deaf or HOH - or associated difficulties.

Example: Anne is in her 70s and, since losing her hearing, avoids going to her friend's crowded coffee morning because she cannot hear or lipread when there are lots of people.

- *Therapeutic challenge: To ask the host if she would mind having an event where she invites fewer people.*
- *Anne's negative hypothesis. 'The host will think I am selfish and rude. She can't put my needs before those of her other friends.'*

Acknowledging how anxiety provoking this is, Anne is encouraged to test out her negative hypothesis and report back.

> *Result from Anne. 'My friend was delighted to be offered a solution to get me back to the coffee mornings. She thought I had stopped coming*

because I disliked her. She was thrilled to be able to help. She asked me how many people would be manageable and I said 4. Now every second week will be a mini coffee morning so I can join in.'

Children adjusting to hearing loss

For children, their perception of hearing loss can be significantly affected by their own experiences, as well as the perceptions of their parents and carers. For this reason, it is particularly important that parents are supported to understand their child's deafness. Parents who experience their child being deaf or having a hearing loss as traumatic tend to unconsciously alter their parenting style (see Chapter C3).

Likewise, the attitude of peers is extremely important to a child's adjustment and consideration must be given to their potential sense of isolation, especially if they are the only deaf child in a hearing mainstream school.

Assumptions of association

Cole and Edelman (1991) found that Deaf teenagers tended to think that all of their problems were because they were deaf. For example, they thought that their hearing peers had no such troubles with relationships or with school being boring. They were not aware that hearing teenagers had the same difficulties and those issues with parents and school may be more associated with their age than their audiological status.

Austen (2004) discussed, using tinnitus as an example, how we can create metaphorical 'Coat Hooks' and 'Smoke Screens'.

Coat Hooks enable us to hang all our problems on one issue and neatly apportion blame and causation (e.g. 'All my difficulties are because I have tinnitus. If my tinnitus was cured all my problems would go away and my social life and marriage would flourish').

Smoke Screens enable us to unintentionally distract from the more important underlying problems that may be harder to acknowledge (e.g. loneliness, marital discord or anxiety).

Community
Shared experience, shared language, shared history and shared social space result in community, which in turn brings a sense of identity and belonging – and ultimately well-being.

However, whereas for BSL users coming together eases communication, for oral deafened people (who may have coped with hearing loss by isolating themselves) it can feel harder, at least in the first instance. Thus, despite shared experience, deafened people do not tend to come together as much and therefore lose out on the benefits of 'community'.

Local and national charities that provide accessible information and promote shared experience are invaluable.

RNID (previously Action on Hearing Loss)
www.rnid.org.uk

Hearing Link:
www.hearinglink.org

Conclusion
Hearing loss can be devastating. Although those with acquired deafness are much less likely than the BSL using Deaf community to welcome their deafness, adjustment is possible with the help of well-resourced services: audiology, community support, and (where necessary) mental health services.

References
Austen, S. (2004). Cognitive behavioural models in deafness and audiology In S. Austen & S. Crocker (Eds) *Deafness in Mind. Working Psychologically with Deaf People Across the Lifespan.* Pp 101-14. Whurr Publishers Ltd

Barthurst, B. (2017). Sound. *Stories of Hearing Lost and Found.* Wellcome Collection

Cole, S.H., & Edelman, R.J. (1991). Identity patterns and self- and teacher-perceptions of problems for deaf adolescents. *Journal of Child Psychology, Psychiatry and Allied Disciplines, 32,* 1159–65

F4 Deaf people and psychosis
Dr Sally Austen and Dr Steve Carney

Psychosis causes similar levels of difficulty and distress for deaf and hearing people. However, some symptoms present differently and can be difficult to assess without understanding the unique needs of each deaf person.

Psychosis symptoms can result from many conditions:
- Severe mental illness (such as schizophrenia, bipolar disorder or severe depression)
- Trauma and stress
- A neurological condition (e.g. Parkinson's disease, brain tumour)
- Physical ill health such as an infection or temperature
- Sensory deprivation

Symptoms of schizophrenia include:
- Hallucinations
- Delusions
- Thought disorder
- Poor motivation
- Dulled reactions or slowed communication

Prevalence of psychosis in deaf people

Deaf people are equally, if not more, vulnerable to psychosis than hearing people. Of deaf people in psychiatric hospitals, schizophrenia is the most common reason for admission. However, this disproportionate presentation is likely to be because psychosis can cause people to behave or communicate in unusual ways, therefore making them more noticeable.

Deaf people generally have great difficulty accessing mental health services (see Chapter G1) so less severe mental health problems go unnoticed.

Grey and Du Feu (2004) suggest that deaf people are at risk of higher rates of schizophrenia, due to heightened biopsychosocial risk factors:
- increased isolation and poorer social support (Chapter F1)
- higher rates of experiencing abuse and bullying (Chapter F2)
- neurological risk associated with cause of deafness (Chapter H1) and inner ear infection

Assessment
As with any client, a background history (life events, access to education, physical health) is needed. Specific to deaf clients, information should be gathered on any health problems associated with their cause of deafness, the client's experience of being deaf or Hard of Hearing (HOH) and their communication preferences and presentation (see Chapter D14).

Even in hearing people the description of psychotic phenomena is extremely personal and requires an incredible degree of caution to understand the client's story. Psychotic symptoms are often assumed to be florid and dramatic. However, sometimes unusual experiences are quietly hidden in a story that, as some point, stops making sense. To allow the person to tell this story, you need to allow additional time, keep an open mind and work with the best language and cultural support.

Each person should be assessed in comparison to their own 'well self'. Therefore, it is important to have information about their premorbid presentation. This usually comes from the client, the family or previous health or care provisions. However, with a deaf client this can be difficult for several reasons:
- *The client:* Many deaf people have difficulty accessing services so they may have a long duration of untreated psychosis and/or have no idea what is required of them in a mental health assessment. Some deaf people have additional language deprivation (Chapter B1), difficulties with time-lines (Chapter B6) and knowledge gaps (Chapter B4) and can therefore be inaccurate historians.
- *Family:* 95% of deaf people come from hearing families, most of whom do not sign. So, a thorough third-party account is not always possible.
- *Services:* A great deal of mental health information is gleaned from a client's communication style. This is difficult for generic (hearing) services, who may not have much experience of working with deaf people.

Diagnosis and misdiagnosis
Under- and over-diagnosis is common. Unless the assessor has experience of working with deaf people in mental health settings, any diagnosis they make must be considered provisional and followed up with a referral to deaf specialist services (see Chapters G3 & G4).

Example: a young man in his early 20s, born in South Asia, came to UK age 8 years with no previous education and no fluent spoken or signed language. Resultant poor language and cognitive development left him with difficulty describing and managing his emotions. After a significant bereavement he was found distressed and agitated, throwing stones at a police station window. He was arrested and assessed by a junior on-call psychiatrist who concluded his incoherence was the result of thought disorder. He was detained under the Mental Health Act and medicated against will. It was 3 months before he was seen by a doctor experienced in working with deaf people, who identified emotional regulation problems triggered by the bereavement and underpinned by language deprivation. The client had been unnecessarily medicated.

Specialist deaf mental health services in the UK, are not currently commissioned to respond to emergencies, so generic (hearing) services are expected to work on their own.

The (almost certainly) hearing psychiatrist, with (almost certainly) no experience of working with deaf people must make the best assessment they can to ensure the wellbeing of the client. They will be able to refer on to a generic psychiatric crisis service, who will also (almost certainly) have no experience of working with deaf people. Each must be very careful not to jump to assumptions. Their diagnosis must be provisional!

It is never appropriate to diagnose mental illness via the medium of writing. BSL has a unique grammar and therefore different word order. In its written form it can incorrectly be considered to represent thought disorder or delusion. Many deaf people also have reduced literacy (see Chapter B3).

Interpreters are essential in any psychiatric interview (see Chapters D1-D6, D11, D13). If a face to face interpreter cannot be booked, use online interpreting services. (see Chapter D7).

Hallucinations
Hallucinations are generally categorised as auditory, visual or tactile. However, this is more complex in deaf people. A 'voice' could be the vision of people communicating in sign language; a memory of a previously experienced noise; or a kinaesthetic sense of physically signing. See Chapter F5 for more information.

Hallucinations should not be assumed to be a communication. It is better to ask 'Is there someone or something there that shouldn't be?'.

Cautious assessment is vital. Other experiences of noise, vision and thought must be ruled out:
- Tinnitus (see Chapter H2). Tinnitus can take the form of virtually any noise: voices, bells, musical instruments. Your client may not know they can experience tinnitus.
- Residual hearing. Make no assumptions about what a deaf person can hear or used to be able to hear.
- Intrusive thoughts (a cognitive symptom of anxiety).
- Some people who have lost their vision (and therefore some deafblind clients) can experience non-psychotic hallucinations, a condition called Charles Bonnet syndrome; their brain making a normal response of filling in the visual gaps.

Approximately 50% of deaf people who are diagnosed with schizophrenia report visual hallucinations. A similar proportion describe tactile/somatic hallucinations. In generic studies, the occurrence of visual and tactile is 15% and 5%, respectively. Since both types of hallucination mostly co-occur with reports of 'voices', this raises the possibility of a direct relationship between these phenomena. (Atkinson, 2006)

Delusions
Delusion are defined as unshakeable beliefs which, when examined rationally, are obviously untrue. These beliefs must be out of context with the client's cultural and religious background.

Clients who are immersed in Deaf culture and who attend Deaf Clubs, may report that 'everyone is gossiping and stabbing me in the back'. Hearing culture may find this statement rather paranoid; Deaf culture would regard this as quite possible. Visual signed information can be seen at a distance (it is harder to 'whisper') so there is little privacy for sign language users across any large space.

Crucially, misunderstanding information is different from believing something that is untrue. Some deaf people who have had difficulty accessing accurate information or who have poor expressive language may use delusional like descriptions, in the absence of mental illness (see Chapter B1).

Example: a deaf client described in sign language that he had argued with his brother because 'the aliens were looking down laughing'. It turned out the argument was real and concerned which brother had the larger portion of mashed potato. The client did not know the word or sign for 'mashed potato' and used a description of the 1980s advert for a desiccated mash potato product called Smash, where indeed aliens are shown looking down and laughing at humans.

Deaf people do not have access to all the same information as hearing people (see Chapter B4). This is because of the lack of captions or sign language on TV and the limited communication skills of their parents, teachers, preachers and bosses. If you do not have full information, you can come up with the wrong conclusion.

Example: a deaf man in his 70s said that the voice of God was punishing his sins. He described this as a commanding noise in his right ear. For a long time, he was considered to potentially have psychosis. It was only when he mentioned that God's voice was louder when he had a cold, that it was realised this was tinnitus. On exploration he reported a strictly religious upbringing with the threat of God's punishment often on his mind. When he started experiencing tinnitus as a teenager, he assumed his punisher had caught up with him.

Thought disorder
Thought disorder describes a change in the way thoughts are presented: loose associations between words or ideas; incoherence; poverty of content of speech; tangentiality; circumstantiality.

Thought disorder is extremely difficult to identify in deaf people due to the crucial role of language. Where assessor and client have different first or fluent languages any translation of thoughts and experiences has the potential to go wrong. The assessor must keep an open mind and allow significantly longer for the assessment. Even hearing professionals who sign fluently should consider involving an interpreter and a deaf professional in their assessment (see Chapter D4).

It is particularly tricky to disentangle thought disorder from language disorder (see Chapter B1) and crucial that written language is not used diagnostically. It is important to establish a baseline: what is this person's language at its best? Has it deteriorated in fluency, style or content?

Secondary symptoms
Secondary symptoms can be harder to spot and treat in deaf people. Whilst many deaf people have sophisticated careers, hobbies and are generally engaged and active, others have a higher rate of unemployment, disempowerment, and overprotection, than their hearing peers (Chapter F1). Thus, establishing what is a 'normal' level of disengagement for each individual is difficult.

Communication idiosyncrasies
Pressure of speech (see Chapter F6)
Each person has a different rate of signing or speech. Signing style and space also varies. Thus, you need to know what is normal for each individual.

Prosody
Prosody refers to the rhythm and pattern of stress and intonation in a person's expressive communication. Unusual prosody in hearing people can be a useful indicator of learning disability, autism or mental health problems. However, unusual prosody in the speech of a deaf or hard of hearing person is more likely to result from their not having been able to hear their or others' voices growing up.

In sign language, features of prosody include use of sign space, duration of a sign, pauses, and facial expression. In hearing and deaf people, assessment must include professionals who share a first language with the client. For deaf people, it is crucial to have a full history of their communication opportunities to have an idea of what 'normal' would look like for them.

Perseveration
Organic causes of psychosis may be related to health conditions associated with the clients cause of deafness (see Chapter H1). For example, perseveration is sometimes associated with thyroid disorders, which are associated with some causes of deafness. However, repeating a word or phrase in sign language is relatively common and can be:
- a language naivety
- a conscious attempt to make sure the other person understands
- a replacement for the hearing hesitation equivalent of 'Um'.

Summary
It is inevitable that hearing clinicians will be required, at times, to assess deaf clients, despite having no prior experience of deaf mental health care. Our advice is to:
- Create working hypotheses rather than fixed diagnoses
- Involve deaf specialists as soon as possible.

References

Atkinson, J.R. (2006). The perceptual characteristics of voice-hallucinations in Deaf people: insights into the nature of subvocal thought and sensory feedback loops. *Schizophrenia Bulletin, 32(4)*, 701–708

Atkinson, J.R., Gleeson, K., Cromwell, J. & O'Rourke, S. (2007). Exploring the perceptual characteristics of voice-hallucinations in deaf people. *Cognitive Neuropsychiatry, 12(4)*, 339-361

Grey, A., & Du Feu, M. (2004). The causes of schizophrenia and its implications for Deaf people *In S. Austen & S. Crocker (Eds) Deafness in Mind. Working Psychologically with Deaf People across the Lifespan.* Whurr Publishers Ltd: London

F5 Do deaf people hear voices?
Dr Elizabeth Wakeland

Introduction
The idea that deaf people can experience auditory hallucinations may appear paradoxical.

There is limited research undertaken regarding the experiences of hallucinations and delusions in individuals who are deaf. That which does exist suggests that hallucinations and delusions are shaped by the individual's own experience of language and their level of hearing loss. For example, those who are born deaf and, as such, have never experienced auditory experiences do not report 'true' auditory hallucinations akin to those of hearing individuals with auditory hallucinations. See Atkinson (2007) for a detailed overview.

The language used by hearing professionals when describing auditory hallucinations involves terminologies that suggest 'true' auditory hallucinations (e.g. shout, loud, quiet). Inadequate examination can lead to a misinterpretation of a deaf person's hallucinatory experiences.

Assumptions are often made by hearing professionals based on their hearing experiences, which risks misdiagnosis or a lack of understanding. A case study will be used to outline a process of coming to understand the hallucinatory experiences of an individual who is deaf.

Case study
Wendy is a 54-year-old female who was born deaf after her mother contracted rubella (German Measles) when she was six-months pregnant. She utilises hearing aids that provide some access to sound. She is the only deaf member of her family and was encouraged to communicate via speech and lip-reading. She began to use British Sign Language (BSL) after attending a specialist school aged five-years.

Considering that an individual's hallucinations are shaped by their experiences of deafness and language, Wendy's developmental experiences are important to understand. Asking questions relating to family dynamics, and communication amongst family members will gather such information.

Wendy has a long history of contact with psychiatric services, commencing at the age of 26-years. Latterly, she was diagnosed with paranoid schizophrenia. She describes experiencing 'explosions' in her head, the voices of various people, seeing hands signing in front of her, and the alien control of her own hands and lips by unknown others in an attempt to convey messages to her. She also describes spirits, noises, and internal and external voices.

The information pertaining to these experiences was gathered using the Atkinson et al., (2007) card sort task. Whilst these are not the only way to assess hallucinatory experiences, the cards provide a language narrative that is not confined by symptoms and diagnostic criteria or language, allowing the client to describe their experiences in their own words.

The card sort task was designed by Dr Jo Atkinson, a clinical psychologist who is deaf. It contains 94 cards for use with deaf clients who are experiencing all forms of hallucinations (auditory, gustatory, taste, tactile and visual). The cards use simple English alongside line drawings to elicit information pertaining to a range of experiences.

They are copyright free and can be found at:

https://www.ucl.ac.uk/dcal/research/voice-hallucinations-deaf-people-schizophrenia

When using the cards, they are sorted into three piles representing 'Yes', 'No' or 'Don't know', according to whether the client recognises the experience as matching their own. The cards include statements such as "the voice is in front of me", "I experience voices even though I am deaf".

Below are copies of some of the cards, printed with permission from Dr Joanna Atkinson.

Sometimes I **smell** things that other people can't smell.

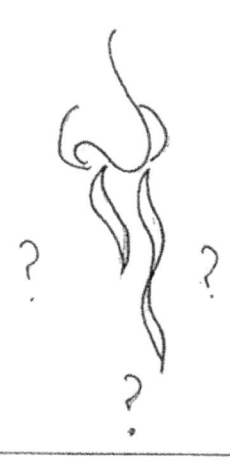

Voice feels similar to my own thoughts.

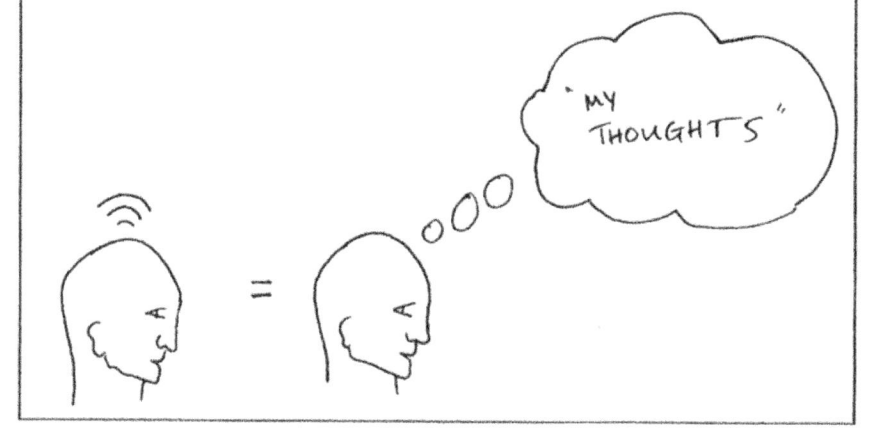

The volume of the voice goes up and down.

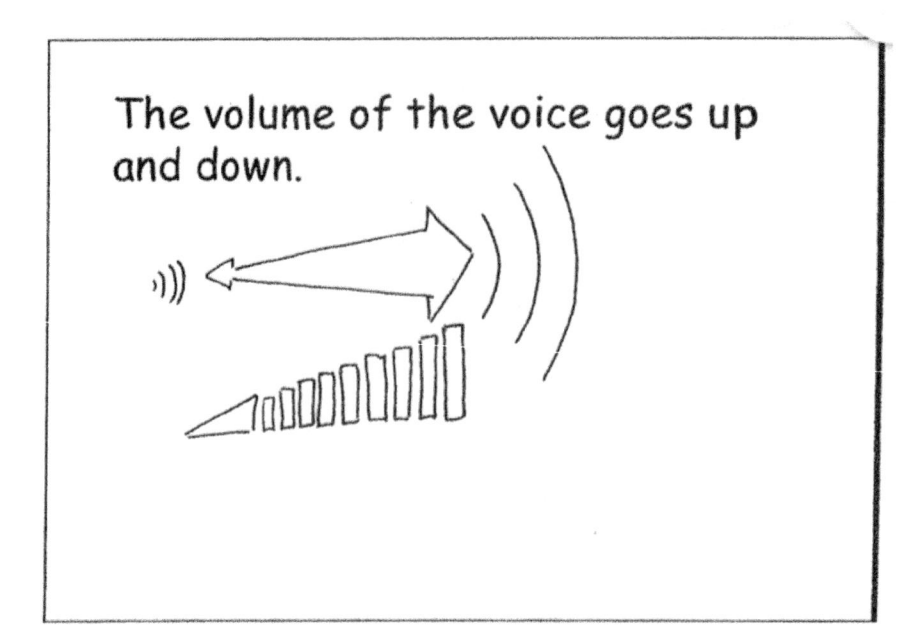

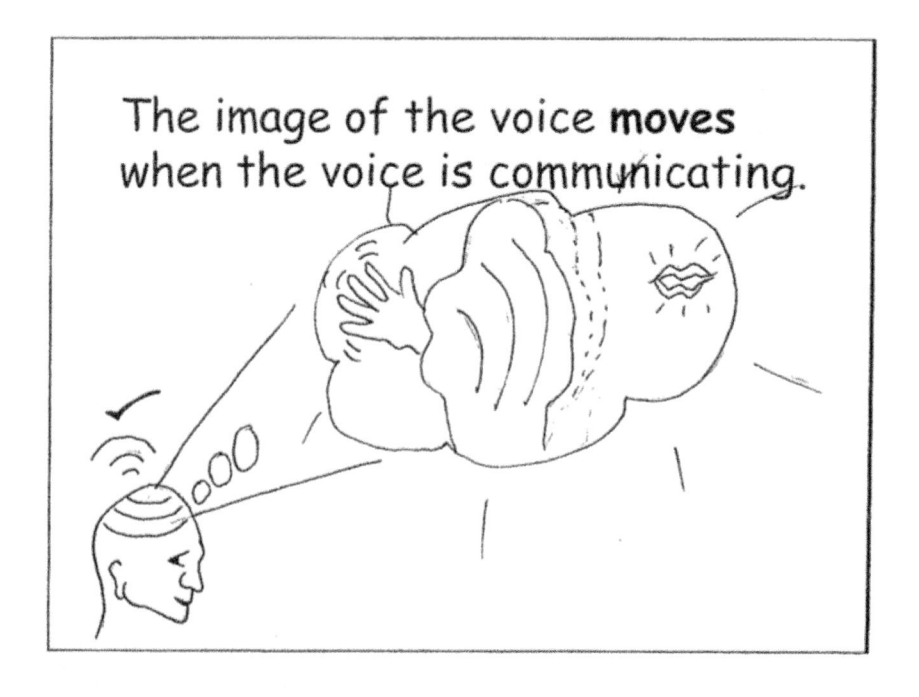

The image of the voice **moves** when the voice is communicating.

Each card allows for discussion between client and therapist/interviewer, which helps to build rapport and engagement. The 'Yes' pile can then be sorted into further piles for different questions relating to frequency, severity and distress experienced, depending on what information the clinician wishes to elicit. The cards can also be used to evaluate treatment outcomes.

The card sort task was used with Wendy facilitating normalising talk, and allowing her to consider that other people had similar experiences to her. Wendy identified seven distinct experiences through the card sort task. These included those she considered 'usual' (i.e. not a hallucination) and those that she saw as 'unusual'. Further clarification was sought, including which experiences were distressing, positive or negative.

Other factors to consider when assessing the impact of hallucinations include the individual's identity, family scripts, cultural and religious affiliations, and social environment. This is not unlike the experiences to explore when working with a hearing individual.

Wendy described being part of the 'hearing world', through her family. However, she had deaf friends and attended a deaf school and so also considered herself to be part of the 'Deaf world'.

Wendy's experiences led to her identity developing in both the hearing and deaf world. She described hallucinations that included people talking to her, or communicating through speech and lip-reading, whilst others used signed language. This mirrors her experiences of communication across the hearing and Deaf world.

The use of the card sort task enabled Wendy to understand, structure and communicate her experiences. It provided a sense of meaning for Wendy and a language with which she could communicate her experiences. This was used with professionals, to identify her different experiences, which were of concern, which were considered 'normal', and which could be understood as part of her family culture. This provided a rich formulation to enable professionals to communicate and work with Wendy, using a shared language about her experiences.

Using the card sort task
The card sort task is a useful tool to gather further information and to aid a professional's understanding of their experiences. The tool is useful for those with cognitive or intellectual impairments. The tool can also be used with interpreters.

There may be situations where the cards still require some explanation, with the picture and simple wording on the card not being enough to clarify what is meant. This may present linguistic challenges as it is difficult to phrase these without projecting the interviewer's own assumptions.

For example, when the cards use the term 'voices', this may not translate to all participants. They may not recognise their experiences as voices, or label them in this way. Alternatively, they may call their experiences 'a voice', but on exploration it is tinnitus, a noise, or self-talk. These nuances require a good working relationship with an experienced interpreter, with thorough discussions prior to and after the assessment to identify differences within the language they use and the experiences described.

Conclusion
When working with a deaf individual who reports hallucinations, it is important to remain curious, be open and aware of our own assumptions. Gathering information pertaining to the age of onset, experiences of hearing, communication experiences within the family and wider community, and their identity is key.

Our assumptions regarding illness and symptoms can bias our view of other people's experiences. Using tools, such as the Atkinson (2007) card sort task, aids in the gathering and understanding of the individual's hallucinatory experiences that can aid both assessment and formulation.

References
Atkinson, J.R., Gleeson, K., Cromwell, J. & O'Rourke, S. (2007). Exploring the Perceptual Characteristics of Voice-Hallucinations in Deaf People. *Cognitive Neuropsychiatry, 12(4)*, 339-361

F6 Pressure of speech or sign
Dr Sally Austen

Communication idiosyncrasy is a feature of mental health changes and shows up in speech or sign. However, the identification of communication difference or changes in deaf people and Hard of Hearing (HOH) people, should be reviewed carefully.

'Pressure of speech' refers to speech or sign that is frenzied, rapid and appears urgent in nature.

It can be symptomatic of several mental health needs, including:
- Mania (associate with bipolar disorder)
- Extreme anxiety
- Psychosis
- Stimulant drug misuse
- Frontal lobe dysfunction
- Attention Deficit Hyperactivity Disorder

Avoidance of receptive communication
Whilst deaf and HOH people can present with symptomatic pressure of speech, caution should be used in diagnosis, as this may be a feature of their communication style, not their mental health and cognitive functioning.

Some deaf people find expressive communication easier than receptive and would rather keep talking/signing than pause to listen/watch. This is particularly common in oral communicators who find it easier to speak than to lipread (see Chapter D8). Some people dread the moment when they will need to lipread, so subconsciously prevent it being necessary (or possible) by developing the habit of filling all communication space with their own expressive communication.

Reflective experience of the professional
The experience of the professional, when faced with this style of communication is important to consider. Erratic or rapid production can:
- make it hard to understand or interrupt
- leave the professional with frustration at not being able to take their turn in what should be a conversation

- a subjective feeling of a weight on their chest (as breathing is altered by the efforts to interrupt) which can be anxiety provoking

Interventions
Physical and visual chairing
Good listening is usually associated with eye contact, gentle nodding, and waiting for a space to respond. This may need to be replaced by:
- Raising your hand to indicate 'stop'
- Changing your body language into a more raised and 'ready' position
- Deliberately dropping eye contact

Structure your appointment
If you know your client does this, it may help to write a list of key points you want to discuss and place between you for repeated reference. This helps give the client structure and context.

For example, a list might say:
- Problems today?
- History of problems?
- Any family problems?
- What you have tried before that has worked/not worked?
- What we suggest you try is...?

Summary
Use caution before considering pressure of speech/sign as a symptom of mental health problems.

Consider how you might alter your communication style to support your client.

F7 Psychological therapies
Dr Sally Austen

For a deaf or Hard of Hearing (HOH) client to receive effective therapy, the therapist must be both appropriately skilled and qualified - and ensure the therapy is fully accessible to the client.

Communication

Communication in its widest sense underpins the relationship building between client and therapist. In any language, therapeutic communication depends on finding the words/signs, meanings and intonation that does justice to the client's experience.

The therapeutic alliance also relies on shared responsibility:
> *We will both work to communicate as best we can*

And shared honesty:
> *I didn't understand that, please can you repeat*

That said, just because two people share the same language and culture, does not mean they will automatically achieve a therapeutic chemistry. A deaf therapist and deaf client may fail to gel, just as a hearing therapist and hearing client might.

When a client is brave enough to come to therapy, they should not be burdened by practical communication challenges, such as limitations in the therapist's deaf awareness or signing abilities.

We are all more able to access our inner most experiences, thoughts and memories when doing so in our first language and with someone who understands our culture. A client who is considering, for example, whether to reveal for the first time their experience of childhood sexual abuse deserves a therapist who has done everything in their power to ensure that communication is maximised.

Whilst any two people naturally adjust their communication to match the style and needs of the other, deaf clients with hearing therapists are often burdened with the greater responsibility for that adjustment. In order to create a safe and useful therapeutic milieu, the hearing therapist must consciously consider their role in communication equality.

Deaf or hearing therapist
A deaf client requires their therapist to have both communication and professional therapist skills. Ideally, the client should be able to choose between a deaf or hearing therapist, and between a signing therapist or interpreter. However, this is not yet the case both because of limitations in financial and human resources.

There are far more qualified hearing therapists than deaf therapists. Just as it not appropriate to have substandard communication with an appropriately qualified therapist, it is not sufficient to have an insufficiently qualified therapist, just because they are themselves deaf. Thus, interpreters are often required.

In choosing a therapist various factors should be considered.
- The client's language pathway: someone who is signing now, may want to explore memories of oral times or their relationship with significant others who are oral. (Fernando, 2004)
- Their need for confidentiality: The very small Deaf community means that clients (or their families/friends), therapists or interpreters could be known to each other.

Therapists' contextual and cultural awareness
In order to fully understand what any person is saying we need to understand the context of what they are saying. To a large extent it is the purpose of this book, to assist in providing the context.

Thus, the therapist (assessing or treating) must prepare themselves to ask the right questions and understand the significance of the answers. For example, the following rather factual points are likely to have great significance to a deaf person:
- Did you go to a deaf specialist school or mainstream school?
- Are you the only deaf person in your family?
- How do you communicate with your family?
- Do you have a deaf/HOH peer group and/or a support network?

A knowledge of the increased possibility of past difficulties is imperative. See Chapters F1 and F2 for more information.

This is similarly important in service-provision for children with deaf parents (see Chapter C4) who benefit from deaf specialist services because they do not have to explain the basics of their upbringing to their therapist. National Deaf CAMHS (see Chapter G3) take referrals for children with deaf parents but the equivalent adult services do not.

Cognitive accessibility
Deaf clients with fluent language will be able to make good use of the available range of therapies. Likewise, if needed, they will work easily with an interpreter.

However, whilst the therapists' choice of intervention may reflect their preference, it must also meet the needs, expectations and abilities of the client. For clients who have experienced language deprivation (see Chapter B1) or knowledge gaps (see Chapter B4) some therapies are less appropriate.

Behavioural reinforcement is one of very few psychological interventions that rely only on the skills of the therapist, not the client. It does not require the client to understand the psychological model or to reflect on their own involvement. However, the areas of its effectiveness are somewhat limited.

Thinking about thinking
Many therapies require the client to think about thinking, which requires significant linguistic skill (in sign or speech). It also requires Theory of Mind (see Chapter B5). For those people with limited language (see Chapter B1 & D3) this might not be feasible.

For example, Cognitive Behavioural Therapy (CBT), requires the client to think about, and identify, whether their experience is a thought or a feeling. Theory of Mind is required to be able to consider whether MY thinking bears any similarities to OTHERS' thinking.

Example: CLIENT A - I waved at my friend in the street but she didn't wave back. I am thinking that my friend ignored me because she hates me – and that thought is making me sad. But if I question my assumption about my friend's motivation, I can see that there are alternative explanations for their behaviour. My friend may have appeared to ignore me but might not have seen me, or she could have been in a rush. In considering the alternative reasons for my friend's behaviour, I feel less sad.

Family and systemic therapy requires the clients to understand that each of us has different roles, different thoughts and different feelings. This requires quite sophisticated Theory of Mind, without which Socratic questioning doesn't work.

Abstract thought (see Chapter B7 for more information)
Many therapies require a client to hypothesise, which requires the ability to use abstract thought. For those deaf people who have grown up in language deprived environments this can be very difficult. Often an abstract question receives a concrete answer.

Locus of control (LoC) (see Chapter B8 for more information)
Locus of control refers to the sense of who should and can take responsibility for any aspect of our lives. Deaf clients who have been overprotected and/or not given responsibility are more likely to have an external LoC (seeing that others have responsibility for outcome). This can affect their ability to see their role in therapy as an active partner rather than a passive 'patient'.

Literacy (See Chapter B3 for more information)
People born deaf or deafened in early childhood tend to have significantly poorer literacy levels than their hearing counterparts. Replacing or simplifying written material may be necessary (e.g. homework sheets, appointment letters, therapy contracts or shared therapeutic formulations). Visual representations are by far the best way to get conversations started.

Autobiographical memory
Many therapies (e.g. psychodynamic and schema based therapies) require significant reflection on how the client's past experience relates to their current situation

Memories tend to be encoded linguistically. Within generic psychological study we consider the first 2 years of life as 'pre-verbal' and accept that these memories are powerful, but linguistically inaccessible. For those deaf people who have acquired language late, the period of linguistically inaccessible memory may be much longer. Non-verbal therapies, such as art or movement therapy, may facilitate other ways of accessing and reflecting on these experiences.

Most sign language users are the only deaf member in a household of non-signers. For those that do not share a useable language with their parents, autobiographical experience may be something that they have never discussed with any shared fluency.

Pre-therapy
Existing therapies tend to be designed for those who already have some knowledge of, and way of communicating, their emotional and cognitive experience. For clients who have some of the difficulties described above, making use of programmed therapies is difficult and 'pre-therapy' may be required. This involves using psycho-educational approaches to enable the client linguistically, emotionally and informationally.

Pre-therapy information is also important for professionals and families. See Section K for a great example of accessible preparation material.

Dr Neil Glickman is an American psychologist in deaf mental health care who has written many books on adapting interventions for deaf people with language deprivation. In his 2017 book, he uses specialised cartoons to enhance his work and makes these available to the reader: https://www.routledge.com/Preparing-Deaf-and-Hearing-Persons-with-Language-and-Learning-Challenges/Glickman/p/book/9781138916937

Outcome measures (see Chapter G7 for more information)
It has become the norm for commissioners to require therapists to use outcome measures, such as the PHQ-9, GAD-7, CORE-OM. However, the majority of standard outcome measures are difficult to access with low literacy, have concepts that do not translate well or just take too long to explain, translate or mark.

These measures have been translated into BSL and are available for free. Research shows the threshold is different for deaf people compared to hearing people. However, even with BSL translation many deaf clients find the fluent signing hard to access. Thus, the author tends to use their own clinical opinion, rather than formal outcome measures.

Summary
Deaf and HOH people deserve equal access to psychological therapies. To achieve this therapists must be prepared to adapt their interventions to meet the linguistic and cognitive needs of the client.

References
Fernando, J. (2004). Psychodynamic considerations in working with deaf people. In S. Austen & S. Crocker (Eds) *Deafness in Mind*. Whurr Publishers Ltd, 75-88

Glickman, N. (2017). *Preparing Deaf and Hearing Persons with Language and Learning Challenges for CBT. A Pre-Therapy Workbook.* Routledge: New York

F8 Group therapy
Dr Sally Austen

Group work has therapeutic benefits – clients sharing experiences and challenging each other to review habits, thoughts or beliefs (e.g Addictive behaviour programs).

Group work is often a cost-effective way to deliver psycho-education and facilitate people completing a 'program' of learning and reflection (e.g. Prison sex offender work).

Therapeutic intervention may also be part of group meetings such as CPA, ward reviews, Experts by Experience interview panels.

Maximised communication
In order to communicate successfully, group members need to be looking at the speaker. This is similar for signers, lipreaders, interpreters, and those needing to redirect their communication equipment (hearing aid, FM pens or microphones; see Chapter D10).

Strong chair or leader
Whether communication is supported by sign, lipreading or maximising residual hearing, a strong group leader is required to maximise effectiveness.

Only one person talks/signs at a time
It is impossible to lipread two people at a time. It is impossible to interpret two people at the same time. Clarity of noise deteriorates if more than one person talks at a time.

The leader must choose a system to ensure only one person talks/signs at a time.

The next speaker/signer doesn't start until everyone is looking at them
The chair acknowledges the first contribution, waits till everyone is looking at them, and then points at who is going to talk/sign next. Also useful is having an object (e.g. a cushion or soft ball) that is passed between contributors, so a person cannot contribute until they are holding the object.

Communication via video conferencing (see Chapter D7)
Covid-19 has resulted in the development of some group therapies being offered by video conferencing. This requires a more controlling chair and encourages all participants to sit face on. Facilities are available for including interpreters and note takers, using captions and sharing a space for writing.

When done well this can improve access for the deaf or HOH client. When done badly (participants facing away, poor bandwidth so that the video is unclear, not booking the right communication professional, no facility for the deaf/HOH person to choose whose picture they would like to enlarge/'Pin') then it is a disaster of depressing, discriminatory proportions.

Relative shared abilities and needs
In running a mixed deaf and hearing group, it is important to be aware that skills may vary. For example, some clients may not have the required fund of knowledge (see Chapter B4) or conceptual understanding. They may need 'Pre-Therapy' (see Chapter F7).

Group therapies often have an inflexibility of number of sessions, style of presentation, or accompanying worksheets that may disadvantage a lone deaf or HOH client. Adaptation may therefore be needed. This can be time consuming and benefits very much from deaf professional involvement.

Any written material should be adapted to the needs of the clients (see Section K).

The therapist's linguistic skills
The right therapist has psychological intervention skills and relationship skills, both of which need maximised communication and cultural awareness. Even fluent hearing signers will be challenged when running a therapy group with deaf people who all may have different signing styles and abilities.

To be both therapist and linguistically vulnerable is daunting. Feeling powerless can lead us to subconsciously control or limit the language usage of those who are superior to us (Schlesinger et al., 1987).

Thus, to run deaf groups, help may be needed in the form of:

- Supervision to reflect on one's signing abilities
- Having a deaf co-therapist
- Having a deaf relay interpreter (Chapter D4)
- Being honest with the group
- Revealing to the group our missed information and ask them if they think it is necessary for them to fill you in – or not

Summary
Ensuring equal engagement for deaf and hard of hearing clients within group therapy requires significant preparation.

Reference
Schlesinger H, Schlesinger, H. S. (1987). Effects of powerlessness on dialogue and development: Disability, poverty, and the human condition. In B. W. Heller, L. M. Flohr, & L. S. Zegans (Eds.), *Mind and medicine series. Psychosocial interventions with sensorially disabled persons,* pp. 1–27. Grune & Stratton, Inc/Harcourt, Bra

F9 Telemental Health (TMH)
Dr Ben Holmes and Dr Sara Powell

The term 'Telemental Health' (TMH) refers to the provision of mental health support through the use of technology. This might, for example, include therapy administered via telephone, text message, email, video call, or self-guided computerised psychotherapy packages.

The field of TMH has been developing over the past two decades or so. With increased access to video call technology, it is increasingly seen as a viable alternative to face to face contact. With the recent experiences of the Covid-19 pandemic, TMH has allowed many therapy appointments to continue that may otherwise have been postponed or cancelled.

For professionals, it provides benefits such as reduced travel time, reduced need for clinical space and it is easier to offer more flexible timings for appointments. Clients, also benefit from reduced travel time in addition to increased access to a greater range of potential therapists. The security of physical distance may be an added benefit for people that do not feel comfortable sitting alone with someone they do not know.

Access benefits
TMH offers a potential solution to a number of problems that deaf people may experience when trying to access mental health services.

For some deaf people, perhaps particularly those that identify as culturally Deaf, there are many reasons why they may wish to see a Deaf therapist or specialist deaf service. This may include wanting:
- someone with a shared cultural understanding
- someone that can empathise based on similar life experiences
- to be able to communicate directly without the need for interpreters
- to avoid repeating previous experiences of oppression by hearing people

These factors are not true for all deaf people but, when they are, having access to a Deaf therapist is often not an option. This is because specialised psychological therapy for deaf people varies according to location and is often centralised to specific regions. The makes deaf people in certain areas, particularly rural areas, particularly vulnerable to lack of access. There is also the issue of the smaller number of qualified deaf therapists nationwide that are able provide the services that are needed. TMH can overcome some of these geographical and access barriers.

For deaf people that meet with a hearing therapist from generic (hearing) services, the use of video calls allows for qualified interpreters to be added with ease (see Chapter D7). This is especially important when the only other form of contact may be via a telephone, which many deaf people cannot use. Here, video calls offer greater equity of access.

Additional benefits of TMH include better access for:
- people who struggle to leave the house because of mental or physical health difficulties
- people who work, that may struggle to fit in with mainstream services that often operate between 9-5
- deaf or hard of hearing people that use captioning or lip reading, that may benefit from video and audio systems that facilitate this
- people who want access to a specific therapy. Online therapy makes it much easier to find this match

Access limitations
Despite these benefits, there is also need for caution and additional planning with some clients. Consideration needs to be given to deafblind clients who may be able to access TMH but may need technological adaptations (e.g. a large screen) or need the therapist to make sure there is good visual contrast (e.g. between background and clothing worn).

Clients who are experiencing active domestic abuse may experience access issues if their safety using TMH cannot be guaranteed. Provision needs to consider how and if sessions can be offered in a safe and neutral space.

Some TMH includes the provision of computerised CBT (cCBT). This can be really useful but it is important to ensure that clients will be able to access this technologically and linguistically. This may be especially the case for deaf clients who have English as a second language to British Sign Language (BSL), or deaf clients who have experienced language deprivation (see Chapter B1). This may impact on the ability to understand information that uses complex or jargonistic wording (see Chapter B3).

Prior to therapy
Technology is not perfect. Just as a car might breakdown on the way to a face to face appointment, there may be disruptions to video calls because of computer problems or internet outages. It is therefore important to agree with a client what you will do if technology fails and disrupts the appointment, especially as the point of disruption cannot be predicted and could potentially come at a sensitive moment. This might, for example, include:
- switching to a different device (e.g. phone) if the computer fails
- using 4G if wifi fails
- trying to call again after 10 minutes to restart the session
- having a number to text to make contact

It is advised that a code word/sign should be established with the client to indicate if the person is in a potentially difficult or dangerous situation and needs help. This is because it is not always possible for the therapist to see who else might be in the room and the client may need to alert you to problems without being able to say what they are. This is particularly important for people experiencing domestic abuse.

It is important to spend more time at the start of an appointment making sure that the set-up is correct. Both people should be able to see the other clearly and should be sat in a comfortable position.

An initial appointment should be offered to determine a client's potential suitability for online therapy. This should largely focus on technological requirements, the client's ability to effectively use the technology and whether the client's needs are appropriately met by providing online therapy (e.g. whether any risk concerns can be adequately managed, and whether the person is living with a currently abusive partner).

Technological requirements
When meeting using the internet, to ensure the highest quality contact possible:
- Use an ethernet cable direct from the router to the computer or device connected to the internet. This reduces the burden of wifi in the house, increasing connection speed and picture quality.
- Clients should check whether their internet provider has a cap on their data allowance prior to meeting so that they know whether they might incur additional costs.

- All other computer tabs should be closed during therapy to prevent interruption by windows spontaneously opening and disrupting the picture.
- A minimum broadband speed of 4mbps is recommended to achieve sufficient video quality for BSL to be visually clear and comprehensible. The download speed, rather than the upload speed, is of particular importance in ensuring good video quality.

Environmental requirements (see Chapter D10)
When meeting with clients via video call it is important that the environment is set up appropriately for any contact. Equipment should be positioned so as to have good lighting. There should be minimal background noise, both auditory and visual. Ideally clinicians should have a plain coloured background behind them. Consideration should also be given to the removal of any confidential, or personal, information that may be visible on the screen.

Security considerations
It is important that all steps are taken to ensure that therapeutic support is provided in a way that offers the greatest confidentiality and security possible. Just as when meeting face to face, this can never be fully guaranteed - people can walk into rooms accidentally; it may be possible to hear through walls or see through windows. However, some internet based communication channels are more secure than others.

Clinicians should make sure that the channel used meets security requirements for their organisation and should not just use an application because it enables electronic contact. Where possible, virtual meeting rooms should be locked when all participants are present (e.g. client and interpreter). Details of the link should be unique for each meeting and should be sent as close to the time of the appointment as possible to minimise the chances of interception.

If a virtual 'waiting room' function exists, this should be used so that it is possible to see who is being admitted before they enter.

Groups (see also Chapter F8 for more information)

Providing group therapy for a deaf person within a group of hearing people is already difficult. This is because there is a necessary delay in information being translated when using an interpreter. This can exclude a deaf person from being able to respond to one point before the next is raised.

Having continued focus on the interpreter also means that a deaf person will miss out on seeing other people within the group and their interactions and reactions. Whilst in some ways the use of TMH might seem to provide greater opportunities for group interventions for deaf people, the problems associated with participation remain even with an interpreter present. Pauses may also be required for the deaf person to be able to 'pin' specific people (e.g. interpreters), especially when there is a change of presenter, so that they can follow what is being said.

Digital poverty and access

It is important to note that not all people will have access to sufficient technology to enable them to make use of TMH. Technological devices may be shared, people may not be able to afford to pay for data usage or it may not be possible to find a large enough, secure space, at home that enables sufficient privacy for TMH appointments to be offered safely. TMH should therefore be seen as an adjunct to other ways of providing therapeutic input and not the standard - otherwise there is a high risk of excluding portions of society, and perhaps particularly those that may be in the greatest need.

Summary

The use of TMH has the potential to provide significant benefits to deaf people wishing to access psychological therapies. However, it should be seen as an adjunct to other forms of contact that increases the flexibility of support options available. Offered correctly, it provides the opportunity for quicker support that is better matched to the needs of individual clients and their circumstances.

F10 Medication and deaf, deafblind or Hard of Hearing people
Dr Sally Austen and Dr Steve Carney

The BNF (British Nationally Formulary) does not differ in the advice it gives for deaf or hearing patients. But the prescriber must take deafness into consideration.

Crucial factors to consider are:
- Side effects: that may affect the deaf person's ability to communicate
- Health conditions associated with the client's deafness.
- Conveying the name of medication in English or BSL
- Conveying the instructions for the use of the medication
- Ensuring the patient can obtain their medication
- Receiving feedback from the client on the efficacy of the medication

Side effects that may affect the deaf person's ability to communicate
Deaf people are not more prone to side-effects of medication but can be more disadvantaged by both by their effects and side effects.

Receptive sign language communication and lip-reading require clear vision and good concentration. This can be impaired by medications that cause blurred vision or sedation such as tricyclic antidepressants or first-generation antipsychotics.

Expressive sign language communication and speech is detrimentally altered by any changes to the movement of the person's hands, body or face. Extrapyramidal side effects include tremors, slow movement, rigid muscles, loss of automatic movements, speech changes, writing changes and impaired posture and balance – all of which can negatively affect communication. Facial immobility and slow movements can be mistaken for unusual emotional responses, which are particularly crucial in the detection of mental health issues.

Of course, there has to be a balance between the risk of long-term chronic movement disorder against suppression of the disabling symptoms of the illness (mental or otherwise).

These variables must be carefully considered in situations where de-escalation has not been successful (see Chapter F13) and PRN or sedation is required as a restraint (see Chapter F14).

Glaucoma is a condition that causes increased pressure in the eye, which can lead to blindness. A variety of drugs can precipitate or worsen glaucoma such as tricyclic antidepressants, typical antipsychotics, occasionally leading to an ophthalmic emergency. Some drugs can produce ocular dystonia, affecting eye movement and blinking, and in the extreme can cause oculogyric crisis.

In British Sign Language (BSL) there is no sign for 'side effect'. The direct English translation will only make sense to someone who already knows what a side effect is. For others, it is important to describe the concept of 'side effects', give some examples, and make sure the client understands the instruction to come back and tell the prescriber if this occurs.

Ototoxic drugs
Ototoxic medications refer to those whose side effects cause hearing loss, balance problems or tinnitus. There are over 200 such medications, some whose effects are temporary and some permanent, for conditions from mild pain to life-threatening infections and cancers.

Tinnitus (see Chapter H2)
Tinnitus affects many people who are deaf and hard of hearing. As with hearing people, it can cause difficulties with concentration in communication. Some drugs can cause or worsen tinnitus (e.g. some antibiotics, diuretics and some chemotherapies). Reports on the effects of antidepressants are mixed: some antidepressants, such as SSRIs, may worsen tinnitus; whilst other antidepressants have successfully treated tinnitus.

Hearing Loss
For clients who have residual hearing it is important to protect what hearing they have.

Where the medication is prescribed for a life-threatening condition and there are no alternatives, hearing loss may be inevitable. As drug treatment improves this will become less likely. However, within the current deaf older-adult demographic there will be a significant number whose deafness is iatrogenic (i.e. the result of the treatment, rather than the illness that was being treated).

The deliberate use of ototoxic drugs to damage hearing is capitalised on by some hearing 'Deaf Wannabees' (see Chapter H7) and Deaf Wannabee website groups share information on drug type, amount and method, for hearing people who want to 'Cross the Bridge' to become deaf.

Health conditions associated with the client's deafness
A client's deafness may be a stand-alone condition. However, for many deaf people the cause of their deafness has other associated conditions (see Chapter H1).

For example, for people who are deaf as a result of Rubella Syndrome, the presence of cardiac issues and diabetes must be considered. For those whose deafness is associated with Cytomegalovirus (CMV), liver problems may require cautious prescribing. Likewise, various syndromes involve Thyroid and renal problems. Syndromes that involve maxillo-facial structures, such as Treacher-Collins, may affect breathing and require sedative medications to be prescribed thoughtfully.

Epilepsy is more prevalent in the deaf populations (likely to be associated with cause of deafness including trauma, infection etc.), therefore medications that affect seizure threshold must be considered.

Conveying the name of medication in English or BSL
The names of medications are tricky in any language. Each medication will have a Generic and a Brand name as well as names that change multiple times as it evolves.
- The majority of these names will be impossible to lip-read
- There are no nationally agreed signs for any medications
- You can write them down, but many prelingually deaf people have low literacy (see Chapter B3)
- The majority of these names are grammatically 'non-words', which means they are very hard to remember
- The majority of these names will be very hard for a BSL interpreter to translate or finger spell in a way that the deaf person understands
- Some deaf people may be more focused on what the medication looks like than it's name

Thus, when you explain the medication, the names may not be fully understood. And when you ask a deaf person to tell you what medications they have been on before, they may not be able to do so accurately.

Example:
Doctor: 'You have been on Chlorpromazine before, is that right?'
BSL interpreter, knowing the deaf person cannot spell well: 'You took tablet name C H L, is that right?'

As the prescriber you need to decide if 'C H L' is sufficient or if you need the full name spelt out. Are you, the interpreter and the patient, all in agreement of the meaning of 'C H L' or is one of you thinking Chlorpromazine while the other is thinking Chlordiazepoxide?

Doctor: 'You have been on Fluoxetine before, is that right?'
Deaf person nodding their head: 'Yes'

As the prescriber you must understand the concept of the 'Deaf Nod' (see Chapter B2), which is when a deaf person nodding appears to be answering in the affirmative, but is in fact, not.

Deaf people, particularly those with impoverished language skills resulting from language deprivation (see Chapter B1), may take more notice of the visual aspects of the medication: colour, shape, logo. This can lead to great confusion if the medication is changed or multiple medications are prescribed. It is frequently the case that patients do not take medication if it comes from a different manufacturer as they believe it is the wrong medication.

Many a specialist in deaf mental health care has searched the BNF for a medication that looks 'right' for certain clients to cope with a medication change.

In areas where deaf people have regular access to deaf-experienced clinicians and interpreters, signs may evolve for various medications. These would tend to be 'Home signs' or regional signs at most (see Chapter C8) and are not likely to evolve at the rate that the actual medication or the prescribing regime evolves.

It is only you, the prescriber, who knows the specifics of the medication – not the interpreter or the deaf person – and you must ask enough questions of both to ensure that you are on top of this. For example, some clinics have developed a sign for Procyclidine as 'P-bicycle' (using the English pun on cycle). Problems could arise from this, for example:

- For deaf people with low literacy or immigrant Non-BSL signers the English pun is of no help and the sign becomes just another 'non-word' to remember.
- The sign will be passed on, through usage, to areas where non deaf-specialists cannot monitor the use of the sign. If the medication were to evolve, for example, to be called Procyclidonate, the sign is likely to remain the same for some time, leading to inaccurate interpretation, until enough deaf-specialist clinicians explain it to the interpreters and deaf patients, such that the corrected sign is passed on through usage.

Conveying the instructions for the use of the medication
Given the paucity of deaf-specialist prescribers and the above difficulties of lip-reading, literacy and lack of nationally agreed signs, it is no surprise that research shows that deaf people are significantly more likely to use their medication inappropriately, to the degree that methods such as oral and suppository may be mixed up.

As the prescriber it would be wise to make no assumption of prior knowledge or competence, and explain each medication, dosage and method (oral, rectal, topical etc) each time. Some aspects of prescribing are counter intuitive to a non-clinician and must be explained thoroughly, (e.g. prescribing a stimulant for ADHD).

It will be up to prescriber to judge how best to convey this information. Some deaf or HOH people may just need a written note. For some clients you will need the support of a language support professional. Use the Communication Assessment (see Chapter D14) to establish what Language support professionals you will need (see Chapters D1-13): sign language interpreter, Lipspeaker, Relay Interpreter, Deafblind interpreter.
Our suggestions would include:
- Type out, print off and give the client a copy of a bespoke description of their prescription. Do not use the wordy drug company version. Cut and paste into this description pictures of the medication.
- Spot and then simplify your own clinical jargon: it might not be comprehensible to others (e.g. topical/oral/rectal, bd, dose, mg)
- Save this document for future use and adaptation.
- Ask the client to take a photo of these instructions on their own phone - so they have hard copy and digital copy.
- Ask the client to repeat back to you their understanding of the prescription. If they haven't understood it, adapt and retry.

Ensuring the patient can obtain their medication:
- Does the patient know where to collect their medication?
- Are they able to get to this venue: hospital, local pharmacy, GP surgery, depot clinic?
- Have staff at the depot clinic or other venue arranged sufficient communication support and access for the patient? e.g. Is there a voice only entry system? Is an interpreter needed?
- A deafblind patient may not be able to identify their medication visually. Use blister packs or dosette boxes designed for tactile recognition, rather than generic strips of tablets.

Receiving feedback from the client on the efficacy of the medication or their clinical needs

Hearing people learn most of their information through 'overhearing'. Deaf people do not. Thus, incidental knowledge from radio, tv, or others' conversations is less available and the deaf client may not know what knowledge gaps they have (see Chapter B4).

Do not assume:
- That the client has any idea what information you might be attempting to gather. They may not know, for example, that sleep problems are associated with depression; that sexual dysfunction may be a side effect of other medications; that experiencing strange tastes are symptoms that one should report.
- That previous clinical meetings, particularly with other professionals, have had effective communication. The client may be well into a long treatment regime and have no idea what they are being prescribed or why.
- That information provided by families is always accurate. Many signing deaf people are raised and live with families who do not sign. Information may need to be gleaned from others who know the client better (e.g. friends, support workers, teachers, other clinicians).

Summary

Prescribing for a deaf or HOH person requires consideration of any associated health conditions, being cognisant of the additional consequence of some side effects and the best means of accurate communication.

F11 Nursing/care co-ordinating with deaf service users: examples of good practice
Jackie Wan Brown, Jennifer Meek and Hannah Whalley

We are all qualified nurses, with decades of combined experience working in specialist deaf mental health services as inpatient and community nurses. We are also all deaf.

Every Deaf person's language fluency, family and educational background is different. This will impact the person's level of communication and abilities in all areas of life and, therefore, impacts their mental health presentation. To ensure that our chapter covers the needs of all deaf people, we have included lots of information on working with deaf people with all levels of ability. You will need to use the information here with discretion.

If working with a deaf service user, our two most important pieces of advice are:

1. Effective communication both ways enables the therapeutic relationship

The therapeutic relationship between you and your deaf service user is underpinned by effective communication. Ensure that communication is mutually effective – that you understand the service user and the service user understands you. This will instill a strong foundation for your work together. Issues in this area are critically disempowering for both staff members and service users.

Support your service user's communication needs in all settings, even beginning with their GP. Ensure that a family member or friend is not being used to interpret. A qualified interpreter must be used. The deaf person can attend their GP appointments with both family and interpreter, the two are not exclusive.

Learn how to book interpreters (Chapter D5) and learn how to work with them (Chapter D2), particularly the boundaries of what they can and cannot do.

2. Contact deaf specialist services

PLEASE get in touch with deaf services if you have any doubts or problems working with deaf service users. We are always happy to chat things through, even if you end up not referring to us! Our services' contact details are found in Chapters G3 and G4.

Deaf people need you to make more time for them
Deaf people will have faced many frustrating barriers in getting to you. The care pathway from their GP to you, and then into the community, is not smooth. It is important that you are prepared and understand, as best as you can (hooray, you're doing it already by reading this book!), how to work with deaf people before you meet them so as not to add to their frustrations.

This may seem like a lot of effort for a busy professional, but the key thing to know is that your deaf service user will likely have fallen through a lot of gaps already before meeting you. Don't become another gap! Being thorough is the best service you can give. This is to ensure the deaf person does not struggle along post-discharge, possibly necessitating re-referral.

Engaging your service user
Deaf people's access to resources is severely hampered by communication issues (notice a pattern here?). You need to ask yourself 'If I don't do it, who will? How would the deaf person meaningfully and effectively access that service?'. If the answer is 'Nobody' or 'They can't', then you will need to do it, or facilitate it. The most important thing that deaf people need is time and information.

Explain your role:
- What you do?
- What you will offer the deaf person?
- Who you work with?

Give the service user as much time to process and engage with you as is needed. Ask questions in different ways, check their understanding gently. You may end up giving lots of information, which may be overwhelming – break it up over several appointments if possible and appropriate.

Check they understand and have the information they need. For example:
- Diagnosis
- Medications
- Stressors
- Coping strategies

Do not assume they have a fund of knowledge or can find resources independently (see Chapter B4). When going through diagnosis and medications with them, ensure that you go through what their diagnosis means. Give examples of what other people with the same diagnosis experience, so they can relate to this.

Make sure they understand what their medication is for, when to take it, how often and for how long; as well as what side effects may happen and what should they do if they experience side effects.

Ensure your communication style is direct. Avoid jargon, as this might not be accessible to the deaf person (see Section K). Work with interpreters.

General deaf awareness tips (see also Chapter D10)
Good communication habits should be a priority for every staff member but nurses are often role models for others so should take a lead in this.

Get to know each individual deaf service user, so that you can start to recognise any changes and variations in their communication as their mental health improves or deteriorates.

Do not be concerned by a deaf person's vocalisations. This is a normal occurrence, though each deaf service user will differ.

To get a service user's attention, do not shout their name. Get into their field of vision and wave at them - or gently tap them on their arm or shoulder (if it is safe to do so).

For inpatient service users, to get a service user's attention in their bedroom, open the door slightly and flick the bedroom lights on and off to indicate you are outside. Then wave. Never just walk in, as you will make them jump. To wake a deaf person asleep in their bed, gently pat their feet or pat the mattress.

Communication is crucial to manage a situation when someone is aggressive. If restraint is required, there is even more need for clear and constant communication. The impact of taking away someone's freedom to move their hands is equivalent to gagging speech (see Chapter F14).

Be aware that all deaf service users have different levels of functioning and language fluency. Some will need extra support with communication via a deaf relay (see Chapter D4), some may have neurological divergence such as autism (see Chapters E4 & E5), language deprivation (see Chapter B1) or cognitive impairment (see Chapter E3).

If the patient's family or next of kin is deaf, check that they have been able to get in touch with service providers. In an inpatient setting, introduce the service user to the staff and other service users; orient them to the ward and how they can access the amenities.

A deaf service user on a hearing ward will be at risk of isolation. They may become frustrated or agitated because of the lack of communication. Make every attempt to communicate with your service user.

Empowerment and independence
Deaf people require assistive technology in their daily lives. This is not always in place for the deaf person, so it is worth checking if:
- They have pagers or flashing lights for their doorbells.
- Accessible fire alarms – if they do not have this, refer to the Fire Brigade for flashing and/or vibrating fire alarms.
- They need to know how to use VRS (Video Relay Service - see also Chapter D7). This is a video interpreting service that allows deaf people to communicate over video call to interpreters who are connected in real time to services that use telephones (e.g. the GP, Banks, utilities companies).
- Make sure deaf service user has been referred to the Sensory Social Work team.

Care co-ordination
If you are the care co-ordinator for a deaf person, you will need to have links with a wider circle of professionals and charities than with a hearing person. This is within your role and will be a great support to your service user. For service users who have had poor access to education and information, lots of psychoeducation is needed, even the basics: personal hygiene, sleep hygiene, mindfulness, diet, exercise, healthy relationships.

Consider how you contact deaf people in the community. Community services need to be willing to use text messaging and/or email not just letters and phones. Not shouting through the letterbox!

Check if they need support with letter reading, attending appointments, family relationships or referrals to other services (e.g. family counselling, independent living skills). Go through easy read information with them, if they want, so they can ask questions. Think about how you can be contacted by the service user – can they read, can they use email, can they text?

Contact your nearest specialist deaf outreach (e.g. SignHealth, Royal Association for the Deaf, Action on Hearing Loss, RNID teams for daily living skills). Isolation is something that many deaf people experience and can have a significant impact on mental wellbeing (see Chapter F1).

Where you need to involve services who do not currently provide adequate access for your deaf service user, point out that they are in breach of the Equality Act 2010.

All About Me: care program
'All About Me' is a recovery package, developed by deaf and hearing people from specialist services to help support deaf people with mental health problems. A booklet is available describing 'All About Me' and how it was developed. It includes a practical step by step guide explaining how to use it and guidance notes for the ten domains chosen by deaf people to be most important to their well-being.

'All About Me' documents can be used to structure recovery planning within Community, Inpatient and Secure settings. It is intended to be a focal point in Care Planning meetings and Reviews of Care between deaf service users, professionals, interpreters, family and carers.

Using a person centred approach the deaf service user may choose to write or draw in the 'All About Me' hard copy. Each domain should be scored from 1-10 so that any improvements can be mapped and targets can be set. The written form of this care plan can be found at :

https://www.cntw.nhs.uk/content/uploads/2018/02/All-About-Me-Deaf-Recovery-Package.pdf
BSL videos explaining the recovery package can be found at:
https://vimeo.com/164432616 (Introduction)
https://vimeo.com/164529931 (Domain descriptions)
https://vimeo.com/159015313 (Sarah's Story - case example)

Crisis plans

Many teams provide services users with telephone numbers for services to contact in a crisis. This is not appropriate for deaf service users and alternative plans must be made otherwise they may be unable to access the help they need at the point they need it most. Familiarise yourself with existing services that might be helpful alternatives:

SHOUT - is a national text message service providing support to deaf people in crisis 24 hours per day. This relies on written English and so may not be suitable for all people (see Chapter B3). Discuss this with your service user and see whether it would be helpful for them.
https://signhealth.org.uk/with-deaf-people/crisis-text-service/

NHS 111 BSL - This is a non-emergency healthcare advice number, equivalent to NHS 111, but provided using BSL interpreters using video link. More information can be found at:
https://interpreternow.co.uk/nhs111

Discuss with your team and attached crisis/home treatment teams how they might be able to adapt their methods of contact to make themselves more accessible. For example, using VRS, text message or email as is appropriate to the service user's needs.

Don't just print off a care plan in written English as this may not be accessible (see Chapter B3). It may be necessary to change language or make it more visual. Ask if the service user can understand their care plan and explain it back to you. If they can't it needs to be changed so they can!

Refer to deaf advocates

Deaf advocates cover gaps that may not have been considered or spotted. Deaf advocates significantly reduce the deaf service user's anxiety (and often the clinician's too) by being a bridge between deaf culture and hearing culture, ensuring that both deaf and hearing parties understand each other.

They find or create resources, taking into consideration the service user's background, upbringing, family communication, skill level and schooling. For example, they may refer to a deaf employment club or deaf counselling services.

The deaf advocate will consider who the deaf service user engages with most and whether there are any dependency issues. There is also always the possibility that the deaf person is experiencing abuse, of any kind.

Deaf advocates will offer in-reach too if a deaf service user is admitted to an inpatient unit. They will support the nursing team to have the information they need to meet the deaf person's needs.

There are several organisations that can provide deaf advocates as well as independent practitioners that may operate in your area. Please check who the most appropriate person for your service user might be. More information can be found about deaf advocates at the following:

British Deaf Association:
https://bda.org.uk/project/advocacy/

Royal Association for Deaf people:
https://royaldeaf.org.uk/services/for-professionals/advocacy/

SignHealth:
https://signhealth.org.uk/for-professionals/advocacy/

Summary
Deaf service users will have experienced many frustrating barriers in getting to you. Don't become another gap in their experience of services. Through making sure you have good communication and deaf awareness you will be able to help make a significant difference to their access to appropriate support. When in doubt, please make contact with specialist deaf services. We are here to help!

F12 Challenging behaviour in deaf and HOH children and adults
Dr Sally Austen

Deaf children have 3-6 times the rate of challenging behaviour as their hearing peers (Hindley, 2000) and this appears to continue into adulthood. However, much of the cause of this is preventable.

For the purposes of this chapter, 'challenging behaviour' includes self-injury, violence towards others and damage to property. The severity of behaviour to be defined as 'challenging' will vary between settings and will depend on the ability of others (family, staff, and authorities) to manage it.

It is arguably the case that low motivation, withdrawal and learned helplessness can be equally or more challenging in other ways. However, the causes of these may have different origins.

Being deaf or HOH is not directly connected with challenging behaviour, but some experiences that deaf people more commonly experience, are:
- Emotional communication: frustration and isolation
- Limited, inadequate, or inaccessible social learning opportunities
- Neurological risk: causing impulse control problems
- Language deprivation: affecting empathy and executive functioning
- Paucity of service provision

Emotional communication
Challenging behaviour occurs in social contexts and may serve the function of drawing attention, escaping attention/activity or gaining something tangible. It occurs when a more effective or appropriate form of communication is not available to the person exhibiting the behaviour. Communication is a two-way process, so a client may be struggling to express themselves (or understand others) due to their own communication limitations – or yours!

Deaf, deafblind and Hard of Hearing (HOH) people tend to experience isolation in a way that hearing people do not. Most are the only deaf person within their family and the only deaf child in their mainstream school. Lack of deaf or HOH peers or role models can affect emotional wellbeing (see Chapter C6).

Furthermore, many deaf children and adults experience some form of discrimination, oppression or abuse (see Chapters I9 & F2).

Soon after I went to school I was sexually abused. I tried to tell my mother but she didn't understand and I got really frustrated and angry. Mum would say 'what is the matter with you?' but I had so much anger inside me that I smashed a table and put my hand through the window (Austen and Two Service Users, 2007, p8).

In contexts where the client and the professional do not share a fluent language, challenging behaviour can be mistaken for the manifestations of mental illness (see Chapter F4).

Social learning opportunities

The beliefs and attributions that parents hold about deafness can influence the way they respond to their child's behaviour (this is also true for parents of children with disabilities or premature babies). Parents who do not view deafness as a tragedy, and share with their child a positive view of being deaf, deafblind or HOH, are more likely to parent effectively and insist upon socially acceptable behaviour, as with any other child (Kentish, 2007).

Diagnostic overshadowing (see Chapter E1) can also result in challenging behaviour being regarded as an integral and inevitable feature of being deaf. Thus, socially inappropriate behaviour is more often accepted, or left uncorrected, by those that should be supporting or guiding understanding. Without adequate role modelling, or explanation about what is expected socially from a situation, a child will not have the opportunity to learn alternative ways of acting or expressing their needs.

My parents would tell my sister and brother off and smack them, but wouldn't discipline me at all. I think they thought I was behaving badly just because I was deaf. And they felt sympathy for me because I was deaf. Even if I was angry and started hitting out at people they reacted with sympathy. I remember once that my father tried to send me to my room in the middle of the day, but my mother said 'Don't be hard on him, He can't help it, he's deaf' (Austen and Two Service Users, 2007, p13).

The combination of an adult feeling deskilled and powerless, with a desire to protect a young deaf person, can result in greater allowances being made. Over time this can reinforce a perception that people other than oneself hold disproportionate responsibility for actions than is the case. This can, in turn, create a lack of agency or sense of responsibility to change actions, which can continue throughout life (see Chapter B8).

Wakeland et al. (2019) demonstrate how this trend continues with similar treatment of deaf adults within the Criminal Justice System with even police officers and professionals believing that deaf people deserve, or should attract, additional sympathy. Information about what is socially appropriate continues to be withheld, and alternatives are not reinforced, meaning behaviour change is less likely.

'On another occasion I went to a football match...a man walking towards my gang...I picked up a bottle, smashed it and lost my head completely. I stabbed him in the face and it took off his nose. As a deterrent, the police said I was no longer allowed to watch home games...' (Austen and Two Service Users, 2007, p9.)

Neurological risk
Cause of deafness may be linked with neurological impairment (e.g. rubella, meningitis, prematurity; see Chapter H1). Between 26-40% of deaf children have additional disabilities (Fellinger et al., 2012). This number is likely to rise in future, as babies are surviving with lower birth weight and following increasingly severe illnesses such as meningitis and CMV.

Neurological impairment can increase the incidence of challenging behaviour directly due to impulse control problems and indirectly due to the exacerbating effect it can have on social communication and parental expectations.

Language deprivation (see Chapters B1 & C2)
Language deprivation, resulting from impoverished access to early language, is associated with poor development of Theory of Mind (see Chapter B5) and poor executive functioning (including attention deficits, working memory, inhibitory control, planning and cognitive flexibility). Thus, even in the absence of global learning disability, or obvious neurological impairment, a deaf person is more likely to display challenging behaviour if they have experienced language deprivation.

Paijmans (2007) reports that it is not deafness per se that is related to increased prevalence of challenging behaviour but that if a deaf person has some disruption in brain function, alongside language deprivation, then they are more likely to have difficulties with self-regulation and goal-directed behaviour.

The merging of language and cognition is essential for higher executive functioning and, without full language reasoning, concept formation, making sense of emotions and planning behaviour is compromised.

Internal dialogue (self-talk) is facilitated by proficient language and is a tool for regulating behaviour. Its absence or delay is likely to interfere with being able to reflect on others' emotions and our responsibility for them; the consequences of our behaviour; the impact of reward or punishment.

Hard of hearing children and adults

Even relatively minor hearing loss is connected to increases in challenging behaviour, although the causal links are complex. Up to 40% of prisoners in the UK and over 90% of Aboriginal prisoners in Australia have some hearing loss (Vanderpoll & Howard, 2012). Associated factors appear to include head injury and untreated childhood ear infections. In such situations hearing loss and socio-economic deprivation are known to be connected via poor access to education and health care.

Whether temporary or permanent, a school child's education and social interactions will be negatively affected if they have a hearing loss that goes unnoticed, untreated or under-resourced. Subsequent deterioration in their behaviour is likely to be a sign of their distress and a plea for help. However, if help is not forthcoming in acknowledging and addressing their needs, the child can assume a negative attitude towards being deaf or HOH (shame, anxiety, feeling that they are 'less able') and then use further deteriorations in their behaviour as a means of distracting from or 'masking' their deafness.

Summary

Language deprivation and neurological risk, experiencing isolation and paucity of service provision, difficulty communicating emotions and impoverished social learning opportunities increase the chance of deaf and HOH children and adults exhibiting behaviour that is challenging. However, five out of these six factors are entirely preventable.

Early intervention by family, social, education, mental and physical health or criminal justice systems could help to alleviate these problems and the associated challenges they bring. However, service provision specific to deaf children or adults, focusing on either prevention or treatment of challenging behaviour, is currently limited.

References

Austen, S. (2007). The deaf service user's perspective of challenging behaviour and restraint *In S. Austen, & D. Jeffery (Eds.) Deafness and Challenging Behaviour: The 360º Perspective*. Chichester: Wiley. Pp3-16

Fellinger, J., Holzinger, D., & Pollard, R. (2012). Mental health of deaf people. *The Lancet, 379 (9820),* 1037-44

Hindley, P. (2000). Child and adolescent psychiatry. *In P. Hindley & N. Kitson (Eds) Mental Health and Deafness*. London: Whurr. Pp 42-74.

Kentish, R. (2007). Challenging behaviour in the young deaf child. *In S. Austen & D. Jeffery (Eds) Deafness and Challenging Behaviour: The 360° Perspective*. Chichester: Wiley. Pp 75-8852-74

Paijmans, R. (2007). Neuropsychological, behavioural and linguistic factors in challenging behaviour in deaf people. *In S. Austen & D. Jeffery Deafness and Challenging Behaviour: The 360º Perspective*. Chichester: Wiley. Pp89-108

Vanderpoll, T., & Howard, D. (2012). Massive prevalence of hearing loss among Aboriginal inmates in the Northern Territory. *Indigenous Bulletin, 7(28),* 3-7

Wakeland, E., Rose, J., & Austen, S. (2019). Professionals' experiences of deaf offenders with mental health difficulties. *American Annals of the Deaf, 164(1),* 137–157. https://doi.org/10.1353/aad.2019.0012

F13 De-escalation of aggression
Dr Sally Austen, Dave Jeffery and Grant Budge

De-escalation describes a series of verbal and non-verbal behaviours aimed at diffusing anger so that it does not escalate into aggression and violence. De-escalation aims to avoid the need for restraint and minimises the need for PRN medication; see NICE guidelines (2015) and the Restraint Reduction Network's (RRN) Training Standards:
https://restraintreductionnetwork.org/training-standards/

Staff should always read the policies and procedures relating to restrictive practice as part of their organisation's induction process.

Understanding the client's distress
Numerous feelings of distress can escalate into anger and then aggression: fear, humiliation, shame, confusion and so on. The earlier the intervention the better the chance of avoiding aggression. The clinician's or law enforcer's role in de-escalation is to find out and change what is making the client angry. Anger becomes more problematic the longer it remains unidentified, unchecked and unchannelled.

Successful de-escalation can only be achieved by knowing the client (or member of the public) as an individual and as a member of one or more cultural groups. The common assumption is that the angry person is the one with the problem. However, by getting to know them as a person and their beliefs about situations it could be apparent that the cause lies with the staff, the service provision or with society. Deaf and HOH people experience oppression and discrimination that may lead to anger (see Chapters F1 & I9).

Example: A deaf man is thrown out of a night club for fighting. It turns out that he was being attacked by 3 hearing men. Adrenalin heightened from trying to protect himself, his animated signing is mistaken for attempts to hit out, and he is arrested and hand cuffed. Now unable to communicate he is both angry and scared.

Numerous preventable events in your workplace could be angering your client. For example:
- Hearing staff speaking, rather than signing or booking an interpreter

- Staff mumbling or talking with their heads turned away, so that lipreading is hampered
- TV programmes with no in-vision signing or captions
- Staff not getting eye contact and saying hello
- Not taking time to include the deaf or HOH client or explain fully

Anger can be transmitted between people. When our clients get angry, we tend to get angry too. Early awareness of anger (the client's and our own) allows us to work collaboratively to diffuse anger at the point at which the individuals have more control and reasoning.

Example: Client S was standing in the corridor clearly agitated. He was pointing at the cleaner's trolley and shouting 'That is mine, it's mine!'. Staff repeatedly told him that it was not his. A tense stand-off developed and, predicting a potential aggressive outburst, more staff approached. The ward clerk was walking past and saw that the client was determined to reach what he thought was in the trolley. She asked him "What do you think is in there?" and the client replied 'Sweets'. This was not correct, but the ward clerk sensed that client S had a hunger need. She replied, 'Do you want some more breakfast? Come with me.' The client immediately relaxed and followed the ward clerk to the kitchen.

In this scenario, the ward clerk was not tasked as senior nurse, psychologist or even kitchen staff – but she knew the client best and saw it as her responsibility (and gift) to be able to figure out what the client's angry behaviour was communicating.

Unequal access and communication breakdown
Communication breakdown is the cause of many disputes in any language or culture. However, where communication crosses cultures and (for one or both people) is not in their first or fluent language, this is exacerbated.

Most often, sign language users are expected to communicate in their second language (speech and lipreading). In addition, lipreading is an imprecise means of understanding (see Chapter D8). In both scenarios, clients are likely to experience heightened adrenaline as both fear and frustration.

Enabling a client to manage their emotions and behaviours is an intervention that, as professionals, we are expected to provide. Consider whether your client can access these equally:

- one-to-one sessions or anger management sessions, in BSL or with a lip speaker/interpreter
- a shouted request to the client to calm down
- an explanation of their rights, leave or care plan
- meetings with those making the decisions relating to their care, such as their consultant and the multi-disciplinary team meetings.
- a relaxing and distracting social activity
- advocacy
- a low stimulus environment
- substance misuse support

Even if the professional and the client are communicating in the same language (as in specialist deaf mental health services or when experienced interpreters are present) there is still the potential for communication breakdown, particularly if the deaf person has minimal language skills (see Chapter B1) or a poor fund of knowledge (see Chapter B4). The fewer deaf staff or fluent signing staff there are, the more likely professionals are to misinterpret a deaf person's innocuous behaviour as challenging.

Example: Within 'grassroots' deaf culture a certain degree of directness is more acceptable. Such as, the statement 'I don't like your new haircut. I preferred it before,' which could be contentious in hearing culture.

De-escalation themes (Jeffery and Austen, 2007)
Communication – knowing your client
Staff should know the client's language style, preferences and nuances, including any disabilities, limitations or idiosyncratic language features. This language match will enable conversations about self-control.

Deaf staff are particularly valuable in this context to identify the intricacies of the emotional content of particular words or signs for the service user. The client's favoured words and terms should be noted.

The same deaf staff member could also interview the service user and their family to find out whether previous methods of aggression management, de-escalation or restraint were successful, or otherwise.

Interpreters
To maximise the effectiveness of the de-escalation, any interpreters should know the service user well, including their particular style of

language. Note whether the client has a preferred or less preferred interpreter.

The interpreter is unlikely to remain emotionally impartial throughout an angry episode. They may (intentionally or unintentionally) tone down the translation of angry material in the hope that resolution can be achieved without aggression - they would not be human if they did not.

It is crucial that professionals have access to the full linguistic manifestations of the client's anger, so that they can use this information in risk assessments. However, an aggressively signing client, seeing their interpreter angrily shouting the voice over, could reinforce the client's heightened emotions. Thus, team discussion including the interpreter should be conducted pre-, during and post-incident, where possible.

Stance and personal space
A deaf or HOH client is more likely than a hearing service user to make use of visual information. Mood and intention can be expressed through stance and posture. Standing with arms crossed or hands on hips can be perceived as authoritative or confrontational. Staff must therefore demonstrate neutral stance to avoid misinterpretation.

Dave Jeffery (Jeffery & Austen, 2007), was a violence and personal safety specialist advisor, in hearing and deaf specialist mental health services for many years. He recommends that staff stand with their body at a side on angle of 45°, and sign at chest height. It allows the staff member to move from a signing position to a defensive position quickly should the need arise – and protect the vulnerable areas from possible assault.

Personal space is incredibly important. As people become more distressed they have an increased need for personal space. The required space to contain a person's anger may be larger than the space required for them to see signing or lipreading, particularly for deafblind people. Optimum distance for communication will need to be balanced with the requirements of staff safety.

Touch
The use of touch during de-escalation requires an intimate knowledge of each individual service user. Although touch is more culturally acceptable within the deaf community (e.g. it is normal to gain attention of a deaf person by lightly placing a hand on their shoulder or forearm) it should be

evaluated consciously and sensitively, recognising the individual's diversity.

Touch is crucial in communication with Deafblind people (see Chapter D11). If the client has some residual vision, it is crucial to get in their visual field before attempting to touch or to communicate. In situations where the client regards staff as a threat, or they are paranoid or anxious, approaching from the outside of visual field is particularly unwise.

If the client has no vision, then discussion is needed on a calm day, to ask how they would like to be alerted to your presence and how you will identify yourself (e.g. a single touch on the left hand...wait for the client to offer you their hand if they want to know who you are... use fingerspelling or an identifiable object (your distinctive bracelet) to identify yourself).

Eye contact
In communicating with an angry person, a balance must be achieved between socially appropriate eye contact and staring with perceived provocative intent.

Poor eye contact may be seen as disrespectful, dismissive or submissive - each of which could trigger an assault. When using BSL, breaking eye contact can be seen as discourteous.

If an interpreter is used, the principal eye contact will be between the service user and the interpreter. However, the hearing professional should continue to look at the deaf person throughout the signed and voiced-over responses. This respectfully acknowledges the deaf person as the source of the message and allows the hearing person to observe the deaf client's non-verbal communication.

Occasionally a client will choose to respond to the interpreter and not acknowledge the practitioner. This may indicate hostility. Even though the client may require the emotional distance from the clinician, it is not appropriate to leave the interpreter as the lead communicator.

To counteract this, and maximise eye contact between the clinician and service user, the interpreter can position themselves slightly behind or to the side of the clinician.

Face
As well as the basic emotion expressed in the human face, BSL utilises the face to underpin grammatical syntax and reinforce verbs. The face expressing a message conveyed in BSL cannot therefore be taken as an indication of intent without a full understanding of the message.

Example: An animated BSL user with a very wide signing space describes a time when they were angry with someone else in the past. They represent some of that anger in their facial communication. The staff member incorrectly assumes that the client is angry, with them, right now.

Voice
Whether in speech or sign, voice refers to the style and content of interaction. Language can convey panic, calm or hostility. Staff need to 'talk a patient down' without talking down to a patient. Therefore, clinicians and interpreters must be aware of the tone of their voice (and signing) and be open to instruction and feedback on communication style.

Environment
Signing requires physical space for arms and bodies to move. Lipreading requires good lighting and lack of visual distraction (see Chapter D8). If a deaf client is aggressive and signing widely or rapidly, it may be necessary to move breakable objects or consider covering unhardened glass windows.

Conclusion
There is no standard approach to de-escalation. An in depth understanding of each unique client is needed, or else we will fail the deaf person at the point of crisis, which may well result in physical intervention.

References
Jeffery, D. & Austen, S. (2007). De-escalation and deafness: seeing the signs. *In S. Austen & D. Jeffery (Eds.) Deafness and Challenging Behaviour. The 360° Perspective.* Pp 159-175. John Wiley and sons Ltd.

NICE (2015). Violence and aggression: short-term management in mental health, health and community settings https://www.nice.org.uk/guidance/ng10

F14 Restraint
Dr Sally Austen, Dave Jeffery and Grant Budge

In this chapter the term 'client' encompasses prisoners and those in a variety of clinical, specialist educational or legal settings.

Restraint is an intervention, applied without the person's consent, that prevents them from behaving in ways that threaten to cause harm to themselves, to others, or to property.

Terminology evolves and varies across professions. In law enforcement the term 'Control and Arrest' (C and A) is used; in care settings it may be known as 'holding' under the guise of 'Restrictive Practices'.

In English mental healthcare settings, Restrictive Practices such as restraint have been determined by NHS England (NHSE) and its implementation monitored by the Care Quality Commission (CQC).

Investigations into restraint related deaths in the general population have questioned both its application and how it is taught.

A national framework to register and monitor appropriate, consistent training standards and content in restrictive practice is being developed by the Restraint Reduction Network (RRN) and BILD (www.bild.org.uk), from the Department of Health (DH) Positive and Proactive Care agenda (DH, 2014) and reinforced by the Royal College of Psychiatrists.

The use of restraint with deaf and hard of hearing (HOH) people adds a layer of ethical and practical complexity and is a requirement of training under the RRN training standards.

Restraint and communication
Restraint must only be used:
- as a last resort
- for the minimum possible time
- with a maximum possible regard for the client or prisoner's safety, dignity and rights

All of which are reflected in communication.

Holding a signer's arms; holding a lipreader's head
A deaf client or prisoner requires either their arms, their eyes or both, to communicate.

Many restraint techniques involve either holding a person's arms such that they cannot sign or holding the person face down such that they cannot see your mouth to lipread. You are in effect gagging them. This would feel the same to a hearing person as being forced to wear a hood, whilst being restrained.

Every effort must be made to allow communication. Where restraint is unavoidable and communication is inhibited due to safety issues, the aim must be to restore communication access as soon as possible: for the client's rights and to facilitate resolution.

Alternatives to prone restraint
Where it is safe to do so, and with team leader agreement:
- use restraints in a sitting position rather than lying down position
- holding the elbow rather than the wrist, so the hands are free to communicate (often described as a level 2 hold rather than a more restrictive level 3 hold)

Communicating during a prone restraint
In allocating roles within a restraint, someone should be put in charge of communication. Where possible work with native signing staff who can identify subtle sign language nuances. In such highly charged events, there is no room for misconception and misunderstanding.

Even if a deaf or HOH client is lying face down on the floor, every effort should be made to communicate with them. If the environment allows and does not increase risk to the staff members, this could involve:
- signing staff or interpreters lying on the floor beside the client to allow face-to-face communication
- a staff member with clear speech patterns lying or sitting so that they have good eye contact with the client
- Writing simple clear messages on paper (being aware that the client may have poor literacy, see Chapter B3)

Glasses may need to be removed or hearing aids/cochlear magnets may fall out during restraint. Both are crucial for communication and therefore de-escalation. Replace as soon as it safe.

If a deaf person is held in wrist locks or fixed mechanical restraints, they can only use their voice. Some deaf people find their voice adds to their frustration and embarrassment, which can cause an escalation in aggression.

Injury to hands or limbs may be evidence of negligence and poor technique and is certainly not in line with the best interests of any client. Specific to deaf clients, injuries to their hands, will have long-term implications on their ability to communicate and may serve as a daily reminder of the event in which it occurred, and then affects future relationships with staff.

Power and autonomy
The restrictive nature of a restraint process automatically introduces the concept of power once it is implied. This can perpetuate the crisis and potentially damage the therapeutic relationship post incident. A therapeutic multi-disciplinary debrief is therefore valuable.

Deaf people experience much oppression and social exclusion (see Chapter F1, G1 & I9). It is important to use physical interventions that acknowledge the need to empower the individual at the earliest opportunity.

Being held by a deaf staff member is arguably no less threatening than being held by a hearing person but may limit the sense of oppression felt by the deaf client.

Touch is a communication
If a client or prisoner experiences restraint as painful or humiliating, or if memories of previous negative experiences such as sexual abuse are triggered, this can create a sense of anger and frustration in some service users that in turn promote further problematic behaviours.

Face up restraint can maximise communication but may, in some cases, remind the client of a sexually abusive encounter. Consider the client's dignity by ensuring that no parts of the body are exposed and face away from the client's genital area if holding their legs in a face-up restraint.

When signing is not possible and touch is the last communication, if the message is one of pain or discomfort the deaf person is likely to interpret the restrainer as uncaring and oppressive.

It is therefore important to consider the impact of physical intervention based upon the unique person under restraint, not the behaviours that they present. Continued de-escalation should always be the goal.

De-escalation during restraint (see Chapter F13)
De-escalation should be taking place even during and after the restraint process, to prevent the need for forced medication or prolonged restraint. An intimate knowledge of your client or prisoner can help.

Example: a 60 year old deaf man with dementia believed a new member of staff was a threat and became violent, very suddenly. He was restrained in a seated position. A staff member who knew him well, from a safe distance, described her experience of mountain climbing (an interest she knew they shared). The man became enthralled in her description and started to forget his paranoid belief. He relaxed and the restraint was gradually released without the need for additional medication. He had no recollection of what had made him angry in the first place.

Chemical restraint (see Chapter F10)
As a last resort, when physical intervention is failing to reduce aggression, PRN and sedation may be utilised in the best interests of all within the environment.

The impact of this has short and longer term consequences. The impact of medication on motor skills is particularly relevant to deaf people. Impairment in the functioning of the deaf person's hands, arms and facial muscles will impair their expressive communication. Any blurring of vision will impair their receptive communication.

In the longer term, unwanted side-effects such as sedation and lack of impulse control from the administration of benzodiazepines may lead to further reliance upon medication to control the behaviours. Repeated use of PRN medication can lead the service user to believe that they are unable to contain their own behaviour and that it is the responsibility of the staff. They are then, less likely to learn to regulate themselves.

Interpreters
Safety
Effective communication and the rights of the client are paramount. However, during an episode of challenging behaviour, the interpreter can be vulnerable.

To maximise their safety, the interpreter should:
- ensure their exit path is clear
- only be present if the professional leading the intervention agrees it is safe to do so
- not be left alone with the client or prisoner
- be thoroughly briefed in advance about the client's need and potential risks
- be given an assistance/attack alarm and be provided with the same personal safety training as other staff

The interpreter should not assist in physical restraint.

Autonomy
Interpreters would usually take their lead from the clinician or law enforcement professional. However, in the heat of the moment staff may not seek to use the interpreter until the crisis is over and the interpreter may need to remind these professionals that, without the interpreter's involvement, the client or prisoner is being prevented from communicating.

During restraint, the interpreter may need to encourage the patient to look at them so they can communicate effectively. If the interpreter thinks they would be best lying on the floor, this should be discussed with the professional coordinating the restraint (who will assess risk and efficacy).

Efficacy
If a deaf signer's hands are restricted, it may not be possible for the interpreter to voice-over the client's speech, which may be, or may have become, unintelligible.

Rights
The interpreter may regard a particular restraint as too rough and feel powerless. However, they do have rights and responsibilities (as does any citizen) to approach the respective management. If this is not satisfactory then they should escalate the concern to the relevant senior executive, complaints department, police or Safeguarding team.

Team debrief
It is good practice to debrief after any restraint, to consider both practical issues (could this have been done differently or better?) and emotional issues (what issues have been raised and what support is required?).

Some additional factors to consider with restraints that involve deaf people are:
- ***Small deaf (BSL) world:*** deaf staff may find they are holding a person they went to school with or someone they know from Deaf Club. The boundary issues need exploring and supporting.
- ***Interpreters:*** The emotional impact of interpreting during a restraint or enforced medication can be traumatic. If deaf staff are in the debriefing team, an alternative interpreter is required to interpret for the debrief, so that the affected interpreter can take part as an equal team member.
- ***Communication reflections:*** Did poor communication play a part in the client's behaviour escalating? Do you have enough deaf staff or hearing staff that can sign? Have you been able to really get to know your client?

Summary
Communication difficulties during restraint can become so marked that deaf or hard of hearing people become effectively 'gagged'. The practical and ethical consequences should be constantly reviewed.

References
Department of Health (2014). Positive and proactive care: reducing the need for restrictive interventions. https://assets.publishing.service.gov.uk/government/uploads/system/uploads/attachment_data/file/300293/JRA_DoH_Guidance_on_RP_web_accessible.pdf

Section G

G1 The Deaf community and systemic failings in health care
Abigail Gorman

The NHS was founded on several core principles. One of which focused on the idea that the NHS should meet the needs of those who use it. The inability to ensure that the NHS is accessible for deaf people has been suggested as one of the main reasons that some deaf people have a reduced life expectancy.

SignHealth's 2014 'Sick Of It' report (Signhealth.org.uk/wp-content/uploads/2019/12/THE-HEALTH-OF-DEAF-PEOPLE-IN-THE-UK-.pdf) cites a patient survey which states that 70% of Deaf people surveyed had needed the services of a GP, but for various reasons, had not gone. Forty-one percent of Deaf respondents said that they had *'not been able'* to access other health services. Over a half (of the 41%) said this was because there was no interpreter available and a third said that they could not easily arrange an appointment.

Many Deaf people reported needing access to health care but could not receive it because of systemic barriers, which culminated in a feeling of 'barrier fatigue', where Deaf people find the system so cumbersome to navigate that they put their health at risk.

Research by Emond et al. (2015) shows that Deaf people's overall health is poorer than that of the general population due to under-diagnosis and inconsistent treatment of conditions.

Within the general population, 12% of hearing people are more likely to experience episodes of depression and poor mental health. When this statistic is compared to the Deaf community, we find that Deaf people are 24% more likely to experience depression and poor mental health. This figure is disproportionately high. By failing to meet this need, services are in direct contravention of the NHS's long-term plan to improve upstream prevention of avoidable illness and its exacerbations.

One of the most significant revelations from SignHealth's Sick of it Report is that deaf people are not only more likely to be misdiagnosed or remain undiagnosed due to poor provision and inaccessible information, but those who have received a diagnosis are also less likely to seek routine follow up appointments or be in a position to manage their treatment effectively.

Many high-risk conditions diagnosed, such as diabetes, cardiovascular disease and hypertension could have been prevented had accessible health care and treatment options been available. The report shone a light on the NHS budget, showing that the NHS spent 30 million per year on issues related to misdiagnosis and poor treatment alone.

Ensuring that Deaf people have access to their health care
1. Ask people for their preferred method of communication - Interpreter, Lip-speaker, etc.
2. Record those needs clearly and in a set way. (see Chapter D14).
3. Highlight or flag the person's file or notes so it is clear they have information or communication needs, and how to meet those needs.
4. Share information about people's information and communication needs with other providers of NHS and adult social care, when they have given permission to do so.
5. Take steps to ensure that people receive information that they can access and understand; and receive communication support if they need it.

Access to mental health services
Deaf people experience barriers to mental health services, at all stages on the pathway. This discrimination can have a profound effect on their mental state.

In order to facilitate a referral to mental health services, the client needs to know that:
a) they are feeling relatively mentally unwell and
b) that there is something that could be done about this and
c) where to approach for help.

This requires access to comparative information which may not be available to all deaf people (see Chapter B4).

If the client is able to access their GP to request a referral, the GP may not know that specialist deaf mental health services are available (see Chapters G3 & G4); or that required assessment or intervention is commissioned by NHS deaf specialist services. Thus, a referral to generic services will be made, which may not consider the deaf person's cultural or linguistic needs.

For example, a deaf person referred to a counselling service where none of the counsellors sign, necessitates the use of a sign language interpreter. This does not make therapy impossible but it can be problematic:

- Interpreters are rarely booked consistently for each appointment. The deaf person, trying to engage with the therapeutic process, may not feel safe with the instability of a new face each week.

- This is compounded by the requirement to relive traumatic events via a third party, rather than directly with the person providing the mental health support.

- This can negatively impact the communication process because the interpreter may not yet be familiar with pre-established signs or the deaf person's communication style, which increases the possibility of unintentional misrepresentation.

- Additionally, the pool of available interpreters working in the UK is relatively small and there is a significant likelihood that the deaf person may know the interpreter from elsewhere; further disrupting the therapeutic process.

- Demand for mental health care and counselling services is high and waiting lists can be long. Deaf people who are already experiencing mental health difficulties may find their wait time extended due to additional barriers related to their deafness.

The importance of referral to a specialist mental health service designed for deaf people's linguistic and cultural needs cannot be understated. Effective therapeutic outcomes can only come from a shared context. This understanding of need provides the foundations required to scaffold interventions in a way that places deaf culture and identity central to the professional relationship, rather than one where the deaf person is constantly required to self-advocate and educate the professional.

References

Emond, A., Ridd, M., Sutherland, H., Allsop, L., Alexander, A., & Kyle, J. (2015). The current health of the signing Deaf community in the UK compared with the general population: a cross-sectional study. *BMJ Open, 5, e006668*

G2 Prevalence of mental health problems
Dr Sally Austen

It is very difficult to be sure about the prevalence of mental health problems in deaf children and adults.

This is because:
- There is little research in this area
- Poor or inconsistent access to health and mental health services (see Chapter G1) means that many deaf people will not receive appropriate diagnoses
- The heterogeneity within deaf communities presents confounding research variables (e.g. language, cultural experience, degree of deafness, age at onset, speed of onset, cause of deafness, presence of associated health conditions, language of parents, education, presence of deaf role models) impacting on the generalisability of research findings
- As there are relatively few specialist clinicians in deaf mental health care, there is a heightened potential for over and under-diagnosis

The Department of Health document, 'Mental Health and Deafness: Towards Equity and Access (2005)', works on the premise that 40% of deaf people will have a mental health problem in their lifetime, as opposed to 25% of hearing people.

http://www.deafinfo.org.uk/policy/Towards%20Equity%20and%20Access.pdf

It seems that this increased prevalence is caused by:
- Increased risk of negative life events
- Increased risk of associated health, cognitive or language difficulties
- Poor access to preventative or responsive mental health services

Recommended reading
Felinger, J., Holzinger, D. & Pollard, R. (2012). Mental health of deaf people. *The Lancet, 379 (9820)*, 1037-44

G3 National deaf child & adolescent mental health services
Dr Constanza Moreno

Deaf children's access to generic child and adolescent mental health services (CAMHS) is recognised as poor (Beresford et al., 2008). The number of deaf children between 0–18 years in England is reported to be 20,160, of whom 42% (8470) are severely or profoundly deaf.

'Forging New Channels' reports that 50.3% of such children will have some mental health problems, with 3.4% at any one time requiring highly specialist services (Hindley et al., 1994) to address complex mental health problems with physical, psychological, neurological or developmental co-morbidities. Contributing factors include:
- communication problems with resultant socio-emotional and cognitive developmental delay
- central nervous system damage
- delays in accessing services
- problems with peer and family relationships
- higher rates of emotional, physical and sexual abuse (ADSS et al., 2002)

Deaf children with mental health problems have difficulties accessing mainstream services. The specialist skills required to meet their needs mean generic services are often not able to provide adequate services (Bailly et al., 2003), mirroring the physical health care experiences of deaf people (see Chapter G1).

Establishing National Deaf CAMHS

In 1991 the first community Deaf Children and Family Service (DCFS) was set up at Springfield University Hospital in London. Corner House, an inpatient ward for deaf children, opened there in 2000. The challenge for this one service to meet the needs of deaf young people nationally, combined with the commissioning of the service across the different care trusts, was considerable.

In 2004 a pilot study commenced with DCFS and 2 CAMHS based in York and Dudley, independently evaluated by the Social Policy Research Unit. Feedback from families and clients was extremely positive with key skills, that distinguished the specialist services from generic CAMHS, were described as:

- meeting the child's communication needs
- expertise in mental health and deafness
- the ability to accept referrals quickly
- liaison with schools
- provision of a range of therapeutic approaches
- provision of outreach clinics which reduces the child/family travelling to the clinics

Parents additionally reported the presence of deaf staff on the team as being important.

National Deaf CAMHS

As a result of the pilot study, 'ND CAMHS' was launched in 2010 and continues to provide services that are highly regarded (Wright et al, 2012). The national services consist of the inpatient ward 'Corner House' and 10 community or 'outreach' centres, based across 4 NHS trusts, covering the whole of England. The shared 'bilingual and bi-cultural' philosophy ensures that: clients (and their families) are acknowledged as deaf and hearing individuals, their linguistic and cultural preferences are respected and met; and their mental health needs are effectively catered for.

Providing services that are linguistically accessible, promote social inclusion and reduce isolation, they also work to promote systemic changes that impact positively on mental health, including:
- safe and inclusive education where communication needs are met
- equitable access to healthy learning and peer relationships
- in-depth understanding and assessments of the child's communication
- awareness and training to generic CAMHS to promote joined up provision of CAMHS for deaf children and young people
- equitable and accessible mental health services at highly specialist levels for deaf children and young people and their families

It should be noted however, that ND CAMHS is **not** an emergency service and any young person requiring to be seen urgently, or in a crisis should access the normal routes of emergency care; namely 999, Accident & Emergency, GP etc.

Staffing
The structure of the teams varies slightly from team to team but generally consists of: Psychiatrists, Clinical Psychologists, Mental Health Nurses, Family Therapists, Speech & Language Therapists and Occupational Therapists. Health Care Assistants are also employed in inpatient settings.

Clinical Specialists, with a range of backgrounds (social workers, play therapists, and art therapists), are employed in some teams. All teams have access to qualified and registered English/BSL interpreters.

Deaf Family Support Workers (DFSW), known as Senior Deaf Outreach Workers (SDOW) in some areas, provide a fundamental role in the work of ND CAMHS. Individual, school and family communication assessment profiles are unique to ND CAMHS and highlight the importance of communication and understanding deaf culture in formulations - both as potential contributing factors to difficulties, and also as potential protective factors, promoting resilience. As well as meeting families and signposting them to useful organisations, the DFSWs explain first-hand what it is like to be deaf, work together with them on communication strategies and work on developing a positive deaf identity. DFSWs receive much positive feedback from families.

The teams have a mix of deaf and hearing staff and while the hope is that in the future more of the professional roles will be filled by deaf members of staff, currently most deaf colleagues are employed as DFSWs.

Service provided
ND CAMHS community teams are commissioned to provide:

Assessment
- specialist mental health assessments of deaf children and young people
- specialist language/communication assessments (including social communication assessments) provided by deaf and hearing clinicians working together

Risk management
- dynamic clinical risk assessments
- and management processes that aim to reduce potential risks posed to both self and others by the individual, through individualised treatment plans

Interventions (direct and indirect)
- delivery of responsive individualised care through multi-disciplinary care planning involving both deaf and hearing staff
- treatment through a wide range of deaf appropriate interventions to address individual's mental health needs
- partnership work with wider agencies ensuring the young person's needs are central to integrated care provision across health, social care, education and the third sector to ensure timely transfer for specialised assessment and treatment.

Consultation and training
- To wider agencies including potential referrers, including schools, mainstream CAMHS, and tier 2 services (see Section K)
- Consultation can also be provided on a discretionary basis for services in Scotland, Northern Ireland or Wales.

Referral criteria
- Below 18 years of age
- Bilateral deafness, at severe to profound level (although those with moderate to severe or unilateral hearing levels are considered if there are additional issues, for example regarding deaf identity).
- Child of Deaf Parent(s) (CODA)
- The service predominantly sees those clients who use sign language, but we also see oral children and young people as well, particularly if it is felt that they are unable to access generic CAMHS
- Consideration is also given to young people with additional communication or language difficulties.
- ND CAMHS requires that clients are registered with an English General Practitioner or are resident in England and eligible for treatment in the NHS under reciprocal arrangements. Patients from Scotland, Wales and Northern Ireland are not part of this commissioned service, although if the young person attends a school in England, they may be able to access ND CAMHS.

Reasons for referral include: mental health; behavioural; social communication difficulties; issues concerned with identity related to being deaf or a CODA.

Team locations
While the teams are generally small (e.g. at the time of writing the London has a whole time equivalent of just over 6 clinicians) all the teams cover a wide geographical area.

The community teams are based in ten ND CAMHS locations:
In the North (Leeds & York Partnership NHS Foundation Trust) teams are based in York, Newcastle and Manchester

For general enquiries e-mail: ndcamhsnorth.lypft@nhs.net

In Central England (Black Country Healthcare NHS Foundation Trust) teams cover West Midlands, East Midlands and South Central regions.

For general enquiries e-mail: bchft.deafcamhs@nhs.net

In the South West (Somerset NHS Foundation Trust) is the Taunton team

For general enquiries e-mail: ndcamhs.taunton@nhs.net

In the South East (South West London & St Georges Mental Health Trust) teams are based in London, Maidstone and Cambridge

For general enquiries e-mail: ndcamhs@swlstg.nhs.uk

Once a referral has been accepted, ND CAMHS offers various models of working:
Sole
- ND CAMHS are the only mental health team working with the young person and family.

Co-working
- Where the young person presents with high risks to self, from others, and to others, then ND CAMHS will co-work with the local generic CAMHS, who can provide risk management.
- Where risk is not considered high, the care plan can be shared across 2 CAMHS teams (e.g. medication managed locally with NDCAMHS offering therapy tailored to the client's linguistic and cultural needs.

Consultation model
- ND CAMHS are not directly involved but consult with agencies (such as local generic CAMHS) who work directly with the young person and family. Consultation themes may include: deaf awareness and deaf culture; mental health presentation in the deaf population; working with BSL/English interpreters; signposting to organisations.

- Consultation can also be provided on a discretionary basis for services in Scotland, Northern Ireland or Wales.

Case study 1
Referral
Marian, a 12 year old girl with moderate to severe hearing level is referred to ND CAMHS by her school. Her parents are both profoundly deaf BSL users. Marian uses both spoken English and BSL to communicate and attends a mainstream school with a Teacher of the Deaf who visits every 4-6 weeks. The referral raises concerns about increasing levels of anxiety since the pandemic. Lockdown has been challenging for the family, as their access to information has been limited. Marian has been brokering for her parents with regards to health appointments and with the landlord. The referral raised particular issues with online learning, which she did not engage with. Now that schools have re-opened she is school-refusing for the first time. Her parents are not clear about the reasons for this. The levels of risk are low.

Referral outcome
Marian's hearing level would not typically be accepted by Deaf CAMHS. However, Marian is also a CODA and the referral indicates that there may be issues linked to her identity and role in the family.

The referral could be accepted solely by Deaf CAMHS or accepted on the basis of joint work with local CAMHS, if the referral met their criteria. Collaboratively, a care plan could be organised whereby some work is carried out by local CAMHS (e.g. individual CBT for Marian) with Deaf CAMHS providing family therapy and consultation for her communication and cultural needs (see Appendix 1). Alternatively, the referral could be accepted by deaf CAMHS for consultation only, with local CAMHS offering both individual and family therapy.

Case study 2
Referral
Anthony is 15 years old and is profoundly deaf. He uses bilateral cochlear implants and spoken English to communicate. He is the only deaf member of his family and attends a mainstream school. He was referred by his family (with the support of their GP) as he presents with low mood and irritability. He has attended his local CAMHS for individual CBT for low mood and anxiety, on two occasions. Some improvements were noted, but difficulties returned soon after discharge from CAMHS. There are

concerns that difficulties are becoming entrenched, with him increasingly isolated in his room with few friends.

Referral outcome
Anthony's referral could be accepted by Deaf CAMHS. It would be helpful to receive copies of reports from local CAMHS prior to meeting with him and his family. While unmodified CBT may have provided Anthony some opportunities to reflect and change, he is more likely to benefit from therapy that is modified to take into consideration his developmental presentation: emotional literacy; language development; knowledge of cultural norms; and incidental learning as well as thinking more about his deaf identity.

Case study 3
Referral
Jackson is a profoundly deaf 7 year old, who became deaf aged 5 following meningitis. He received a cochlear implant shortly after. He is the only deaf member of the family and uses spoken English to communicate. There are reportedly significant delays in his language. He attends a mainstream school with provision for deaf children. He was referred by his audiologist because he is refusing to wear his processors, which impacts on his language, social and academic development.

Outcome
Based on the referral information above, ND CAMHS would not accept this referral as the mental health needs are not clear. In the first instance it may be more appropriate to refer to the Clinical Psychologist or hearing therapist in the audiology/implant service.

Inpatient services
'Corner House' is a 6 bed inpatient unit based in Springfield Hospital (South West London & St Georges Mental Health Trust) for young people up to 18 years. Commissioned by NHS England, referrals are accepted from within the UK. For referrals outside England funding is agreed with the local team prior to admission.

Referrals can be made by CAMHS, paediatricians, audiologists, social services, schools, GP's and national deaf outreach service.
Exclusion criteria include:
- Severe to profound Learning Disability

- Conduct disorder and/or unstable Personality Disorder, unless there are additional co-morbidities
- Dependence of admissions on current patients.
- Corner house is not a Psychiatric Intensive Care Unit

Where deaf young people need urgent, and acute inpatient care, or present with some of the exclusion criteria, they may need generic inpatient admission. We nevertheless recommend contacting Deaf CAMHS as assessments and admission can be supported by Corner House and/or ND CAMHS community teams, through consultation. Furthermore, it may be appropriate to refer to ND CAMHS as part of the discharge plan once the crisis has been managed.

References

Association of Directors of Social Services, British Deaf Association, Local Government Association, National Children's Bureau, National Deaf Children's Society, Royal National Institute for Deaf People (2002) Deaf Children: Positive Practice Standards in Social Services

Bailly, D., Dechoulydelenclave, MB, & Lauwerier, L. (2003). Hearing impairment and psychopathological disorders in children and adolescents. Review of the recent literature. *L'Encephale, 29(4)*, 329-37

Hindley, P. A., Hill, P. D., McGuigan, S. & Kitson, N. (1994) Psychiatric disorder in deaf and hearing impaired children and young people: a prevalence study. *Journal of Child Psychology & Psychiatry, 35(5)*, 917-34

Beresford, B., Greco, V., Clarke, S. & Sutherland, H. (2008). An Evaluation of Specialist Mental Health Services for Deaf Children and Young People. Working Paper No. DH 2259 05.08, Social Policy Research Unit

Wright, B., Walker, R., Holwell, A., Gentili, N., Barker, M., Rhys-Jones, S., Leach, V., Hindley, P., Gascon-Ramos, M. & Moore, K. (2012). A new dedicated mental health service for deaf children and adolescents. *Advances in Mental Health, 11(1)*, 95-105

G4 Specialist mental health services for deaf adults
Dr Ben Holmes

Research shows deaf people experience significant inequalities in accessing physical and mental health services (SignHealth, 2014). This extends from reduced provision of accessible information and self-help material, to the literal access to buildings and appointments (e.g. voice intercoms, being called for an appointment from the waiting room) (see Chapter G1).

Deaf people are already at risk of greater prevalence of mental health problems (see Chapter G2). The effect of poorer access compounds this with limited availability of appropriate treatment and support which, in turn, can mean that by the time an appropriate intervention is identified it becomes either less effective or is required more intensively. This is one of the factors that contribute to deaf people having a greater length of stay in psychiatric hospital (see Chapter G5), for example.

Mental health services for deaf people
There are two ways of providing mental health services for deaf people.
- Devise specialist deaf centres of excellence. Given the relatively small numbers of deaf people with mental health problems in the general population, these services will tend to be limited in number and therefore require service users or their families to travel long distances.
- Train service providers in mainstream (hearing services) to work with deaf people which, given the cost of sufficient training, may prove untenable or result in a somewhat diluted service.

Currently within the UK, several specialist Deaf mental health services exist. However, these are not commissioned to provide services to all deaf people, to meet the full range of mental health needs. Furthermore, these services can vary by region. Thus, most deaf people who require support from mental health services will need to access mainstream services. However, in many cases support can be supplemented by input from specialist services.

This chapter aims to highlight the specialist services that do exist for deaf adults, to help guide professionals in knowing where to seek support.

Primary care
At the time of printing there are no nationally commissioned primary care mental health services for deaf people. However, there are different charities and organisations that provide primary care level psychological interventions in British Sign Language (BSL). Currently, the only organisation that offers an equivalent stepped care model to mainstream Increasing Access to Psychological Therapy (IAPT) services is Sign Health.

Interventions are provided face to face or online and are subject to funding being agreed by GPs and Clinical Commissioning Groups (CCGs) on a case by case basis. The organisations that offer these services are often able to help in the completion of funding applications. Alternatively, people are able to pay for their own therapy.

Locally commissioned specialist services
There are currently specialist deaf mental health services in some areas of England (Bristol, Nottingham, North East England and South Yorkshire). These are often funded via local arrangements between health and social care and provided by NHS Trusts.

The input provided by these services varies according to which professionals form the teams. The aim of the services is to support and supplement the work of local community mental health services; for example, by providing advice about how interventions might be adapted for deaf people. Therefore, ongoing input from local mainstream mental health services is required. In some cases, direct therapeutic input can be provided in BSL (e.g. psychological therapy, nursing interventions).

Referral criteria vary according to each service, although service users would typically access this level of support when there is greater complexity of mental health need than primary care services might be able to meet. This might include clients with higher levels of risk or more complex mental health needs. Some services are provided free at the point of access and in other areas additional funding agreements must be made through GPs or CCGs. Please see below for contact details.

National specialist services
Tertiary, national, mental health services accept referrals for deaf people with severe and enduring mental health problems where individuals are

unable to access mainstream hearing services. Typically, this is for service users where there is a significant and long-standing risk history and multiple, complex mental health needs.

The level of input provided by tertiary services will vary on a case by case basis. For some clients, the majority of clinical input can be provided by the specialist team. For others, input may be limited to supervision, consultation and liaison. This can be agreed following initial joint assessment.

Crucially, it is a commissioning requirement that in order to access this level of specialist support service users must already be supported according to the Care Programme Approach (CPA), with a named care coordinator, by a mainstream secondary care community mental health team or community learning disability team. Ongoing input from local secondary mental health services will be required for the duration of specialist input.

As tertiary services are centrally funded, no additional funding agreements have to be arranged with CCGs. Once the service user has been accepted by a secondary care service, tertiary services can become involved where it is appropriate to do so.

Currently, NHS England centrally commissions specialist national mental health services for all of England, both community and inpatient. Northern Ireland and Scotland also have specialist tertiary community services, although no specialist inpatient services. At the time of print there are no equivalent services in Wales although efforts are being made to establish these services.

Each service has a multidisciplinary team consisting of professionals that include nurses, psychiatrists, psychologists, occupational therapists, social workers and speech and language therapists, although not all teams have professionals from each discipline. There are also some subtle differences in the types of support that each service might be able to provide (e.g. different therapeutic models, or the ability to meet specific additional needs).

Contact details
National specialist community services

England
Birmingham Deaf Adult Community Team
https://www.bsmhft.nhs.uk/our-services/specialist-services/deaf-mental-health-services/

London Deaf Adult Community Team
https://www.swlstg.nhs.uk/our-services/specialist-services/national-deaf-services

John Denmark Unit (Manchester)
https://www.gmmh.nhs.uk/john-denmark-unit

Scotland
Scottish Mental Health Service for Deaf People
https://services.nhslothian.scot/mhdeafservice/Pages/default.aspx

N. Ireland
Mental Health and Deafness Team
https://belfasttrust.hscni.net/service/mental-health-service-for-deaf-people/

National Specialist Inpatient Contact Details:
Bluebell Ward (London)
https://www.swlstg.nhs.uk/our-services/specialist-services/national-deaf-services

Jasmine Suite (Birmingham)
https://www.bsmhft.nhs.uk/our-services/specialist-services/deaf-mental-health-services/

John Denmark Unit (Manchester)
https://www.gmmh.nhs.uk/john-denmark-unit

Regional specialist community service contact details
Bristol
http://www.awp.nhs.uk/services/specialist/deaf-mental-health/

North East
https://www.cntw.nhs.uk/services/north-east-mental-health-deafness-service-walkergate-park/

Nottingham
https://www.nottinghamshirehealthcare.nhs.uk/deaf-services

South Yorkshire
https://www.rdash.nhs.uk/services/south-yorkshire-service-for-deaf-people-with-mental-health-needs-main-page/information-for-health-professionals-off-main-page/

References
Baines, D., Patterson, N., & Austen, S. (2010). An investigation into the length of hospital stay for deaf mental health service users. *The Journal of Deaf Studies and Deaf Education, 15(2)*, 179-184

Sign Health (2014). *Sick of it: A report into the health of deaf people in the UK.* Sign Health https://signhealth.org.uk/wp-content/uploads/2019/12/THE-HEALTH-OF-DEAF-PEOPLE-IN-THE-UK-.pdf

G5 Length of inpatient stay and delayed discharge
Dr Sally Austen and Adele Cockerill

Deaf inpatients in specialist deaf mental health services tend to stay approximately twice as long as hearing people on general acute wards (Appleford, 2003; Baines et al., 2010).

Whereas less than 10% of the hearing cohort stayed for longer than 1 year in inpatient services, this could rise to 50% of the Deaf cohort (Appleford, 2003).

This appears to be due to deaf clients requiring a longer time to be ready for discharge and then not having appropriate community facilities to support their discharge.

Longer time to be ready for discharge
Complexity of presentation
Deaf people are more likely to have co-morbid conditions that make treatment more complex, for example: language deprivation (see Chapter B1), isolation and poor social networks (see Chapter F1), trauma (see Chapter F2), conditions associated with their cause of deafness (see Chapter H1) and physical health conditions that have worsened due to poor access to health care (see Chapter G1).

Longer duration of untreated conditions
Deaf people struggle to access mental health care (Chapter G1) and generally have fewer informed contacts with whom they can communicate or ask for advice. Particularly in relation to psychosis, delay in starting treatment, significantly affects treatment efficacy.

Possible previous misdiagnosis
Where deaf people have not been able to access specialist deaf mental health care, rates of misdiagnosis are high. Re-assessment and altering interventions (e.g. changing a medication regime) take time.

Paucity of move on and community support services
Paucity of move on services and availability of community support services increase a patient's length of stay within mental health inpatient services. This is often referred to as 'Delayed Discharge' and used to be

called 'Bed blocking'. Without the support in the community, a deaf patient is more likely to spend longer, and return sooner, to an inpatient hospital setting.

Work environments, school, day services, 'half-way houses', probation services, support groups, churches, hobby groups and healthcare are far less available and accessible for deaf people. Significant cuts have been made in social services, housing and rehabilitation charities, and funding for personal support, reducing the options for discharge.

An audit of one of the National Deaf Mental Health Services, showed that in October 2017 patients considered to be 'delayed discharge' had risen to 64%. Seven out of eleven patients were considered ready for discharge with regard to their mental wellbeing but discharge was being delayed by specific inactions (often resource gaps) of the secondary level (mental health and learning disability) services and social care services.

Summary
Improvements in deaf people's access to health services and better availability of support in the community will be required in order to reduce the number of days deaf people stay in inpatient mental health care settings.

References
Appleford, J. (2003). Clinical activity with a specialist mental health service for Deaf people: comparison with a general Psychiatric service. *Psychiatric Bulletin, 27*, 375-377
Baines, D., Patterson, N., & Austen, S. (2010). An investigation into the length of hospital stay for Deaf mental health service users. *Journal of Deaf Studies and Deaf Education, 15 (2)*, 179-184

G6 Deaf research hubs – past and present
Dr Kate Rowley

Research that focuses on deaf people is relatively sparse. This has been largely to do with resources and relatively small numbers of experienced researchers; and partly to do with the heterogeneity of the 'deaf cohort' (see Chapter G7).

However, since the 1970s there have been several UK research hubs exploring deaf people (their language, educational attainment, cognition and psychological well-being) and the number is growing.

Such research began in the 1970s, first with Mary Brennan establishing that the signs that deaf people were using to communicate, was indeed a bona fide language with its own grammar and vocabulary. Mary Brennan also coined the term, 'British Sign Language (BSL)'. Brennan worked closely with deaf people, including Lillian Lawson and Gerry Hughes, to conduct research into sign language. Without them providing insights into BSL, subsequent research would not have been possible.

The Centre for Deaf Studies (CDS), at the University of Bristol, opened in 1978. It coined the term 'Deaf Studies' in 1984. Sadly, CDS closed in 2014 due to University cuts. CDS was seen as the gold standard for interpreting training and led the field of research into deaf people and sign language. Many deaf people worked at CDS as lecturers in Deaf Studies and also led the department.

Between 1977 and 1979, several research projects into BSL were set up at the Universities of Bristol, Edinburgh, and Newcastle. In the 1980s, the BSL Teaching Academy was set up at the University of Durham. This was to train deaf people to become qualified teachers of BSL and this course was entirely deaf-led by Clark Denmark, Frances Elton and Dorothy Miles. This course produced many BSL teachers and empowered them. Today, many speak highly of this course and how it gave them pride in their language, BSL. During this time, Durham University worked with the British Deaf Association (BDA) to develop the BSL Dictionary, which was finally published in 1992.

In the 1990s, several interpreting programmes were developed, at the Universities of Bristol, Central Lancashire (UCLAN) and Wolverhampton, producing the first fully qualified and trained interpreters to translate between English and BSL. These Universities also provided Deaf Studies programmes which enabled both deaf and hearing people to learn about deaf history, deaf education, linguistics of sign language and BSL arts (poetry, storytelling). This was particularly empowering for many deaf people who had never been taught about their language, culture or history due to strict oralist educational policies. Furthermore, the mixture of deaf and hearing people attending such programmes gave hearing learners of BSL a fully immersive BSL environment enabling them to develop good sign language skills, producing some of the best sign language interpreters in the UK. Such training programmes for interpreters still exist now and now Heriot-Watt University also delivers interpreting training.

In 1990s, research into deaf education grew, mainly at the University of Leeds and City, University of London. At Leeds, a training programme for 'teachers of deaf children' (ToD) was set up and at City, University of London, new assessment tools were set up to track and assess deaf children's sign language development. City, University of London still continues to carry out research, mainly focusing on deaf children's language and literacy development. There is also an assessment clinic for deaf children to measure their language and cognitive abilities, mainly for the purposes of providing educational reports.

In 2006, the Deafness, Cognition and Language (DCAL) Research Centre was set up in London, providing more information about how deafness and sign language shapes cognition; and how deaf people process language and what atypical language looks like in deaf people – whether developmental or acquired.

Social Research with Deaf People (SORD) was also set up in Manchester, around 2008 focusing on the socio-emotional well-being of deaf people, as well as developing psychometric tools appropriate for deaf people using sign language (see chapter G7). During this time, research at Heriot-Watt University has also branched out focusing on interpreting, translanguaging and how such practices can ensure deaf people achieve full citizenship equal to that of their hearing peers.

At the University of Central Lancashire (UCLAN) the International Institute for Sign Languages and Deaf Studies (iSLanDS) was set up in 2006 and this research facility focuses on sign languages and deaf studies on a global scale, looking at several sign languages and deaf cultures across the world with an aim to empower deaf people.

Deaf researchers
Deaf researchers were extremely pivotal in setting up several of the deaf research hubs. Their intrinsic knowledge and lived experience of being sign language users ensures accuracy and authenticity in research published on sign languages, deaf people and deaf communities.

During the 1970s and 1980s, at the launch of these hubs, very few deaf people were university graduates. Thus, most of deaf researchers worked as research assistants, collecting and analysing data with the guidance of qualified hearing researchers. Nowadays, access for deaf people to further and higher education has vastly improved and significantly more deaf researchers design, lead and commission research.

It is vital that hearing professionals reflect on their motivation to approach other hearing, rather than deaf, professionals for advice or leadership on issues in relation to sign language, deaf people and deaf communities. This motivation may potentially be audist (see Chapter C10) and their deaf colleagues may be best placed to provide the advice and guidance they need.

G7 Using standardised assessment measures with Deaf people
Dr Kevin L. Baker and Dr Katherine D. Rogers

Introduction
Standardised assessments are usually developed for the general population and are rarely designed with Deaf people in mind. Gathering statistical norms often excludes Deaf people in samples (see Chapter E2). Some assessments may include instructions for adapting an assessment for use with Deaf people (e.g. WNV and ABAS-iii) but scoring and thresholds are rarely presented separately.

Many professionals who work with Deaf people, adapt their assessments and therefore use a non-standardised approach. They use their expertise to apply clinical judgment to interpret a Deaf person's performance. It is good practice for professionals without experience of working with Deaf people to consider:
a) whether the use of a standardised assessment is necessary and appropriate for their client; and
b) involving or co-working with d/Deaf specialist services where possible and desirable (see Chapter G3 & G4).

If appropriate, also consider which option the Deaf person prefers. However, even adapted measures may not be suitable to use with all clients or in all situations. And where adaptations are possible, this can be extremely time consuming.

This chapter provides information on some adapted measures that can be used when assessing the mental health of a Deaf client. Many of the observations and comments also apply to other measures and assessments in medical, legal and educational contexts.

Factors to consider for using standardised assessment measures with Deaf clients
The communication checklist (Chapter D14), provides a simple way of starting conversations and gathering information about a client's communication preferences, literacy skills and level of competence. It is then for the professional to consider whether their intended assessment is accessible to the client, is worth completing, and if the scores will be meaningful.

It is important to note, as part of the assessment, whether the d/Deaf person was poorly educated and/or had inadequate access to early language (see Chapters B1, C2 & C6). If so, they are likely to struggle to understand both the concept of a measure and the concepts used in the measure. This can partly be addressed by working closely with an experienced Registered Sign Language Interpreter (see Chapter D3) and a Deaf Relay Interpreter (see Chapter D4).

Most assessment measures are provided in written form, which creates barriers for d/Deaf people who might have insufficient literacy skills to self-report appropriately (see Chapter B3) or those who prefer to respond in British Sign Language (BSL). How the person responds will depend on their communication style, their conceptual understanding and the cultural appropriateness of the measure.

The benefits of standardised assessments are to focus questions on the topics that have been shown to be important in a structured manner. It is tempting to rely heavily on standardised assessments but taking a more conversational approach can build a client's engagement and rapport with a professional, yielding more useful and relevant information.

Deaf clients who have not had much opportunity to develop their literacy skills, may have never completed a questionnaire before (see Chapter B3). Similarly, they may have little experience describing and understanding different emotions, and may have a reduced vocabulary to describe and reflect upon them (see Chapter F1). One study found differences between Deaf and hard-of hearing people compared with hearing young people on items measuring depression symptoms (Bozzay at al., 2017) which suggested that the differences are due to the experience or expression of depression.

Motivation is also an important cultural consideration. Poor motivation can be a sign of depression, however for the Deaf population this can be dependent on social context, such as being in a hearing environment (Rogers et al., 2013a). For example, connecting with others is one indicator of well-being but, if a Deaf person lives in a neighbourhood where no one can sign, then their ability to connect with their neighbours is determined by cultural experiences, not by degree of well-being.

There are significant challenges to consider when translating written assessment measures into signed languages. There are some specific concepts that might need to be clarified. For example, in English the word "anxiety" covers a range of concepts including physical, cognitive and emotional angst. Whereas, in BSL the sign for "anxiety" involves multiple features that denote slight differences in meaning, the sign occurs simultaneously with facial expression and the intensity of this can alter its precise meaning. Another challenge is the use of visually motivated signs without giving specific examples which in their nature are suggestive, such as the signs for "suicide" and "violent" (Rogers et al., 2013b).

For professionals with little or no experience of working with Deaf people, working with an interpreter and/or Deaf Relay Interpreter can take some time but is invaluable. With careful thought and planning, it will be possible to gather detailed information for the assessment over and above the scores given in the standardised version. Clinical judgment can also be used to record something mentioned by a client that might not immediately relate to the assessment but that can be used as a baseline to compare with future results.

Some assessments provide clinical cut-off scores to help determine 'caseness' and clinically significant change. Crucially, these may be different for Deaf people, and any interpretation of the assessment using standardised scoring must refer to the evidence. For example, the PHQ-9 BSL and GAD-7 BSL have been found to have different cut-off scores for Deaf people when compared with their hearing counterparts. The cut-off scores for hearing people are ten and eight for the PHQ-9 and GAD-7 respectively. For Deaf people, following rigorous analysis, the values have been found to be lower, at eight for the PHQ-9 BSL and six for the GAD-7 BSL (Belk, Pilling, Rogers, Lovell & Young, 2016). For other assessments where the clinical cut-offs have yet to be established, bear in mind that standard clinical cut-off scores may not be an appropriate metric to use with Deaf populations.

Using a mental well-being, mental health and/or health-related assessment in BSL with a Deaf person
Many mainstream services are commissioned to use standardised assessments with every client. However, virtually every clinician is aware that adaptations to standardised assessments are often necessary. Many standardised assessments offer spoken language translations, but few provide translations into sign language with validation studies to support them.

Below are descriptions of BSL mental health and health-related assessments, which could be used by mental health professionals and academic researchers. Their psychometric properties, reliability and validation have been examined and are reported in the referenced articles. The BSL assessments can be used alongside the paper version or computer software to record responses whilst watching the BSL video clips. These accessible mental health assessments are available in BSL and are freely available to non-commercial organisations.

CORE-OM BSL and CORE-10 BSL

The Clinical Outcomes in Routine Evaluation – Outcome Measure (CORE-OM), measures global distress and is part of a system developed to help the management of large numbers of cases over time. The assessment was designed to be short and accessible. A BSL translation has been created using strict and standardised protocols developed by the CORE System Trust.

There are two BSL versions available: The CORE-OM contains 34 items which can be aggregated into four domain scores: well-being, commonly experienced problems or symptoms, life/social functioning, and risk. The CORE-10 is a short version with 10 items.

The BSL version of the CORE-OM was produced with the UK Deaf population and found to be valid and reliable (Rogers et al., 2014). Both assessments, along with a guide on how to use the CORE-OM BSL can be accessed via the Social Research with Deaf people website (https://sites.manchester.ac.uk/sord/resources/core-om-bsl/) and via the CORE System Trust (https://www.coresystemtrust.org.uk/translations/bsl/).

EQ-5D-5L BSL

The EQ-5D-5L measures health-related quality of life and was developed by the EuroQol Group. It contains five domains of health: mobility, self-care, usual activities, pain/discomfort and anxiety/depression.

The findings from a validation study of the EQ-5D-5L BSL with a Deaf population, confirmed that it was a good health status measure for Deaf people (Rogers et al., 2016). Findings indicated that the health-state values for Deaf people were 10% lower than that of the published norms for the hearing population and that Deaf people with depression have poorer health statuses (Sheilds et al., 2020).

The EQ-5D-5L BSL is available from the EuroQol website. Register for permission to use the EQ-5D-5L BSL via this link, selecting the British Sign Language version (https://euroqol.org/support/how-to-obtain-eq-5d/).

PHQ-9 BSL, GAD-7 BSL, and WSAS BSL
These assessments are often used by primary care mental health services such as Improving Access to Psychological Therapies (IAPT). The Patient Health Questionnaire 9-item scale (PHQ-9) measures depression (Spitzer et al., 1999), the Generalised Anxiety Disorder 7-Item Scale (GAD-7) measures anxiety (Spitzer, et al., 2006), and the Work and Social Adjustment Scale (Mundt, et al., 2002) measures functioning.

BSL versions of PHQ-9, GAD-7, and WSAS have been piloted with the Deaf population, with good levels of reliability and validity (Rogers et al., 2013a). The BSL versions with guidelines for their use can be accessed via the SORD website: https://sites.manchester.ac.uk/sord/resources/phq-9-bsl/ for PHQ-9 BSL; https://sites.manchester.ac.uk/sord/resources/gad7-bsl/ for GAD-7 BSL; and https://sites.manchester.ac.uk/sord/resources/wsas-bsl/ for WSAS BSL).

SWEMWBS BSL
The Short Warwick and Edinburgh Mental Wellbeing Scale (SWEMWBS) measures positive mental well-being, which contains 7 items including mental and emotional well-being; and psychological functioning. SWEMWBS BSL has been validated by Rogers et al. (2018). To use the BSL version of SWEMWBS, register via this link: https://warwick.ac.uk/fac/sci/med/research/platform/wemwbs/using/non-commercial-licence-registration/. Further information and a guide on how to use SWEMWBS BSL is available: https://sites.manchester.ac.uk/sord/resources/swemwbs-bsl/.

SDQ BSL
The Strengths & Difficulties Questionnaire (SDQ) is widely used in CAMHS services. It is a behavioural screening questionnaire for 3-16 year old children and their families. There are three versions: parent, teacher and self-report version (for 11-16 year olds). It explores 25 attributes about the child and their perceived difficulties; provides an impact supplement and follow up questions.

The BSL versions have been piloted with parents of Deaf children, teachers and Deaf young people; it was found to be valid (Roberts et al., 2015). The parent, teacher and self-report versions are available in BSL translation from the SDQ website (https://www.sdqinfo.org/py/sdqinfo/b3.py?language=BSLqz).

Summary
Using BSL mental health assessments that have been validated with Deaf populations is important and assists in the early identification of mental health difficulties which is crucial given their higher prevalence amongst Deaf people. It should be possible for a clinician experienced in carrying out mental health assessments to adapt their assessment with a Deaf person, providing they are cautious about their interpretation and clinical judgments. It is recommended to seek advice from specialist clinicians experienced in assessing Deaf people to prevent inaccuracies in the identification of mental health difficulties and consequent impact this may have on their long term recovery.

References
List of the relevant articles by Rogers and others can be found at: https://www.research.manchester.ac.uk/portal/katherine.rogers.html

G8 Media walls
Dr Rachel Lever

To ensure that all deaf service users have the same experience and access to information as hearing people The John Denmark Unit, a specialist Deaf mental health service in Manchester (see Chapter G4), has enhanced their deaf inpatient experience with 'media walls'.

What are media walls?
A media wall is an interactive, touch screen that has built in speakers, camera and microphone. It is particularly useful in spaces with high security requirements and tends to be constructed in such a way as to resist extreme violence.

How did we get started?
We used a company called Recornect (https://recornect.com/en/) to install a media wall in each bedroom and one in each communal area of the ward. They are approximately 33inch in size. A yearly fee is paid to Recornect for service and maintenance costs.

How does it work?
All media walls are controlled from one central computer, where all information is stored behind local firewalls. The information is then streamed to each device.

The streaming of information allows control over the content available on each device. The information is delivered via apps, which contain information in either video or PDF form and are created by the unit. This allows accessible information to be provided to each service user in their preferred language. This might be British Sign Language (BSL), subtitles or pictorial form.

Who do you need to work with?
To achieve this aim, a technological solution was required that would fulfil the needs of, and work with:
- the service users
- the unit's staff and environment

- the Trust's information governance staff and policies
- IT department
- other local and national polices.

How is the media wall content created?
All information is scripted and filmed. The filming is done via a Surface Pro, as this fits with our Trust's policies and procedures (other Trusts may prefer and use different devices for filming). The films are then uploaded to the central computer where they are edited and subtitled. Once ready they are then placed on the media wall server via specific software provided by Recornect. They are then placed into a specific bedroom or streamed to all devices.

For such a project to be maintained and kept up to date it requires a dedicated person to do all the scripting, filming for inpatients, editing and subtitling. It also requires a good working relationship between the clinicians and the Informational Governance team, to prevent policy breaches. Multidisciplinary professional and service user involvement is required to ensure all information is correct and accessible for each individual person on the unit.

Security
Personalised information allocated to a specific device, via the central computer, is kept secure via the use of a passcode ensuring that no other service user has access to that information.

What type of information is made available?
By using media walls, all inpatients are provided with access to their information in a format that they can understand:
- welcome information about the unit
- care plans
- medication information
- review meeting minutes
- ward rounds
- rights
- advocacy
- community leave

Additional functions

The media walls have additional functionality and pre-installed Apps, (e.g. Freeview TV, games, BSL Zone, relaxation Apps, drawing Apps, and music Apps (where applicable)).

Benefits to service users

The service user benefits are limitless. Each person can have information available to them in a format that is accessible to meet their communication needs. Having information at their fingertips means they are not reliant on others to translate the information for them, as it is there when they want to access it.

Using the additional apps provides the service users with features that can aid their inpatient journey in terms of distraction, entertainment, mindfulness and relaxation; as well as pleasurable activities such as playing games and drawing. This encourages them to take responsibility for their own recovery and participation in activities. It also ensures the service users have some space from others, can spend some time alone - but without being totally isolated.

Section H

Aetiology does matter: causes and consequences of deafness
Dr Lindsey Edwards

Deafness is considered a rare condition, and therefore many professionals only come into contact with deaf clients a handful of times. Many deaf people may not know, or have not been told, the cause of their deafness, even when investigations have identified the aetiology.

For some in the Deaf community, asking about aetiology can cause discomfort and suggest adherence to a medical model of what it means to be deaf. Nevertheless, since deaf people represent a highly heterogeneous group, knowing the cause of an individual's deafness has important implications for providing appropriate support and interventions. This applies both in relation to their deafness and any conditions that are associated with the cause of deafness. It is therefore arguably something that is important to know.

Conductive v sensorineural deafness

In general, it is permanent sensorineural deafness, rather than temporary or fluctuating conductive hearing loss, for which it is important to be aware of the cause, although the conditions can co-exist.

Sensorineural deafness is the result of damage to the hair cells of the inner ear or the auditory nerve that transmits sounds from the ear to the brain.

Conductive hearing loss is the result of sounds being unable to reach the inner ear due to blockage of the ear canal or middle ear. Although it often results in a mild hearing loss, it can be permanent and profound (as in conditions such as microtia-atresia where the ear canal is malformed or absent). Conductive hearing loss is very common in young children as a result of 'glue ear', a build up of fluid behind the ear drum meaning sound is poorly transmitted.

Genetic v non-genetic deafness

There are many different causes of permanent, sensorineural deafness. Around 80% of congenital hearing loss is genetic. In around 20% of genetic cases, deafness is part of a syndrome associated with a wide range of additional medical and cognitive/learning disorders. However, there are more than 400 genetic syndromes alone that have hearing loss as part of the constellation of difficulties. Since many of them are expressed to different degrees in different individuals there is an almost infinite number of clinical presentations.

The most common cause of non-genetic, congenital deafness is Cytomegalovirus (CMV). Other prenatally acquired infections include rubella, toxoplasmosis and herpes. There are many other infections that can cause hearing loss at any time, the main one being meningitis. Prematurity and birth complications, often associated with cerebral palsy, can also lead to deafness. Finally, a number of medications, particularly some chemotherapeutic agents, can cause damage to the hair cells of the cochlea (ototoxicity) leading to permanent hearing loss.

Thus, clearly, it is not possible to provide information on each and every aetiology of hearing loss, and their likely implications for any one child. The following are the ones professionals are most likely to come across.

Syndromes
Usher syndrome
There are three main types of Usher Syndrome varying in the degree, and age of onset, of deafness:
- Type I is associated with profound deafness from birth, vestibular (balance) problems and deterioration in vision that starts in childhood.
- In Type II, hearing loss is usually in the mild to severe range, there are no balance problems and vision typically begins to deteriorate when the individual is in their teens or twenties.
- In Type III, both hearing and vision loss tend to occur later in life, importantly, after spoken language has developed. However, while the degree of hearing loss is often mild, it can be severe.

In all types, vision loss occurs as the light-sensing cells of the retina gradually deteriorate. Night vision loss begins first, followed by blind spots that develop in the side (peripheral) vision. Over time, these blind spots enlarge and merge to produce tunnel vision.

The problems with balance that lead to delayed motor milestones in babies and infants may be the first clue for professionals that Usher Syndrome is a possible aetiology. Genetic testing is not universally offered to families when their child is diagnosed as deaf, and therefore a diagnosis of Usher Syndrome is sometimes not made until the child starts to experience deteriorating vision.

For parents, the implications of Usher Syndrome, particularly Types I and II, are largely around coping with, and understanding the diagnosis, and then accessing appropriate support for their child. Some may wish to protect their child from knowing that they are going to lose their sight (to a greater or lesser extent), and do not tell them until visual problems occur. This may come at a time when the young person is making decisions about their future in terms of exam subjects and career choices, so knowing their diagnosis is crucial.

The implications of vision loss for communication are profound if the young person relies on sign language to communicate. As their sight deteriorates this will become increasingly difficult and adaptations to communication will be needed (see Chapter D12). Restrictions imposed by deteriorating vision on access to education, activities of daily living, relationships and so on may also affect mental health and wellbeing.

CHARGE, Waardenberg, Crouzon, Branchio-Oto-Renal, Treacher Collins, Alport, and Down's Syndrome

Many syndromes are associated with multiple physical and medical conditions, some of which may be life-limiting. Some are also associated with global developmental delay and cognitive disabilities with great variability in the extent to which children are affected, both within and across diagnoses.

Children with these syndromes may need support from a very large number of services (see Chapter H5) including health, education and social services, placing strain on families due to the number of appointments they are expected to attend, the number of different professionals they need to engage with, and often the financial burden. Therefore, it is important to be mindful of the needs of parents/carers and siblings as well as the child themselves.

Deaf children are at greater risk than their hearing peers of all forms of abuse, particularly where there are additional disabilities (See Chapter F2). This group of children are often unable to communicate effectively through either signed or spoken language (but may do so through their behaviour), so are unable to report abuse. Neglect is the commonest type of abuse and frequently concerns are first raised when there is repeated non-attendance at hospital appointments or poor school attendance.

Infections
CMV
CMV is a member of the herpes virus family, and is very common, although most people are not aware that they have been infected.

Infection leading to deafness is typically acquired in utero or very early in life. Associated hearing loss is frequently progressive and may fluctuate. It therefore may not be diagnosed until the child is in their second year of life, or even later. This is exacerbated by the wide range of other consequences of the infection and their severity, such as visual problems and developmental delay. The progress of children whose deafness is caused by CMV may therefore need closer monitoring than other deaf children, especially their general development in the early years.

Ongoing, regular monitoring of communication, academic progress and social development will be essential throughout childhood and adolescence. Other more subtle difficulties may not emerge until later but could still have a significant impact on development and well-being.

Meningitis
Bacterial meningitis leads to sensorineural deafness in around 10% of cases. Most commonly, as the infection spreads it damages the hair cells of the cochlear, but it may also cause inflammation of the auditory nerve.

Degree of hearing loss can vary significantly but it is nearly always permanent. A common complication of bacterial meningitis is ossification (hardening) of the cochlea that usually occurs in the first few weeks or months following the illness. It is crucial that this is monitored by CT scanning of the ears as, if cochlear implantation is being considered, ossification can result in surgical complications when inserting the implants and therefore poorer outcomes.

As with other infections, the severity and impact of meningitis can vary enormously between individuals. The younger the child is when they have the illness, the more severely their development may be affected and the longer it may take them to recover. Meningitis can commonly affect balance (leading to delays in sitting and walking), cause tinnitus (Chapter

H2), and may result in a wide range of cognitive deficits ranging from very subtle processing difficulties to significant learning disabilities.

Where the cognitive sequelae are less obvious, the impact may still significantly affect a child's learning and academic progress. Teachers should be particularly alert to the possibility that the child will need adaptations to teaching methods as well as consideration of classroom acoustics.

Children deafened by meningitis are at significantly greater risk of problems with attention. They often have difficulty focusing on and completing tasks and may:
- be excessively fidgety
- have difficulty waiting their turn
- have problems regulating their emotions (e.g. temper tantrums that are more severe and last longer than the typical "terrible twos").

All these behaviours will have an impact both at home and school, sometimes requiring specific interventions from educational and mental health professionals.

Cerebral palsy
Cerebral palsy is caused by brain injury or brain malformation that occurs before, during, or immediately after birth and while the infant's brain is still developing. It is frequently associated with prematurity and birth complications such as anoxia but may also be the result of genetic factors or infections. How the brain injury affects a child's motor functioning and intellectual abilities is highly dependent on the nature of the injury, where the damage occurs, and how severe it is.

Probably the most important consequence of cerebral palsy for a deaf child is the impact on their ability to communicate and learn a language. Problems with motor control mean they are less able to use sign language and, if the muscles of the face are affected, they may also be unable to develop speech. However, it is entirely possible for a child with severe motor disabilities to have normal intellectual ability. It is therefore crucial not to make assumptions about their capacity to learn and develop based on appearances. It is equally essential to find a way of communicating that is tailored to their specific needs. This will require highly specialist services and equipment, such as eye-tracking devices.

It is also very important to attempt to assess the individual's intellectual ability in order to guide expectations for learning and development. Again, this will require highly specialist services and professionals with expertise in this area.

Ototoxicity

Ototoxicity is the property of being toxic to the ear: the cochlea, auditory nerve or vestibular system. Hearing loss caused by ototoxicity can range from mild to profound, and occur at any age, although the impact is typically more severe the younger the child. The medication (and radiotherapy) used for treating childhood cancers may also result in cognitive deficits with implications for learning.

Children may spend long periods of time in hospital for treatment, often leading to changes in parent-child relationships, as parents struggle to maintain normal routines and boundaries. Children may start to exhibit low mood, anxiety and behaviour problems that do not necessarily resolve after treatment has finished. Hearing loss may be perceived as 'the least of their worries', which may lead to reluctance to follow advice regarding the use of hearing aids as these are perceived as further making the child different from their peers.

Sudden hearing loss can cause difficulties for adolescents as this is a time when identity is forming and friendships, social interactions and 'fitting in' are increasingly important. The impact on schooling, further education and career choices may be significant. Awareness of the psychological needs of these young people by all professionals involved in their care will be fundamental in ensuring they receive the support they require.

Conclusion

Although not always the case, these diverse causes of deafness may be associated with many other cognitive, physical or psychological conditions, in deaf children as well as adults.

When working with a deaf child or adult, consider with them whether exploring this would be of benefit.

H2 Tinnitus
Dr Sally Austen and Nikki Stephens

Tinnitus refers to the myriad of unexplained and unwanted noises that people can experience in their ears or heads. They are probably the result of a misfiring nerve, responding to an inappropriate stimulus. People with a hearing loss are more likely to pick up tinnitus as the auditory system seeks to pick up sounds it is missing.

The noise is often perceived as a random whistle, or screech, drum, buzz, pulsatile noise, and can even be heard as voices or music.

There are two types of tinnitus:
Subjective tinnitus is the most common and only the individual can hear it. Objective tinnitus is a very rare kind of tinnitus that is caused by a blood vessel problem or a middle ear condition and can be heard by a doctor through a stethoscope.

Most of us have experienced temporary subjective tinnitus. For example, after leaving a noisy concert. It can be triggered or worsened by tiredness, stress, a cold, general illness or loud noise.

The effect of tinnitus
There is no 'cure' for tinnitus as it isn't a disease. For most people tinnitus will come and go - staying long enough to be briefly annoying. But it can also take over the lives of many other people, especially those with a tendency to experience underlying anxiety.

For a minority, whose jobs or hobbies depend on the discernment of different noises, tinnitus can affect their everyday activity (e.g. musicians, piano tuners, music producers, radar, pulsars and military operatives).

Is tinnitus dangerous?
Tinnitus is almost always harmless but people with persistent tinnitus should see their GP or audiological professional to rule out anything sinister, such as tumours (this is very rare affecting only 1 in 100,000). One sided tinnitus and asymmetrical hearing loss are 'red flags' and many patients will be referred for an MRI scan to rule out an acoustic neuroma. A negative result can help the patient deal with the tinnitus more easily.

Health anxiety
Despite medical reassurance some people remain unconvinced and worry that their tinnitus is the sign of a missed brain abnormality. Once a reasonable number of investigations have failed to reassure the client, then Health Anxiety may be identified. Early multidisciplinary collaboration between Ear, Nose and Throat (ENT), Audiology, and psychological professionals can prevent health anxiety escalating.

At this stage further physical investigations are discouraged, as they tend to perpetuate the health anxiety. However, for medical and audiological practices, this can prove difficult to apply because:
- they either have automatic appointment systems that send out further appointments
- they do not have time or skill to counsel distressed clients, so authorise scans or other investigations to placate the client and bring the session to an end

Chronic tinnitus
1-3% of the adult population have chronic tinnitus, meaning that it disrupts daily function by negatively affecting mood, concentration and sleep. Chronic tinnitus has been causally and incidentally linked to depression and anxiety. However, where it is has been linked to suicide, the person tends to have a pre-existing mental health condition.

"I never thought I would miss silence, but I really do. The tinnitus fills everything that should be peaceful"

Those people who find tinnitus hardest to manage tend to feel that the tinnitus has taken over control of their lives and that they have lost the 'old them'. Negative ruminations and over-generalised thinking lead to difficulties adjusting to the tinnitus.

"I shall never hear silence again. I will never be happy again"

Chronic tinnitus sufferers often report difficulty getting to sleep, which can lead people to develop unhelpful coping mechanisms such as:
- overuse of alcohol or sleeping medications
- checking behaviours, such as measuring the qualities of tinnitus and the amount of sleep, which can lead to increased arousal and distress

Traumatic causes of tinnitus
Some people can date the onset of their tinnitus to a particular event: usually a loud noise or illness. For some the memory of this event takes on the form of trauma and appears fuelled by anger and blame.

My tinnitus started when I walked past a busker with a trombone who deliberately blasted me with a silly tune to make me jump. Because of this, I can't sleep and am at risk of losing my job. I will never forgive him.

Noise induced hearing loss is causally linked to tinnitus and is more common amongst certain professions: those that have worked in the military, musicians, factory and construction workers. Improvements in tinnitus experience may not be noticed if litigation is still in progress.

Treatment of tinnitus
Discussing tinnitus treatments with a client should be done thoughtfully. Whilst the professional may try to explain that there is no recommended medication or surgery, the patient often takes home the message 'there is nothing you can do about it'. On the contrary, with the right interventions most people with tinnitus can make significant progress.

Treatment often involves:
- supporting clients to give up cure seeking
- teaching management techniques
- addressing other issues, that tinnitus may have been psychologically masking

Resisting 'cure seeking'
Despite much research and debate it is still not clear exactly what causes tinnitus or whether it will ever be 'cured'.

Cure searching is usually unsuccessful and can make the tinnitus worse in that the sufferer gives it more attention. Investing time and money in alternative and untested interventions can be both physically and financially risky. Some 'alternative' treatments such as hopi ear candles have been proven to be dangerous.

The extreme efforts put into finding cures or treatments can become a full-time job and for some people tinnitus becomes the focus of blame for all their difficulties (work, relationships, finances etc).

Understanding and managing tinnitus

Having a sense of being out of control, or controlled by the tinnitus, increases anxiety and hypervigilence. This makes the client more likely to notice their tinnitus. Providing a model that helps the client understand the tinnitus mechanism often means that they can begin to predict when the noises will be more troublesome (e.g. in times of stress, in silence, or on retiring to bed). They can then plan ahead and use the distraction tactics they have learned to achieve a more measured response and regain some sense of control. The final page of this chapter is a copyrighted explanation and model that can be photocopied.

Where is it possible, distraction is by far the best intervention. Even the most severe tinnitus goes unnoticed when the client is fully engaged in other tasks. In contrast, a client who monitors their tinnitus constantly will experience louder and more varied tinnitus (and even hear their own pulse).

White noises generators and other sound enrichment can be very successful in tinnitus management. White or pink noise is broadband sound, a bit like a 'shushing' noise (pink is a softer, rounder sound than white). White/pink noise allows the tinnitus to become part of the broadband sound. This helps the client 'habituate' to the tinnitus. 'Wearable' white noise generators, where a program is provided through hearing aids, may be available via the NHS. This can be beneficial but is used much less often nowadays.

Nature or environmental sound enrichment may be presented from an App on a mobile device via a pillow speaker, SleepPhones, or from standalone devices. These are widely available to purchase. None of these devices or methods of accessing sound enrichment should be used to 'drown out' the tinnitus. The sounds should be played at a just audible level. At bedtime, listening to a choice of sounds, alongside mindfulness or thinking about happy times or places, doing breathing exercises and using other relaxation techniques, can help reduce sleep delay. Improving sleep hygiene can also help.

Factsheets, online shops for equipment can be found at:
RNID   www.rnid.org.uk
British Tinnitus Association   www.tinnitus.org.uk
Helpline number: 0800 018 0527

Psychological intervention
Many people do live with tinnitus without becoming (or remaining) troubled. Pre-existing psychological resilience, personality and coping style contribute to the client's ability to live healthily with tinnitus.

Cognitive behaviour therapy is highly recommended for learning to live with tinnitus:
- to identify and challenge unhelpful thoughts (e.g. *"Now the tinnitus has started, I definitely won't get any sleep."* or *"This tinnitus is controlling my life. I will never get better."*)
- CBT also helps clients to recognise the cycles of tinnitus and worry/depression/anxiety (e.g. *Worrying makes the tinnitus worse – And – Tinnitus make the worrying worse*)
- to reinforce and recognise the areas of life that the client does have control over

Unfortunately there is a shortage of psychological practitioners who have experience in working with people with tinnitus and other audiological conditions.

Hearing loss
Tinnitus is experienced by individuals with no difficulty hearing, right through to profoundly deaf people who have never been able to access useful sound. There does not seem to be a bias towards one gender or the other, but incidence does increase with age.

Some people find, that despite not having any kind of hearing loss, that they struggle to hear speech above the sound of their tinnitus.

Children
Children also experience tinnitus. They can find it scary and, in the absence of a clear explanation, they can interpret their ear noises as monsters or the voices of their nightmares. Children may cope better if they are helped to identify and then name their noises.

Example: Boy Age 7 "I have noises in my ears. I have a Grunt and a Hiss. Sometimes the Hiss is funny. But sometimes the Grunt makes me jumpy, so then mum puts some music on, and I ignore Grunt."

Mental health and 'Voices'
In assessment of mental health in deaf people it is important to clarify whether the client is reporting noises that are the result of residual hearing (i.e. they really can hear something), tinnitus or noises that are the result of mental health hallucinations (see Chapter F5).

Iatrogenic causes of tinnitus
Certain iatrogenic (negative side effects of a medical treatment) causes exist, such as certain prescription medication. In the majority of cases these medications are life-saving. Tinnitus resulting from lifesaving treatment leaves some clients appraising their situation positively: feeling so relieved to be alive that they view the resulting tinnitus as a relatively benign side effect. Others regard the tinnitus is a constant reminder of their mortality and a negative sign that their illness might return.

Summary
Tinnitus will be experienced by many individuals in one form or another during their lifetime, including deaf and hard of hearing people. Everyone copes differently with tinnitus, as they do with other physical and mental challenges, but commonly a fear of the unknown 'cause' can block habituation and rehabilitation. Increasing understanding of the tinnitus and how to manage it is beneficial at an individual level. Research, such as that funded by the British Tinnitus Association, is crucial on a national scale.

Recommended reading
Tinnitus in Children Practice Guidance: British Tinnitus Association
    https://www.tinnitus.org.uk/practice-guidance
Andersson, G., Baguley, D., McFerran, D. & McKenna, L. (2013). *Tinnitus. A multidisciplinary approach*. Oxford: Whurr

TINNITUS

Awareness of tinnitus can be triggered in different ways in people with normal hearing and also in people who have some deficit in their hearing which affects the filtering process in the inner ear and brain.

Tinnitus occurs when the neural activity, which is happening naturally in the brain all the time, is perceived as a potentially dangerous signal, and thus undue attention is paid to it. Sounds are also generated in the nerve cells in the cochlea itself.

Because it cannot match the pattern of the tinnitus sound to any of the 'normal' sounds, the auditory memory is unable to label the sound. In turn, the limbic system which controls our emotions is over-stimulated by the unfamiliar nature of the sound.

The result is that more attention is paid to these *internal* sounds than to the normal *external* sounds, particularly in people with impaired hearing. The stress caused by straining to hear and the stress set up by the limbic system's reaction to the tinnitus can become a vicious cycle.

Tinnitus
↙   ↖
↙   ↖
Normal sound èèèèè Auditory memory →→ Limbic System→ filter out →
↙↗
↙↗
↙↗
STRESS

We need to change the way the tinnitus is being perceived so that it is no longer a threatening signal. The focus needs to be shifted away from the tinnitus and when it is no longer perceived as a threat, much less attention is paid to it consciously or unconsciously. It is important to reduce stress levels and avoid silence too.

Copyright Nikki Stephens © 2021

H3 Balance and dizziness in people who are deaf and hard of hearing
Dr Anne Easson

Our balance is made up of several different systems, which help to keep us standing up. In broad terms these are:
- Vision, 80% of our overall balance
- Information from our joints, tendons and muscles (called proprioception), approximately 15% of our overall balance
- Information from the balance organs in our inner ears, 5% of balance

You have a balance organ on each side. If one or both of these balance organs is functioning poorly or not at all then the body compensates for the loss by relying on the other systems that are functioning.

A balance problem tends to mean that a patient is unsteady, or falls and often feels uneasy because of this. It can also mean that they have an abnormal sensation of movement.

Dizziness is a descriptive term that can mean many different things. To some people it can mean light-headedness. To others, a sensation of spinning or movement, either within their head or their environment (vertigo). Yet for others, it means a sensation of imbalance like being on a boat or a sensation of motion. Many other descriptions can fit under this banner so clarification of what the patient is describing is always the most important factor in taking a history from a dizzy patient.

Many systems of the body can cause dizziness, for example cardiac problems and neurological problems. Dizziness can also be a symptom in anxiety and depression or due to medications.

Incidence of balance problems in deaf people
Deafness can be due to structural changes in the inner ear. Therefore, if there is a problem with the hearing part of the inner ear there may also be a problem with the balance part of the inner ear. Hence deaf patients can be more likely to have balance problems. Equally deafness can be due to a range of syndromes which can cause also cause problems with other systems in the body that can affect balance.

Deafness itself causes balance issues as we know that we use our sense of hearing to tell us where we are in the world and if hearing is impaired this information is decreased. Patients may have become deaf due to treatment such as medications (for example platinum-based chemotherapy), or surgery (such as cochlear implants), which may also have affected their balance organs.

Children with balance problems

Approximately 1 in 1000 children are born with a severe to profound hearing loss. Of these, 40% will have complex health needs involving several other conditions requiring medical care, such as: cerebral palsy, epilepsy, renal impairment or Down's syndrome. In some cases, these additional health needs can impact on the patient's balance.

Published reports have identified balance problems in 30-70% of hearing-impaired children. This is under-recognised. These children have delayed motor skills or may be described as 'clumsy'. Referral to Audiovestibular Medicine, or a dedicated ENT balance clinic, for a balance assessment can help with access to interventions such as physiotherapy or safety advice.

Elderly people and balance

As we get older our vision deteriorates and we may develop cataracts. As 80% of our overall balance involves our vision this can cause a significant effect on our balance. Simple steps such as ensuring that patients have had a regular eye test (2 yearly for the general population and more frequently for the deaf population) can significantly help.

As we age, we may develop osteoarthritis, are more prone to develop type II diabetes (which causes nerve damage and hence less information to return from our peripheries) and may have joint replacements. All of these factors can impair the information returning to our brains about where we are in a 3D space (proprioception). Therefore, the aging process itself can impair our balance.

We also are more likely to be on medications which have side effects including dizziness, which can impair our balance. Finally, we are more likely to develop hearing loss associated with increasing age which further limits the information we receive about where we are in 3D space.

Why is knowing about a balance problem important?

If you have balance problem you may appear clumsy, bump into things and walk as if you were drunk. This has social implications as well as affecting function. Deaf children with balance deficits may have delayed motor milestones such as walking late.

There are also safety implications to a balance deficit. In patients who have no inner ear balance function they rely on visual input and proprioception. In environments where these inputs aren't available such as swimming or diving a patient with an inner ear balance deficit won't be able to tell which way is up and may be at risk of drowning.

If you have an inner ear balance deficit then treatment is available in the form of vestibular rehabilitation. This therapy is provided by an audiologist or a physiotherapist. The balance deficit will not be regained so the therapy requires the patient to do guided exercises to try to improve the other parts of their balance to provide compensation for the loss.

How to establish if a deaf patient has a balance deficit

There are certain questions that may help to establish if anyone has a balance deficit. Simple questions such as do they veer to one side when they walk, do they fall a lot, do they feel dizzy on movement, do they struggle with their balance in the dark.

If you or the patient thinks they have a balance problem then the best course of action is to get them to see their GP who can refer to an Ear Nose and Throat (ENT) specialist or an Audiovestibular Physician.

Dizziness in deaf people

Dizziness is a common symptom in the general population and more so for deaf people. This may be due to an underlying inner ear balance deficit but may also be due to other factors associated with their deafness, such as syndromic problems with their heart or nervous system, or other systems of their body (e.g. visual loss in Usher's syndrome).

There is a wide list of common causes of dizziness which may not be related to deafness so the first course of action is to make a GP appointment who will rule out the common causes of dizziness and if necessary, refer them on to ENT or Audiovestibular Medicine.

Meniere's disease

Meniere's disease is a triad of ear symptoms, vertigo and hearing loss. To have a definite diagnosis of Meniere's (according to the 2015 criteria) a person must have 2 or more spontaneous episodes of vertigo lasting between 20 minutes and 12 hours associated with a hearing loss and fluctuating aural symptoms (hearing, tinnitus and/or aural fullness).

Meniere's patients tend to get a warning of their symptoms by increased tinnitus (see Chapter H2) or pressure sensation in their affected ear (50% of Meniere's patients will get the disease in both ears). These episodes are often perceived as very disabling and they may experience severe vomiting.

Meniere's is less common in people over 50 and is very over diagnosed. Vestibular Migraine is around 10 times more common as a cause of vertigo. 30% of the female population and 20% of the male population get migraine and of those 20% will get balance symptoms as part of their migraine and 20% don't get a headache.

Summary

Balance problems can affect many people, with deaf people at greater risk. Understanding the causes of balance difficulties is important to identify potential risks and access interventions that may be of help. If balance problems are suspected, then a GP appointment should be sought so that onward referral can be made to specialists if required.

H4 Genetic counselling
Dr Sally Austen

The topic of genetic counselling for people who are deaf and hard of hearing should be approached thoughtfully.

Some people who are deaf or hard of hearing see this a disability that they wish they did not have and would not wish on their offspring. In contrast, some deaf people see being deaf as core to their identity, enabling their relationships, language and life choices.

There are some campaigners for the Deaf community who believe that clinicians, whose job is to prevent or reverse hearing loss, are diametrically opposed to understanding Deaf Culture and its roots in British Sign Language (BSL). Consequently, they are uncomfortable with the concept of genetic counselling, assuming its purpose is to eradicate deafness.

Professionals within the field of genetic counselling aim to provide objective information to individuals so they can understand their own situation and make informed decisions. They are looking not just at genetic information about deafness but collate information on a myriad of associated life changing or life limiting conditions. Their job is only to offer this information: not to enforce decisions or to shape the gene pool.

However, Eugenics is fresh within the narrative of many deaf people. Started by medical researchers in America, and then continued by the Nazi regime in Europe in the first half of the 20th century, eugenics resulted in thousands of deaf people, alongside people with mental or physical disabilities, being murdered, sterilised or prevented from marrying.

There are families where many generations have been deaf, happy and healthy such that discussion about deliberately changing this would be seen as offensive – as well as utterly pointless.

However unintentional, discussions between a caring professional and an emotionally robust client about 'improving' the health and welfare of their offspring, can often be received as a message that the deaf adult is defective and that, if they were a potential embryo in today's world, decisions may have been made to prevent them being born. It is important for professionals to be aware of this so that these conversations can be approached thoughtfully.

H5 ENT multidisciplinary working and onward referral
Dr Anne Easson and Dr Sally Austen

Which professionals are required in the diagnosis, treatment and management of deafness or hearing loss? The answer is complex. The obvious focus is on the clients' ears and hearing, but many more perspectives and professionals may be needed.

Aetiological investigation
Deafness is usually picked up by the New Born Hearing Screen (see Chapter C3) but it may be picked up later by parents or other medical professionals. A child will then be referred for diagnosis and explanation - followed by aetiological investigations into the cause of their hearing loss. This will either be by an Audiovestibular Physician, a paediatrician with a special interest in audiology, or an Ear, Nose and Throat (ENT) surgeon.

The purpose is twofold:
   a) to ensure that the appropriate audiological services are offered
   b) to identify and manage any associated health conditions

Geneticist/Genomic counsellor (see Chapter H4)
If it is clear that the client's deafness is non-genetic (e.g. caused by meningitis or anoxia) the involvement of a geneticist is not required.

Where there is a family history of hearing loss a referral to a geneticist may be recommended by the medic. The geneticist's role is to collate information about the deaf individual and their family in order to help predict the likelihood of future offspring being deaf and, if their deafness is syndromic, the likelihood of other associated conditions.

Clients are empowered to use this information to make decisions. For example, mutation in the Connexin 26 gene is associated with a non-syndromic deafness. As it is a recessive gene, both parents need to be carriers, the chances of which increase if the parents are related to each, as in consanguineous marriages (e.g. first or second cousin).

Paediatrics
Any child with complex health needs should be seen by a Paediatrician as they can co-ordinate care for the child and ensure that the child is developing in all aspects at an age appropriate level. This is often performed by the Community Paediatricians.

Occupational therapists
Deaf children who have complex health needs may have problems with vision, co-ordination and balance. Occupational therapy can be very helpful in adapting a child or adults' home, work or school environment to help them.

ENT (Ear, Nose and Throat) surgeons (also known as Otolaryngologists)
In patients with glue ear causing deafness they may need grommet surgery for conductive deafness or cochlear implant surgery for severe sensorineural deafness. ENT surgeons are routinely involved in the care of many children whose deafness is syndromic. For example, many children with Down's syndrome are likely to have Glue Ear.

Audiologist
The audiology department will frequently test a child's hearing and fit appropriate hearing aids.

Ophthalmology
Any child with a severe to profound hearing loss should be referred to an Ophthalmologist for visual assessment. With one existing sensory impairment, the importance of the other senses is heightened. Some syndromic conditions affect both hearing and vision (e.g. Usher's Syndrome, Alport syndrome), so it is important that the Ophthalmology team monitor this.

Speech and Language Therapy
Deafness can affect acquisition of language and the production of speech. Any child with a delay (in spoken English or BSL) should be referred to the Speech and Language therapists.

Speech and language therapists are also involved in swallowing assessments and training, which are relevant for people whose difficulties are associated with facial structural and muscular difficulties. This would be a very rare referral for children, but more common in older adults.

Vestibular service (see Chapter H3)
Many syndromes will have hearing or balance problems associated with them. For children and adults with balance problems, the client may be referred to an audiovestibular physician or an ENT surgeon; and they may refer onto a vestibular scientist.

Cardiology
All children and adults with a severe to profound hearing loss should have an ECG performed to rule out cardiac abnormalities. For example, Jervell and Lange-Nielsen syndrome associates hearing loss with heart arrhythmias (Long QT leading to fainting, seizures or sudden death); or people with Rubella who may also have congenital heart disease.

Learning disability services
Clients may need referral to services for cognitive or behavioural challenges. For example, people with Down's syndrome have a very high chance of both hearing loss and learning disability.

Endocrinologist
Some syndromes require specialists in the endocrine system (a series of glands that produce the body's hormones) such as Pendred's syndrome, which can affect the thyroid gland and the balance system.

Nephrologist
Some syndromes require input from the Nephrologists (kidney doctors). For example: Alport's syndrome can cause deafness, problems with vision and kidney abnormalities; Branchio-oto-renal syndrome can cause defects in the development of the tissues in the neck and malformations of the ear and kidney.

Maxillofacial team
Where deaf people have structural or facial differences this can affect confidence. Referral on to psychological services to support their adjustment to their identity and development might be useful. However, structural differences may be far more important in affecting breathing, sleep (and therefore concentration and cognitive ability) or living with pain, (e.g. Stickler Syndrome or Treacher-Collins syndrome).

Mental health professionals (see Chapters G3 & G4)
Deaf adults and children have a higher prevalence of mental health and behavioural problems. Co-working with educational psychologists or mental health professionals may be useful.

Conclusion
Although it varies with a person's cause of deafness, and whether they have associated health conditions, it is likely that their care team, over the years, will be made up of a great variety of health care professionals. The potential need to involve other professionals should be considered.

H6 Non-organic hearing loss (NOHL)
Dr Sally Austen

Non-organic hearing loss (NOHL) refers to the state where a person is reporting a greater degree of hearing loss than is described by their formal hearing test.

Alternative names (in no particular order and without judgement on their accuracy) include: pseudo hyperacusis, factitious hearing loss, functional hearing loss, conversion disorder, malingering, and feigning.

Diagnosis
Audiological
The hearing test administered, called a PTA (Pure Tone Audiometry), usually requires the client to listen to a variety of frequencies, in decreasing loudness, indicating when they have heard something (either by raising their hand or clicking a button).

If the client reports a greater degree of hearing loss than their hearing test indicates, it is important to check the validity of this result, and rule out:
- Impairments in the technology being used. Were the headphones plugged in? Is the room sufficiently soundproofed?
- Has the person understood the instructions fully or answered inaccurately for another legitimate reason (e.g. they thought they should only press the button if they heard the noise loud and clear).

If a discrepancy remains, then an Objective Hearing Test may be suggested (Otoacoustic Emissions, Auditory Brainstem or Cortical Evoked Response Audiometry). In these tests either a small probe is put in the client's ear to measure the response from the ear, or sticker electrodes are placed on the client's head to record brain response to sound. Either way the client is not responsible for responding to noise.

Before NOHL is diagnosed, two further conditions need to be ruled out:
- Auditory processing disorders are where the brain receives the noises passed through the ear but cannot make full sense of it, so the client's perception is that they are not hearing clearly.
- Auditory neuropathy (AN) is a hearing disorder in which the outer hair cells of the cochlea are present and functional, but sound

information is not transmitted sufficiently by the auditory nerve to the brain.

Behavioural
The most useful and obvious indicator is when the audiological professional observes the client responding to conversational speech at a level that would be impossible to according to their audiogram.

Other behavioural factors, important in the early stages of the identification of NOHL are:
- Exaggerated 'listening' movements, such as holding their hand behind their ear, or leaning excessively forward
- Showing inconsistent receptive skills that are not explained by tiredness, stress or environment
- Not saying 'pardon' or asking for repetition very often
- Sabotaging attempts to correct hearing loss or help communication (e.g. refusal to wear hearing aids because of an unproven allergy to the mould; finding multiple reasons why the interpreters are not suitable; repeated prevention of assessment or intervention)

Motivation
The presence of NOHL is diagnosed by an audiological clinician. However, to devise treatments or interventions, it is necessary to understand the clients' underlying motivation, which may require the involvement of other professionals such as mental health teams (Austen & Lynch, 2004).

Malingering
Malingering describes a deliberate behaviour to mislead, for the purpose of external gains such as benefit money, work sick days, or avoidance of something (e.g. nerve-wracking exams or army conscription). The person is only likely to behave as deaf for the duration of relevant assessment days or hospital appointments. They are likely to stop when 'caught out'.

Conversion
Conversion, the other end of the spectrum, describes an unintentional deafness that creates a strong psychological protection of which the client is not aware. Conversion disorder is often associated with severe trauma. For example, a child who is being abused may unconsciously present as deaf in order to draw the attention of protective professionals or family and reduce unaccompanied access by the abuser.

Someone with conversion deafness is likely to live as deaf most of the time. Being 'caught out' is not necessarily helpful for someone with a conversion deafness. Their genuine perception of deafness may mean that they are unlikely to believe the newer diagnosis and/or be psychologically distressed by it. Time and co-working between audiologists and mental health professionals is needed.

Factitious hearing loss
Factitious deafness is the largest category of NOHL and describes consciously feigned deafness. Motivation may be for psycho-social benefits such as:
- company
- attention
- physical contact (including fetishist attraction to deafness and/or hearing aids)
- medical investigation (formally known as Munchausen's Syndrome)
- control (of communication environment - often associated with high functioning Autistic Spectrum Disorder)
- an attempt to dupe the clinician, which may be linked to a personality disorder (this is discussed further in Chapter H7)

For those whose Factitious deafness is serving a psycho-social purpose, their being 'found out' can result in their finding alternative ways to achieve the same psycho-social ends. In this instance, they may replace a non-organic hearing loss with, for example, non-organic skeletal, neurological, or gynaecological disorder.

Feigning
Feigning means a deliberate pretence or exaggeration of deafness; this could be associated with Malingering or Factitious deafness. Thus, someone with conversion deafness would not be feigning their deafness.

Movement between these categories is very possible. For example, a client could start with a consciously exaggerated deafness to avoid difficult school exams (malingering) but then find the care and attention they receive rather comforting and thus continue with a factitious deafness.

Treatment
In the author's experience, NOHL is extremely difficult to treat. The client's deafness may be non-organic, but it may be their best way of coping with their other issues.

Thus, our attempt at 'treatment' often means taking away that person's coping strategy. This means we are offering them something that is for our benefit not theirs. Our only recourse to treatment must include helping them to find different ways of coping that are more attractive to them. Thus, us finding other more orthodox ways of coping with social anxiety, narcissism, loneliness, may help the client replace the symptom.

Within a clinical mental health setting, it is rare to see the 'hearing loss' wane. Other aspects of the mental health and social functioning may improve but clients often hold on to their 'deafness'. This is particularly understandable in that giving up their deafness may also mean giving up **you** – the clinician who has understood and helped them.

Example: Client A was on 32 medications a day, was unable to function in daily life and had NOHL. After a year of psychological intervention, he was down to 16 medications, was virtually independent – but was still 'deaf'. The mistake was made of suggesting their deafness might also improve. All the progress made reversed in a matter of days. The client appeared to regard the support they received as dependent on them being deaf and that if they 'gave up' their deafness they would lose the support. They were probably right!

Working with clients with NOHL can have a powerful effect on the clinician. Many clinicians experience anger and resentment. Some have a blanket response to deception: if the deafness is not genuine, they will not believe that the client's other presentations or complaints are genuine.

Professionals benefit from open team discussion to counteract 'splitting' and reduce distraction. The variation in motivation of clients with NOHL is complex and varies enormously. However, a shared feature in these clients is the time and effort they will put into trying to distract or derail therapeutic conversations onto hearing and communication issues. Time that clinicians would prefer to spend exploring the genuine mental health difficulties underpinning the NOHL.

To challenge or not?
To choose to carry on providing support, while leaving their NOHL alone is intellectually and emotionally challenging.

Within Deaf specialist mental health settings, we don't challenge our clients on their NOHL, and we don't even mention that we know they are less deaf than they are presenting. We accept that the deafness is offering them some sort of psychological protection and it would be counterproductive to attempt to remove this.

It is important to remember that NOHL is usually an overlay to a lesser genuine deafness, so the client probably does need communication support. However, it is also important to remember that the client may be able to overhear your conversations, in a way that your other deaf clients cannot.

Children with NOHL: a graceful recovery model
Within an education or child mental health setting, it may be more feasible to replace the motivation behind NOHL with effective alternatives. The younger the child, the more flexible their chosen identity remains, and the more alternative support resources are available.

For example, if the child's 'deafness' is helping them to avoid difficult schoolwork, then provide tutoring; if the NOHL is communicating something about fear of abuse or bullying, look at what protection the child needs.

A 'Graceful Recovery' is often orchestrated by multidisciplinary co-operation, such as between teacher/therapist and an audiologist or SALT. Explanations can be given that open doors for recovery (e.g. 'Your latest test show that you've got the sort of deafness that can improve gradually'. 'It seems your ears are clearing - maybe because it is the end of the cold/hayfever season.' 'I think we measured your deafness wrongly. We have some better headphones now and it looks like your hearing is not so bad. Sorry about our mistake').

Deaf identity
In my experience discussion of NOHL within the audiology and oral worlds is welcomed whereas such discussion within the sign language using worlds is not. It appears that discussion of NOHL may cause a sense of threat to those who use sign language but have some residual hearing.

This should not be the case. Excluding those with conversion disorder, where the client has no knowledge of their maintained hearing, NOHL incorporates a conscious attempt to deceive. Deaf Community members who have effective hearing may choose to sign and may choose not to broadcast their PTA, but the assumption that they have no hearing is made by others, not offered by them.

Protective exaggeration

The concept of NOHL may seem alien or extreme. And yet it has relevance to most of us. When visiting the GP with a virus, we may all exaggerate a sore throat in the hope of getting antibiotics that we believe will magic us better – or when feeling guilty about taking sick leave and letting colleagues down, we exaggerate the description of the causative illness.

There are many times when being deaf is exhausting: the eye strain, the concentration, explaining environmental and communication needs to others. Severely deaf people may not volunteer that they have some useful hearing because the hearing other will then require them to speak and lipread perfectly – instead of putting the onus on the hearing person to take responsibility for communication. Greater hearing loss gives 'permission' to get an interpreter or palantypist and not have to worry about the background noise/tinnitus/bearded speaker. It is not deception but an appropriate request for support.

This has raised concern in cochlear implant teams with clients who are saying they are profoundly deaf and need an implant but who are found to be exaggerating their severe deafness. On asking, the clients have honestly described their deafness as severe but say they are tired and just want a 'cure'. Although the threshold for implants is lowering, it is still relatively high to balance out the risk of losing any residual hearing if the implant is not successful. Some severely deaf people are so weary that they are willing to take that greater risk.

Summary

Working with clients with any non-organic or self-inflicted disorder is extremely challenging. However, whilst the symptom (NOHL) may be specific, the underlying cause is one that is well known to practitioners who specialise in psychosomatic presentation: same pain, different symptom.

Reference

Austen, S., & Lynch, C. (2004). Non-organic hearing loss redefined: understanding, categorizing and managing non-organic behaviour. *International Journal of Audiology, 43(8),* 449-457

H7 Deaf Wannabees
Dr Sally Austen

Deaf Wannabees is an online community of people who find deafness attractive in some way. This includes:
- People who want to present as more deaf than they are (see Chapter H6)
- People who are interested in deafening themselves or advise others on how to deafen themselves (referred to as 'Crossing the Bridge')
- People who have a sexual interest in people who are deaf or who wear hearing aids

How group members share their motivation is varied. Some are explicit both inside and outside of the group; others are only explicit within the group; and a third group practices municipal deception.

Whilst the potential for explicit and deceptive group communication has increased with the rise of online social media, the overall number of Deaf Wannabees, internationally, is relatively small. This results in the group having to include people whose motivation varies widely. Some sympathise with the values of the deaf communities; some exploit them. For some, membership can be harmless and supportive; for some, membership can leave them vulnerable.

'Crossing the Bridge'
The choice to deafen oneself, either partially or wholly; either temporarily or permanently is an extraordinary one. It may be a decision made with full Capacity; in the vulnerable it may reflect an absence of better options. It is achieved through noise damage, poisoning the nerve cells or physical damage to the structures of the ear.

Body Integrity Identity Disorder
Some people believe that they are a deaf person born into a hearing person's body. This is referred to as Body Integrity Identity Disorder and overlaps with the TransAbled conditions (and their websites).

They believe that deafening themselves will release them from their mismatched unhappiness (dysphoria) to a state that integrates mental and physical comfort. There is not sufficient longitudinal studies of transitioning into deafness (or other physical conditions such as amputation) to draw general conclusions.

When people choose to feign or facilitate deafness, the benefit to their overall wellbeing, must outweigh the risks. This may be because other options and opportunities are either unavailable or the person is unable to make use of them.

Loneliness and adjustment issues
Some people see the Deaf community or deaf communities as having social value to them. Through loneliness or low social confidence, they believe they have more chance of being accepted within these communities, than other communities they might otherwise belong to.

Deaf Wannabees websites declare that their rights to act as deaf or to deafen themselves should be respected. However, it could be argued that a person who is willing to deafen themselves in order to gain social belonging, needs support to gain such belonging in a less drastic way and perhaps with a more immediately accessible community.

Autistic Spectrum Disorder
Some people find noise and/or communication unpleasant and use a presentation of deafness as a way to control their environment. In the author's experience, the people in this group often have high functioning autistic spectrum disorder. This may also reflect the fact that the client with ASD does not have the sophistication of Theory of Mind to know that their portrayal of deafness is not entirely convincing.

A person with ASD who is considering deafening themselves in order to get peace or privacy, should be helped to find alternative coping strategies (e.g. desensitisation, environmental changes, head phones).

Exploitative
Certain benefits are afforded members of the deaf community but not the hearing community (e.g. disability benefit money, educational support, access to recreational or professional opportunities). Some people use feigned deafness, or deafen themselves, to capitalise on these benefits. However, even where the behaviour is primarily illegal or unauthorised, it is possible it also represents a diagnosable co-morbidity or vulnerability.

Narcissism
Some people believe they have more chance of 'succeeding' within the deaf communities and take leadership roles. As well as having the

advantage of more communication methods, they may have an educational advantage. They capitalise on being a 'big fish in a small pond'. Although therapy for personality disorder is difficult, and requires the client to be motivated, there is scope for the promotion of solutions that don't resort to feigned or self-inflicted deafness. There is benefit to interventions that emphasise the individual's own and original value and that promote the use of less duplicitous opportunities.

Psychopathy

For some people is seems that they are motivated by wanting to feel superior to clinicians and find 'tricking' the audiological professionals in some way satisfying. These people will have detailed knowledge of the workings of the ear, the resources and the testing procedures. They share methods for duping clinicians. They tend to take the lead in offering advice on getting a diagnosis of deafness, being prescribed hearing aids, or on methods to deafen oneself. The need for this type of relationship shares features with a presentation of Psychopathic Personality Disorder.

Fabricated and Induced Illness (FII)

Previously called Munchausen's Syndrome, the person fabricates or induces the illness in themselves or someone they care for (this used to be called Munchausen's by Proxy).

Motivation seems to result from a sense of physical comfort in the actual medical interventions, however painful - an emotional comfort of being cared for and a sense of social value gained from the respectful relationships shared with the clinicians. Whilst the person has Capacity and is consciously facilitating these medical assessments and interventions, it is possible that these behaviours are indicative of underlying need for support.

Sexual fetish

Another group sharing the Deaf Wannabee sites are those with a sexual fetish for people who are deaf and/or hearing aids, either in themselves or others.

Summary

Those people who identify as Deaf Wannabees have hugely varying motivations, behaviours and commitment. Their relationship with the deaf communities is complex and variable.

H8 Sleep disturbance
Dr Sally Austen

Sleeping problems affect up to two-thirds of all deaf children and adults.

Cognitive and communication effects of poor sleep
People who are deaf or hard of hearing must work harder to distinguish one sound from another and to lipread. These are skills that involve central auditory processing and concentration: both of which are negatively affected by poor sleep.

Adults
Deaf adults are often asked if they sleep better than hearing peers because of the absence of noise disturbance.

In fact, deaf adults are at risk of poor sleep quality, waking more often throughout the night, despite sleeping for the same length of time overall. Research has also shown that they experience less time in 'Delta sleep' - the stage that resets the body's feeling of needing to sleep - so they often report feeling exhausted and as though they barely slept at all. Delta sleep is also thought to play a role in memory formation and mood regulation.

Sleep and depression (see also Chapter F1)
Poor sleep (specifically, difficulty dropping off and early morning waking) is associated with depression. Depression is more common in deaf people (those who are congenitally deaf and people with acquired hearing loss) However, poor sleep can also cause low mood and depression, thus creating a vicious cycle.

Sleep and anxiety
People who are anxious or traumatised may ruminate (repeatedly think things over) at night. Interventions often involve psychological therapy, which can be hard for some deaf people to access (see Chapter F7).

Noise Induced Hearing Loss (NIHL) may be acquired during military activity or other work-related experiences. The experience often co-exists with trauma reactions.

Tinnitus (see Chapter H2)
The rate of sleep problems among tinnitus sufferers is estimated to be as high as 77% and is part of a vicious cycle:

- The noise of tinnitus makes it difficult to sleep
- Tiredness worsens tinnitus
- Tinnitus sufferers have a higher risk of depression and anxiety, which is also connected to poor sleep

In hearing people, noise (either white noise generator, or gentle music) is considered a useful mask and distraction from tinnitus. This may be useful for people with milder hearing loss but is unlikely to be of any benefit to profoundly deaf people.

Medication
Anti-depressant medication often improves sleep by treating the depression. Medication specifically to help people sleep is cautiously prescribed.

Benzodiazapines (informally known as the old fashioned 'sleeping tablets', such as valium) are highly addictive and rarely prescribed for more than a few days.

Non-benzodiazapine sleep related medications, such as Zopiclone, are less addictive and may be used for a few weeks to get the client back into a sleep pattern.

'Sleep hygiene'
This refers to behavioural interventions such as:
- a good night-time routine
- reducing screen time
- meditation
- relaxation
- avoiding daytime naps
- avoidance of drug and alcohol
- using the bedroom for only sleep and romance, so that the bedroom is not associated with stress

Deaf children's sleep
Once a profoundly deaf child has closed their eyes at night, they are without hearing and vision. This can be frightening or unsettling. Whereas hearing children can be soothed by their parents' voices or other sounds (e.g. music) this is not possible for deaf children.

Balance (see Chapter H3) relies on the inner ear and vision, so in the dark the child may feel particularly disorientated. It may help to tuck them in tightly so that they feel 'grounded'.

Children who get some benefit from hearing technology (e.g. hearing aids, cochlear implants) during the day may not like taking them out at night.

Tinnitus (see Chapter H2)
Some deaf children have tinnitus, which can be intrusive or scary at night:
- Get a check-up from the child's GP or audiological provider
- Ensure the child has the opportunity to discuss their experience of tinnitus, to know it is harmless
- Use mindfulness techniques to help them predict the experience and direct their own reaction to it

Interventions
Environmental
- leaving a small light on or using glow in the dark stickers
- Leave a piece of your clothing with them so they are left with your familiar smell

Behavioural
- Stick to consistent bedtime/morning routines
- Tell them when you are leaving the room, so they don't get worried when they realise you have gone
- Have clear and consistent strategies for what they should do if they cannot sleep or wake in the night

Technological
- Leave hearing aids or cochlear implant processor on the bedside table so they can put it back in if they wake up and feel scared
- (Short term) letting the child fall asleep with the technology in, and then take it out for them

Medication
- Melatonin can be very effective treatment for sleep problems in children, particularly short courses to give parents respite. However, sleep hygiene and behavioural approaches should be used first.

Conclusion
Congenital and acquired deafness can be associated with sleep problems through interactions of tinnitus, balance, anxiety and depression. There are various interventions that can be used to help with this although some may need adaptation to make them accessible to deaf people.

Section I

I1 Deaf people in the Criminal Justice System: guidelines
Dr Sue O'Rourke

Deaf people are vulnerable throughout the criminal justice system pathway. Awareness of this is important because:
- Unfair treatment is traumatic for the person concerned
- This can complicate and compromise the case

Arrest: guidelines when you come to arrest a deaf person
- If the arrest of a British Sign Language (BSL) user is planned, you should book a BSL interpreter. This will make the arrest much easier to carry out, the person will know why they are being arrested and there is more chance that they will understand the police caution (Miranda warning in the US).

- If the arrest is not planned, there will inevitably be no interpreter and significant communication difficulties.

- Be aware that if the deaf person seems to be 'ignoring' you they may in fact have not heard. Get their attention by waving or tapping them on the arm or shoulder.

- It helps if there is good lighting. Stand in front of the deaf person so they can see you. The light needs to be on your face (see Chapter D8 for tips on communication)

- Do not assume that the person can lip read – this is a difficult skill at the best of times. Lipreading is liable to error, even under optimal conditions. In some situations it is practically impossible: high emotion, intoxication, poor light, or the general chaos of arrest.

- If you are using writing, use simple English and keep questions and answers to a minimum. The deaf person may use their phone to communicate with you in 'text speak'.

- Even with an interpreter, the police caution is linguistically complex, particularly the concept of adverse inference. The deaf person may 'nod', which makes it appear that they have understood the caution. However, this may well not be the case (see Chapter B2). The caution needs to be repeated as soon as an interpreter is available.

- Deaf sign language users find being handcuffed behind their back particularly aversive, as this effectively deprives them of language. It is preferable if this can be avoided.

- Be aware that if the deaf person cannot see you, they cannot communicate. Always try to have someone in line of sight to communicate.

- Sometimes hearing people misunderstand sign language as aggressive and misinterpret the person 'waving their arms around' which escalates the situation. Be aware of this.

- Try to learn a few signs, such as deaf, calm down, arrest, please, thank you, name. This can go a long way and give the impression that you are 'deaf aware' and attempting to communicate.

Police interview
Once you are back at the police station, be aware that the deaf person is likely to be very anxious about not being able to communicate. The most important thing to do is to book an interpreter for the police interview (see Chapter D5 & D6). This may take a while and can cause considerable delay. Meanwhile, if you are attempting to communicate, use the basic communication tactics above and provide pen and paper for simple messages.
- Never use pen and paper for a quasi-interview. Many deaf people have lower literacy and this can cause difficulties in the case later.

- If you are concerned about the person's mental health, be aware that the police doctor is unlikely to have any deaf awareness or BSL and will need an interpreter in order to communicate to carry out an assessment.

- One option for interviewing a vulnerable deaf person is to book a Deaf Intermediary (see Chapter I8) in addition to the interpreter.

The interpreter is likely to let you know if there are obvious vulnerabilities, for example by letting you know if the deaf person does not appear to understand even simple questions. If so, an Appropriate Adult should be used. However, many 'Appropriate Adults' are actually inappropriate as they too cannot communicate in BSL, and therefore have no means of monitoring communication. The deaf person may have a social worker or support worker who could assist. The most appropriate adult is someone who is able to communicate in BSL.

All interviews with deaf people need to be video recorded. This protects the person and the police. Without a video recording the original interview is lost, as the interpreter's voice over is not a direct translation of the interview. The recording allows for a future challenge of the interpretation.

When video recording, it is important that both the deaf person and the interpreter can be seen on screen in order that any challenges to interpretation can be made at a later date.

Example: a video recording of a police interview was badly set up so that the interpreter could not be seen on the screen and therefore the defence argued that it was unclear exactly how the questions were signed, putting the person at a disadvantage as the interpretation could not be challenged and inferences could not be drawn from their responses.

Going to court
- Probation – if probation are required to assess and produce a report on the day that a deaf person is in court, they can be guided by their own toolkit. This advises that, if a BSL interpreter is not available, an adjournment should be requested.

- Court Liaison and Diversion schemes will not necessarily pick up mental health needs in deaf offenders or be able to carry out their assessments reliably. Again, an adjournment can be requested, in order that specialist assessment is obtained.

- There should be a team of BSL interpreters in court; usually two or three people, separate from interpreters for the defence, in order to maintain their independence. There may also be a Deaf Relay and/or an intermediary (see Chapters D4 & I8).

- It is often BSL interpreters in court who pick up that the deaf person may lack capacity in proceedings or may have additional needs. Interpreters also tend to be able to direct legal professionals to experts who could assist. Deaf mental health services are a source of advice (see Chapters G3 & G4) and a specialist website to access experts in mental health and deafness is www.deafexpert.co.uk.

It is arguable that any deaf BSL user in court is vulnerable and certainly this should always be considered. Even without any additional needs such as mental health concerns or language impairment, a deaf person is likely to be unfamiliar with court related concepts and require additional support.

The mismatch between the highly jargon-laden language of the court and the visual language that is sign language, often leads to confusion. In such cases, the use of BSL interpreters alone is not sufficient to ensure understanding. The risk is that the deaf person does not fully understand the concepts used and the court does not know what it does not know.

The illusion of understanding can be created by the competence of the BSL interpreters in court; despite the fact that the deaf person is confused and disadvantaged. In recognition of these difficulties, the use of Deaf Registered Intermediaries (RI) is becoming more common in relation to deaf defendants (see Chapter I8).

Another benefit of engaging an Intermediary is that he or she will assist the court at a 'Ground Rules Hearing', for example in terms of the layout of the court, timing and breaks and how questions are put to the deaf person.

Example: a deaf man with little sign language who was relying on lip reading went to the initial hearing and sat in the dock in the back of court, therefore making it impossible to lipread counsel who had their back to him. Unsurprisingly he had no idea what happened at the hearing.

Managing the hearing
A Deaf case can feel 'hijacked' by issues of language, leaving the court somewhat bewildered by people signing and arguing over a particular sign for something. The legal professionals usually come to the case with little idea of language and culture of the Deaf Community and with misconceptions about deafness and deaf people. To prepare, it is recommended that all involved, including the Judge, read the Toolkit 11: Planning to question someone who is deaf (www.theadvocatesgateway.org/toolkits).

Counsel are often understandably resistant to revealing their questions in advance. However, doing so to the Intermediary can allow for a smoother cross examination. The Intermediary can advise which questions would be difficult for the person to answer and how these can be reframed.

Asking a deaf person about something they said earlier can often lead to great confusion. If a previous response has been video recorded (e.g. at police interview) it is often more effective to play the video section and then ask a question about it, rather than referring to it in the abstract (which may be interpreted into English in a way that is not exactly how the deaf person remembers what was said).

An effective means of reducing the amount of argument in court regarding language and interpretation is to video record all evidence provided by deaf people. This is in fact the equivalent of audio recording evidence of hearing people, which is the norm.

If a deaf person's evidence is only audio recorded, it is in fact only the interpreter's interpretation which is captured and not the original. This leaves the deaf person vulnerable as there is no way to challenge the interpretation. The case at Snaresbrook Crown Court[3] attests to the fact that this can be achieved, although many courts seem to think it is too difficult or cumbersome. An application to do this prior to the hearing (rather than on the first day) is recommended.

Sentencing
Whilst, the same sentencing options are open to the court for deaf as for hearing people, the impact and efficacy of these may differ.

Prison
The impact of a custodial sentence on deaf people has been called a 'double jeopardy' due to the additional difficulties that communication problems cause a deaf person in prison. This affects everything from casual encounters with prison staff and peers, to more serious matters such as psychological assessment and offence work.

---

[3] https://www.lawgazette.co.uk/practice/sign-language-trial-big-step-forward/5041926.article

Deaf prisoners are often subject to bullying and abuse. This combined with the extreme isolation puts them at risk for developing mental health problems, in a system ill-equipped to assess their mental health needs.

Probation

Probation services have traditionally not taken account of the needs of deaf people and have been unable to meet their needs or carry out the required supervision and monitoring to the same standard as with hearing peers. However, a recent project in the North West of England has provided a model for training Offender Managers in Deaf Awareness and all probation staff in the UK now have access to a Toolkit on Deafness. Following feedback from deaf offenders and Offender Managers, further developments in making probation more accessible are being considered, including a project to train Deaf Link Workers to work alongside probation staff.

Example: a young Deaf man breached his probation conditions, explaining that he needed to travel to meet people in the Deaf community. He felt the probation officer did not understand his needs, neither did he understand the compulsory nature of the probation order.

Mental health disposal

Those deaf offenders with a mental disorder are appropriately diverted to mental health services, which are discussed elsewhere in this book. The concern is that, whether in court or prison, a lack of specialist knowledge on the part of professionals may mean that serious mental health problems are not identified, indicating the importance of instructing deaf experts to advise the court or prison.

12 Forensic mental health services for deaf people
Dr Sue O'Rourke

Introduction
Forensic mental health services for deaf people are a relatively new speciality. Historically, deaf people who committed offences, and were deemed to have mental health needs, would be detained under the Mental Health Act (1983, amended 2007). This was either in secure services, with hearing people and staff who had no specialist deaf expertise, or in open deaf mental health units without specialist forensic provision. There are some startling historical examples of deaf people admitted to secure services for minor offences and remaining there for the rest of their lives.

By contrast, practitioners in deaf mental health care are aware of offenders who have been 'let off' by the criminal justice system as a result of their being deaf and a sense of sympathy - only to go on to commit more serious offences. This attitude of tolerating minor offences is likely to contribute to an ongoing 'lack of learning', which prevents the person reflecting on their crimes and developing an understanding of responsibility and consequences.

In the last 20 years there has been development of Forensic Deaf Services including in High, Medium and Low secure conditions. With this has come consideration of specialist assessment and treatment approaches. The problem of small numbers remains, meaning that whilst forensic services for hearing people are further specialised, those for deaf people take all offenders. This can lead to an unfortunate mix of patients, for example those more vulnerable people mixing with higher functioning offenders, who may seek to exploit them.

Deaf forensic services
Adult
Currently in the UK, specialist forensic services for deaf people only exist in England. These are:
- Rampton Hospital (high secure) in Nottinghamshire
- St Andrews Hospital (medium secure) in Northamptonshire
- St Mary's Hospital – Elysium Healthcare (medium secure) in Warrington
- All Saints Hospital - Elysium Healthcare (low secure and open forensic) in Oldham, Greater Manchester

- Cygnet Hospital (low secure – male and female wards) in Bury, Greater Manchester
- John Denmark Unit, Prestwich Hospital (open unit with forensic pathway) in Greater Manchester

Child
There are no specialist forensic services for deaf children or adolescents. This makes finding an appropriate placement difficult. Secure adolescent services are not used to taking account of deaf children's needs. In contrast, placing a deaf child with severe challenging or risky behaviour in a deaf (non-forensic) mental health ward may be inappropriate in terms of managing risk.

Role of forensic services
The main focus in a forensic setting is the assessment and management of risk, with an overriding public protection duty.

Risk must be understood in the context of the deaf person and their experiences. In practice this means taking account of:
- the deaf person's communication needs
- the impact that being deaf has had on their development
- understanding the relevance that being deaf has had on their offence

Before a deaf person reaches a Deaf Forensic Mental Health service, it is likely that they will have been assessed within services that have not considered these factors. This casts doubt on the reliability of assessments, which will have often been carried out by non-specialists.

Risk assessment and risk management
Assessment (and intervention) is likely to take roughly twice as long as with hearing people. Whilst it is always essential to obtain some specialist advice, beyond this some points to consider are:

Communication (see also Chapter D14)
- Engage the correct communication specialists. This may be a British Sign Language (BSL) interpreter (See Chapter D2), a relay interpreter (see Chapter D4), a deaf advocate or a Deaf Intermediary (see

Chapter I8) depending on the language fluency and cognitive ability of the offender.
- Where possible book the same interpreter each session so they become accustomed to the patient's language and difficulties.
- Do not abdicate your assessment responsibility to the interpreter - this is not their role and their code of conduct dictates that they advise on matters of language and communication only.
- Be 'deaf aware' - enrol on a Deaf Awareness course and learn a few signs, to show you have a positive attitude to deaf people.
- Do not assume your patient can lipread or read (see Chapters D9 & B3).
- Once you have completed your risk assessment, you will need to book an additional session(s) to explain the results to the deaf person. Use an interpreter as they are very unlikely to be able to read and understand your report.

Cognition and learning
Make no assumptions about your patient's cognitive ability. Some hearing people assume that being deaf equates to a learning disability; others assume that deaf people are the same as hearing people but for 'broken ears'. Deaf people's developmental trajectory is often very different to their hearing peers. The engagement of a specialist assessor is recommended.

- Different developmental experiences can result in deaf people having reduced access and consequently significant information gaps and poor literacy (see Chapters B3 & B4).
- Lack of access to learning may significantly impact risk. Even for those with intellectual ability within normal limits, missing or misunderstanding information can have massive consequences (e.g. understanding the law, age of consent, nature of consent, what is risk).
- Those deaf people who grew up in overprotective families may have little experience of acting independently or taking responsibility for their actions.
- Neurological factors may play a role in understanding the behaviour and offending of a deaf person. Ask about cause of deafness (see Chapter H1), some of which may also be linked to cognitive impairment (see Chapter E3) or Autistic Spectrum Disorder (see Chapters E4 & E5), as a mediating factor in increased risk.

Assessment tools
Psychologists in forensic services tend to be particularly keen on using psychometric assessments. This is fraught with difficulty and as a rule of thumb should be avoided (see Chapter E2). In particular, questionnaire measures are often not valid, even when translated into BSL (see Chapter G7).

Assessments which provide a Structured Professional Judgement approach, such as the HCR20 or RSVP have greater face validity and are not subject to issues of translation; however, reliability and validity still need consideration (see O'Rourke & Grewer, 2005 for further discussion).

When considering static/historical risk factors, which may have predictive value in hearing people, be mindful that they may have less predictive power for deaf people. For example, challenging behaviour is more prevalent in deaf children (see Chapter F12) and as such may be less discriminatory in predicting future risks. Dynamic risk factors, such as lack of insight or denial need to be considered with an understanding of difficulties in acquisition of knowledge and information in deaf offenders (see Chapter B4).

Deaf and hearing community experience
When considering risks in the community, seek advice about the local Deaf Community as there may be a supportive and resourceful peer group. However, this could also inadvertently provide access to victims; or create additional stress to the deaf person in the form of victimisation of deaf ex-offenders.

Be aware that deaf children are particularly vulnerable to sexual abuse (see Chapter F2). This is relevant to thinking about potential victims but also points to the fact that the deaf adult you are working with is more likely to have been a victim also.

In some cases, the dynamics of deaf/hearing issues are relevant, for example a deaf person may justify violence against a hearing person if they feel hearing people have discriminated against them. Be mindful that you too are a hearing person and may be at risk for this reason.

Be aware that a Deaf offender in a hearing environment is vulnerable for many reasons. His or her mental health is likely to be affected by being isolated in a non-communicating environment. In addition, staff are less able to assess risk on a day to day basis, which can increase risk to self and others. Teasing and bullying of deaf people in hearing environments is common and staff need to check this when an interpreter is available.

Intervention
Many of the issues that affect assessment are also relevant to intervention. Adaptation of programmes (e.g. sexual or violent offending) require much more than the addition of an interpreter and often require specialist skills to rewrite from a 'deaf perspective'. If the person is to remain in a non-specialist environment, co-working with deaf staff is recommended.

Assuming the therapist cannot sign and is working with a BSL interpreter and (hopefully) a deaf co-worker, there will need to include:
- time before to prepare sessions to clarify purpose of the session and to discuss issues of language
- time after for a debrief. As a visual language, the disclosure of offences in BSL can be very graphic and traumatic for the interpreter or deaf co-worker, who may require further support

Sexual offending
One often cited research finding is the increased prevalence of sexual offending in the deaf population. However, the conclusion that deaf people are more likely to offend sexually than hearing people would be premature. An alternative explanation of this finding is that deaf people are charged with sexual offences more than with other offences, because:
- Either they may be less likely to offend in other ways
- Or they are less likely to be prosecuted for minor crimes but will be prosecuted for offences that are considered serious (such as sex offences).

The efficacy of sex offender treatment programmes generally has been questioned in recent years. Since the existence of specialist forensic services for deaf people, clinicians have attempted to develop or adapt programmes to treat sexual offending. There is no standardised or agreed approach across services, all of which offer such intervention on a group or individual basis. What is clear is that offenders trying to take part in groups for hearing offenders, even with an interpreter, have been left confused and derived little benefit. Hearing groups with an interpreter are not truly accessible and for most deaf people are not effective.

Treatment groups for deaf sexual offenders need to consider cognitive and linguistic factors. Deaf offenders are more likely than hearing offenders to have:

- language deprivation and dysfluency
- not learnt about the law, age of consent and nature of consent
- poor social and emotional understanding
- lesser empathy and poor Theory of Mind
- lower levels of literacy

Desistance

Understanding what leads to an offender desisting from further crime involves an understanding of subjective/internal factors and societal/engagement factors. Research relating to desistance in deaf offenders has not been carried out. However, difficulties in accessing work and educational activity, isolation from the community and a lack of accessible support are self-evidently relevant. In considering helping a deaf offender desist from further crime, his or her place in the wider community needs to be considered and issues of access and discrimination addressed.

Conclusion

Arguably, deaf offenders with mental health problems should be referred to a specialist service. This is not only due to access to appropriate risk assessment and interventions, but also in order to benefit from the therapeutic milieu that a signing environment allows. However, there may be reasons why this is not possible or desirable, in which case efforts must be made to minimise the isolation and exclusion that the deaf person will inevitably feel in a non-communicating environment. This has considerable cost implications and it is important that senior managers, those holding the budgets and commissioners acknowledge the need to make reasonable adjustments in order that the person can be properly assessed and access, not only therapy, but also social activity and day to day life on the ward.

References

O'Rourke, S. & Grewer, G. (2005). Assessment of Deaf people in Forensic Mental Health Settings: A Risky Business! *Journal of Forensic Psychiatry and Psychology, 16 (4),* 671-684

13 Capacity to parent assessments with deaf clients
Dr Andy Cornes

Parenting assessments are ordered when there are child protection concerns in a family. They are generally conducted before the matter is in the family court (pre-proceedings), as a means of assisting the social workers, but may be conducted within proceedings.

Deaf specialist Expert Witnesses (Deaf Experts)
Expert parenting assessors tend to be social workers or psychologists but the necessary training and experience is not profession-dependent.

A Deaf Expert is a professional (deaf or hearing) who is sufficiently trained and experienced in working with deaf people, to conduct parenting assessment with deaf clients. A generic assessor does not become a Deaf Expert merely by working through a sign language interpreter.

Currently, there is a national shortage of Deaf Experts who can assess parenting. Training is required to address this deficit.

Assessment frameworks
Some Expert assessors use the Parent Assessment Manual (PAMS) when assessing deaf clients. It is not recommended in its pure form as it concludes with a 'score', which has not been normed or validated for use with deaf clients. Furthermore, it was originally devised to assess parents who have an intellectual disability (ID), thus inadvertently giving the impression that the deaf person being assessed has an ID.

What is assessed?
There is no standardised template for a parenting assessment, but following the elements drawn from the Department of Health Framework of Assessment for Children in Need and Their Families (2000) is recommended. For each of these elements the appointed expert must answer the following crucial questions:

1. Can the parents provide good enough parenting for the child or children now and throughout their childhood and adolescence?
2. If not, what are the gaps and can the parents make the necessary changes (i.e. bridge the gap in their parenting) within timescales?

3. Do the parents understand professional concerns?
4. Do the parents have the ability to protect the child from risk?
5. If the child or children are not living with the parents, what are the placement options and what level of access is appropriate?

Assessing the parenting chronology
The role of the parenting assessment is not only to consider whether the parent currently has good enough skills. If the parent is 'failing', the assessor must also determine at what stage of the person's pathway did the failure occur, what contributed it and whether they were provided with appropriate reparation opportunities.

For example, if the client is reported to have refused to attend parenting classes, but it turns out that they were not provided with an interpreter, they will likely need another opportunity to attend with an appropriate interpreter/relay/intermediary before a conclusion can be drawn about their willingness to engage and ability to learn.

Examples of good practice in Deaf Expert assessments
Assessing a deaf parent requires more than just an ability to sign. (Hence, providing a generic assessor with an interpreter is not sufficient). Some deaf parents may use sign, speech, residual hearing, lip reading, or a combination of all of these. Each aspect of the parenting assessment needs to be adapted in relation to specialist deaf knowledge about language, cognition, development, culture, and attachment.

Assessing language and understanding - not speech
It is crucial for the assessor to appreciate that it is fluency and functionality in a language that is required for good parenting, not that the language be spoken English.

Hearing people tend to make negative assumptions about dysfluent speech. Quality or fluency of a deaf person's speech does not indicate their intelligence, functional skills or fluency in sign language. If there is a concern about intellectual ability or linguistic understanding, then further referral for cognitive assessment or language assessment should be made.

Hearing children raised in a deaf family may experience delay in their acquisition of spoken English. Assumptions that this is a sign of neglectful parenting, should be resisted. If the child is fluent in sign language, they, like other bilingually raised children, will most likely catch up when they start nursery school. Ongoing concern should be addressed with specialist speech and language therapy assessment.

Language dysfluency
Some deaf parents being assessed will have impoverished language in both British SIgn Language (BSL) and English (see Chapter B1), and literacy (see Chapter B3). In this case, co-working with experienced sign language interpreters (Chapter D2) and Deaf Intermediaries (Chapter I8) is vital.

Visual cues and clues
It is always important to be ready to use visual supports in your communication. Props may include, for example, pictures of Calpol bottles, healthy and unhealthy food, and tick charts/scales to represent degrees of emotion. Not knowing a word or sign does not rule out the parent being able to succeed functionally.

Client A does not know the word Calpol but recognises a photograph of it and knows that it is necessary for pain and fever relief in children. They are not able to read the instructions but have successfully sought support from a friend and a pharmacist to check the dosage.

If a parent is accused of having injured or neglected their child, ensure that there are photos of the injury or a copy of the 'body map' available for the assessment, as a visual aid for conversation.

Crucial and hard to translate concepts
Many of the concepts that are vital to good parenting are actually very hard to translate into BSL (e.g. boundary setting, stimulation, safety, parental responsibility). If a deaf parent appears to be failing to achieve a target, then the most crucial responsibility of the assessor is to ensure that the failure is not, in fact, one of being able to communicate their success. This might require you to give multiple examples, to use visuals or even to role play.

Example: A deaf mother is asked 'How would you keep your child safe in the home?' but seems unable to answer. The Expert assessor discusses this with the Deaf intermediary and it is decided to use role play. The Deaf intermediary crawls on the floor pretending to be the child, trying to put his finger in an electricity socket and reaching for a candle on the mantelpiece. The mother immediately understands the concept and lists the various measures she takes to keep her child safe in the home.

Gaps in knowledge (see also Chapter B4)
A deaf parent may have a gap in knowledge that is the result of lack of opportunity, not lack of ability. Where hearing people learn much from 'over hearing' (e.g. conversations around them, on TV or radio), access to incidental learning is restricted for deaf people. Simple education may provide the necessary knowledge.

Example: Child A has been slapping his sibling and appears to be being rewarded by his parents, who sit with him on the 'naughty step' and give him sweets. They say their social worker advised them to do this. After a short explanation about the difference between rewarding good behaviour (e.g. giving sweets when the child plays nicely with his sibling) or punishing bad behaviour (i.e. leaving him on the naughty step if he has slapped his sibling) the parents can demonstrate how to use this strategy effectively.

Theory of Mind (ToM) (see Chapter B5)
Theory of Mind is the ability to think that others think and feel differently to us and may have different information to us. Its development is dependent on good language skills.

Using an interpreter, to elicit information about ToM can be tricky, as much is given away in the translation. The hearing professional ideally needs to have fluency in sign language themselves, even when using an interpreter, to be able to lead the mode of questioning.

For example, when a client does not appear to be understanding a question, it is common for interpreters to give a list of possible answers, as an explanation to the client of the style of the assessor's questioning.

Assessor: How do you think your child felt when you hit him?
Interpreter: You hit your child. Did your child feel: Sad, happy, frightened?

A feature of sign language called 'role shift' (where the signer takes the role of each person) makes it difficult for the interpreter to sign 'frightened' without also enacting showing that it is the child being frightened in response to being hit by the parent.

The assessor needs to be experienced in working with interpreters so that they can discuss the methods and styles of interpreting appropriate at each stage of the assessment.

The use of photographs of adults and children experiencing different emotions, and Likert scales to express the degree of emotion, is recommended.

Attachment
Attachment is the quality and nature of the bond between the child and its parents/wider family. Given that many families that include a deaf person have experienced early health related trauma, lack of information, isolation and lack of shared language, it is important to consider whether attachment issues are present.

Whilst this is not routinely assessed in parenting assessments, it should be viewed as a crucial element when the child, parent or both are deaf. To do this, the Expert parenting assessor requires deaf specialist knowledge and experience.

Issues such as assessing the level of communication between the parent and child (including the degree of fluency or dysfluency), and how this impacts on their language, development and behaviour are relevant; particularly setting boundaries and establishing logical consequences.

Examples of bad practice in parenting assessments of deaf parents
The ruling and guidance handed down in the case Re C (A Child) [2014] EWCA Civ 128 changed the way Deaf clients are assessed in pre-proceedings and in family court proceedings.

In the case Re C, the local authority was severely criticised. According to the court record, the mother 'had a low level of cognitive functioning and a speech and hearing impediment', whilst the 'father is disabled by reason of profound deafness and who communicates via British Sign Language (BSL)'. Concerns included their having:
- Used the mother as an interpreter for the father, when they sought Section 20 consent

- offering the mother an 'ordinary parenting assessment' to be conducted by a generic social worker, with a BSL interpreter, which commenced 4 weeks before the final hearing.
- using a generic parenting assessment of the father, which disadvantaged him greatly as it did not take into account his communication needs.

The full care order and placement orders were successfully appealed. The child who was incorrectly removed, was reunited with the father. The father's claim for compensation under the Human Rights Act was not opposed by the local authority.

The Court of Appeal judgment also set out the necessity for
- early resolution of funding arrangements for BSL interpretation
- consideration as to whether a deaf relay interpreter or Intermediary should work alongside the BSL interpreter

As a result of this case it is now against case law for Deaf clients to be assessed by generic assessors. If this is ignored, then the case is likely to go to appeal. Unfortunately, it will take some time for all within the legal professions to be fully aware of this ruling and there are still a number of clinicians attempting such assessments, unaware of their own limitations or working outside of their competence.

Risk to child and parent

Even the most cognitively and linguistically able deaf person may not receive an accessible and equitable parenting assessment. Access to interpreters is sketchy with professionals sometimes inappropriately using family members to interpret or forcing a deaf person to work with them in their non-preferred language (e.g. lipreading or reading/writing). Social workers may do spot checks without interpreters, excluding deaf parents in favour of hearing parents, or necessitating the use of their children as quasi-interpreters which is highly inappropriate. This results in them failing to use the time to provide equitable information or reassurance to the deaf parent.

Assessments (and court proceedings) may take place in poorly lit or noisy (distracting) environments. Inappropriate and invalid cognitive or mental health assessments may be proffered by inexperienced 'experts'. There is a risk that deaf parents, who do not know their rights, 'agree' to their children being taken into care without interpretation or explanation.

Summary
The purpose of a parenting assessment is to analyse the needs of the child(ren) and to assess risk. Currently, there is a problematic shortage of Deaf experts who are suitably qualified assessors, as the demand is so high. Many professionals consequently end up taking on parenting assessments without suitable knowledge or experience. This is potentially highly damaging to deaf parents and children and is against established case law.

I4 Mental Capacity Act assessments
Dr Ben Holmes

Assessment of deaf people under the Mental Capacity Act (MCA, 2005) carries the same legal considerations as assessment of any other person under the Act.

This chapter does not consider the Act itself but instead provides guidance on how the process of completing MCA assessments may differ, or need to be adapted, when working with deaf people.

Language
Being deaf, in itself, does not impact on an individual's ability to make capacitous decisions. Equally, simply using an interpreter (see Chapters D2 & D3) or lip speaker (see Chapter D9) may not always be sufficient in itself to guarantee a person can access and respond to questions.

When a capacity assessment is completed this should always be in the best language, or form of communication, for the individual being assessed (see Chapter D14). Deaf people vary in their communication preferences and may use sign language, lipreading, residual hearing, speech or written communication. Alternatively, a mixture of multiple channels of communication may be used and these may change according to the circumstances or context of the assessment.

Example: A deaf adult with ASD, who lost her hearing as a teenager, uses speech to give answers, and lip reading and sign language to receive information. However, for people she has not met before, looking at their face can be anxiety provoking. She therefore relies on signs to a greater extent with new people until she is comfortable with them even though she takes less meaning from this than lipreading and sign combined.

Assumptions about what is best must not be made based on casual observations (e.g. the person can read and write therefore it is okay to use written communication). Instead, all efforts must be made to provide the best communication and language match for the individual according to their needs and preferences. In some situations, an assessment of the client's communication by a deaf specialist, such as a Deaf Intermediary (see Chapter I8), may be needed first.

Use of interpreters

If the professional completing the assessment does not have fluency in the same language as the person they are assessing then it is highly likely an interpreter will be required. Some, limited, knowledge of a language is not sufficient for important decisions such as capacity assessments. Nor is pen and paper a valid substitute just because the person is able to read and write some words and an interpreter is not available (see Chapter B3).

Getting a good match between interpreters and the deaf person being assessed is essential (see Chapters D2, D3 & D13). Regional variations within signed languages mean that time may be needed for the interpreter and deaf person to 'tune in' to each other. It is also important to remember that there are many different sign languages from around the world and simply booking 'a sign language interpreter' does not guarantee it is the correct language for the assessment. This should always be checked with the person being assessed.

Example: A deaf woman moves to the UK as a refugee. She is fluent in her country's native sign language and has some knowledge of British Sign Language (BSL). However, use of a BSL interpreter does not give full opportunity to understand or participate in assessment in the same way.

Fund of information (see also Chapter B6) and access

Even when using an interpreter, other adaptations may still be needed. Some deaf people have had reduced opportunities to access information or learn from experience because of factors that may include: limited educational opportunity, reduced opportunities for incidental learning, and over-protection from significant others. None of these factors is equivalent to the inability to make capacitous decisions. However, the presence of these factors could impact on a person's decision making.

Fund of information deficits could result in a person appearing to lack capacity when actually they need to be provided with information first in order to aid their decision making process. Where this is the case decisions about capacity should be postponed until the individual has had the opportunity to acquire this information wherever possible.

Where urgent decisions need to be made, consideration should be given to the possibility of a person gaining capacity at a later date which may necessitate a repeat assessment in the future.

Variable profiles and assumptions about ability
The inconsistent opportunities to access different types of information that some deaf people have mean that particular skills in one area, or difficulties in another, should not lead to global assumptions about ability (see Chapter E2).

For example, someone that has experienced severe language deprivation may have lifelong difficulties understanding certain concepts but still function in the average range intellectually (see Chapter B1).

Equally, someone who presents as functionally very skilled in certain tasks, because they have been encouraged to repetitively practise them, may still require significant support in other aspects of functioning that they have never been given the opportunity or encouragement to develop.

Example: a chatty, sociable man holds down a job as foreman of a factory. He does his job, and instructs others, well. He receives a wage, pays his bills and has not been in debt before. When involved in a family financial dispute about a legacy the solicitor queries his financial understanding. On thorough assessment it is identified that he has difficulties with basic numeracy and cannot tell the difference between £2000 and £200,000. He is also unaware that he has the same rights, as his hearing brothers, to dispute a will.

Making things more visual
For deaf people with minimal language, additional intellectual difficulties (see Chapter E2) or that have experienced language deprivation (see Chapter B1), any assessment will require working alongside interpreters experienced in working with clients with non-fluent sign language (see Chapter D3). A Deaf Relay Interpreter (see Chapter D4) or Deaf Intermediary (see Chapter I8) may also be required.

Limited early language experiences can result in difficulties with conceptual understanding, and abstract thought (see Chapter B7). Coupled with any fund of information deficits that may exist, this can mean that abstract conversations about things that have never been experienced can leave the person unable to meaningfully participate in the assessment for reasons other than their capacity to make a decision.

In these instances, the assessment may need to rely more on pictures, videos, role play, props or gesture to aid discussion. The person may need to visit places being discussed (e.g. accommodation). Or, it may be necessary to use more concrete examples and provide fixed options to facilitate conversation. Discussing the assessment in advance with any interpreters and Deaf professionals involved will help to make the assessment as accessible as possible.

Example: A deaf adult that has experienced significant language deprivation is asked where he would like to live. He has only ever lived in one house, so replies 'home'. He is taken to look at alternative accommodation and then later shown pictures of his current house and the alternative accommodation. When subsequently asked the same question in different ways after this visit he consistently indicates a preference for the new accommodation.

Use of advocates
Consideration should always be given to the use of an advocate when completing a capacity assessment with a deaf person, preferably a Deaf advocate. Many deaf people have experienced some degree of oppression or disempowerment, some significantly so, and particularly at the hands of powerful hearing people.

It is possible that a deaf person might agree with something because they either do not realise they have the right to challenge it or because the effort involved in doing so seems significant and potentially overwhelming (see Chapter B2). Advocates can help a person to express their preference and to provide a fuller answer that indicates the full extent of their understanding of a situation.

Inadvertent restrictions
This is particularly pertinent when considering admissions to hospital wards where the Mental Health Act (MHA) might apply. According to MHA, if a person consents to their admission then they can be admitted on an informal basis to a ward and the MHA will not be used to enforce the admission. However, if consent is given it is essential to then check whether the person has the capacity to give that consent - something that is very easy to assume (see Chapter B2).

In this instance, there is a risk that the person being admitted may continue to remain as an informal patient for an indefinite period of time, with professionals assuming they are happy to stay. The reality may be that they did not understand the reasons for admission in the first place or realise that they have a choice to challenge the decision.

This may be further complicated if a deaf person is admitted to a hospital to an unfamiliar area. Their lack of knowledge about routes home and local transport links, distance from family and support network, coupled with a communication environment that does not facilitate access to that information may further encourage a perceived need to accept staying in hospital because there does not seem like an obvious alternative.

Not assessing capacity to consent to admission at the point of admission can create difficulties later on. This is particularly true if a person does in fact lack capacity to make this decision but this is only queried when they ask to leave the ward. The sudden use of an MCA assessment and subsequent Deprivation of Liberty Safeguarding (DoLS) application may leave the person feeling confused, further disempowered and as though they have been tricked. The ethics of doing so is also questionable.

Summary
Being deaf in itself does not impact on an individual's ability to make capacitous decisions. However, when the need for a mental capacity assessment is identified, greater consideration must be given to adaptations that may be required, particularly for professionals that are new to working with deaf people. Where possible, deaf professionals or advocates should be involved and for more complex decisions involvement of specialist services may be required.

Capacity assessments for deaf people are likely to require more time and may require adaptations to your approach in addition to booking an interpreter. Care must also be taken not to make assumptions that could lead to deaf people being unable to participate fully in an assessment or, potentially, inadvertent restrictions being imposed.

I5 Mental Health Act assessment, sectioning, Tribunals and Lay Managers' Hearings
Dr Steve Carney

Mental Health Act (MHA) assessment
This chapter refers to MHA for England and Wales, but similar laws apply in Scotland and Northern Ireland.

Assuming the assessor and the client do not share a fluent language, anyone conducting a Mental Health Act (MHA) assessment with a deaf person must work alongside appropriate registered and experienced sign and/or spoken language interpreters. Where there is language dysfluency, a Deaf Relay Interpreter may also be needed (see Chapters D2, D3, D4 & D13).

The interpreters should be prepared with sufficient background information to enable them to recognise names, terminology and the expected language style.

The client's 'nearest relative' must legally be informed. However, most signing deaf people have hearing parents who do not sign and may have little deaf awareness. A more accurate picture of the client's background may be additionally provided by other friends and carers. It is important to engage people who know the patient, their signing style and what is 'normal' for them.

Prior to MHA assessment, consult with your nearest Deaf Mental Health service for advice or support – and to see if co-working is feasible (see Chapter G4).

If your client is detained once the MHA assessment is completed ensure that this good communication continues to admission. It is preferable that the interpreter stays for the admission process to enable the deaf client to understand what is happening and their rights. Deaf carers and family members will also need interpreters to understand the process.

Mental Health Act powers
Sectioning laws are the same for deaf and hearing people. In the author's clinical experience, Section 2 (up to 28 days assessment) tends to be used

more than Section 3 (up to 6 months assessment and treatment) because of additional time it takes to gather knowledge about the clients' language and background information. Section 3 is more often used with patients with an established diagnosis who are likely to need a longer period in hospital.

The use of Section 5(2) is to briefly detain those who are already in hospital and who are deemed unsafe to leave due to their mental disorder, often due to agitation, distress or aggression. This may be used in physical or psychiatric hospitals, by a registered medical practitioner.

In a generic health facility, it is unlikely that you will get a face to face interpreter in the time before the client attempts to leave the ward. Online interpreters (Chapter D7) are crucial in such situations. An assessment for section 2 or 3 must be carried out within 72 hours.

Once detailed, the client must be advised of their rights with an interpreter (face to face or via video). This is always hard in any language. If your deaf client also has problems with literacy or language deprivation (see Chapters B3 & B1 respectively) this will need to be repeated on numerous occasions. The use of a deaf advocate is recommended.

Tribunal
Clients are allowed to appeal against section. They will need to be supported to make this decision and to instruct a solicitor.

They will need an explanation of what to expect and what the process of the Tribunal is. Currently, during Covid-19, these Tribunals are being held online.

A Mental Health Tribunal is a branch of the Court system and has set procedures, which can be very formal. There are 3 Tribunal members: a Judge, a Psychiatrist and a Specialist Lay Member. They may have little knowledge of deafness or sign language.

The interpreters required will have unique legal/court training. Whilst they will try to be personable, the client will need to be informed that these interpreters are appointed by the Tribunal service and will therefore be rather formal.

A minimum of 2 interpreters and a Deaf Relay Interpreter (see Chapter D4) should be booked. If any of the interpreters are not present, the Tribunal cannot go ahead.

Lay Managers' Hearing
When a section is due for renewal, the client must be seen by a consultant psychiatrist for a Lay Managers Hearing. This is less formal and uses interpreters who are more likely to be known to the patient, which can be more reassuring for them.

Consent to treatment
Whilst someone is on section, they are required to accept treatment whether that be medication, nursing interventions or psychological assessment. At all stages, communication in the clients' best language is of paramount importance for both their Human Rights and their benefitting from engagement in their own treatment.

Under Section 3, treatment can be enforced for the first 3 months. If there is a lack of capacity regarding treatment (see Chapter I4), or if the patient refuses consent, there will be a referral to a Second Opinion Approved Doctor (SOAD) who should hold an interview with the patient using an interpreter. The SOAD will also need to interview a nurse and other clinician regarding the decision.

Resources
A BSL video explaining the Mental Health Act can be found at:

https://www.swlstg.nhs.uk/news-and-events/video-wall/bsl/56-the-mental-health-act

I6 Representing a deaf person in court
Clare Wade QC and Christian Wasunna

The Criminal Justice System is complex and primarily designed for hearing professionals and court users. The needs of deaf defendants and witnesses have largely been overlooked. However, if hearing legal professionals bear the following communication factors in mind, then court hearings can be adapted to accommodate the needs of deaf defendants and/or witnesses.

Sign language
Forensic significance of non word for word translation
Hearing professionals in court rooms commonly and erroneously assume that that there is a 'word for word' translation between BSL and English.

British Sign Language (BSL) has its own grammatical structure and word order, which is different to that of spoken English (see Chapter C8). The unit of interpretation is not the individual word or phrase but one of meaning. Some matters that are easily expressed in spoken English are not easily interpreted in BSL, and vice versa. Thus, the BSL/English interpreter must make lexical choices consistent with meaning. The choice of sign/word used by the interpreter will depend on his or her understanding of the overall context. An interpreter may therefore seek clarification before interpreting.

Example:
Hearing barrister: Mr Brown hit Mrs Green
Interpreter: How did he hit her? With his hand or with an implement? What implement?

Literacy (see Chapter B3)
For many deaf BSL users, English is their second language. The hearing lawyer should not assume that information can be communicated in writing. Simple written statements such as "we can meet tomorrow" may be reliably understood but the difference in structure, vocabulary and syntax between the two languages is likely to lead to misunderstanding and unreliability when written information is more complex.

Knowledge gaps
Most deaf people are of average intellectual ability but have been disadvantaged by a lack of access to information. They may therefore require additional information to be provided. See Chapter B4 for more information.

Interpreters
Pre-trial interviews require the booking of a registered BSL interpreter from The National Register of Communication Professionals (NRCPD) or the Regulatory Body for Sign Language Interpreters (RBSLI). If the best or preferred language of the defendant is another sign language, such as American Sign Language (ASL), then the appropriate sign language interpreter must be provided. In the case of oral deaf communicators, a registered lipspeaker may be needed (see Chapter D9).

Court interpreters are engaged by the court. At trial, the court interpreters will work in teams of three, with one person interpreting, a second assisting and the third will rest: rotating every 30 minutes. They will only interpret in court.

The deaf defendant will require their own BSL interpreter not least, because they will be giving their lawyer legally privileged instructions whilst at court.

Proceedings in the police station
If instructed from the outset of the investigation, the solicitor attends the police station when a deaf client is interviewed under caution.

Most police forces are moving towards conducting visually recorded interviews. However, this is still not guaranteed so police station representatives should insist that the interview is visually recorded - even if this causes the interview to be delayed or requires the interview to take place in an alternative police station. It is important that all signing can be seen on the recording. This ensures that any disagreement at trial about what was said and translated, can be resolved.

ABE interviews

Police officers conducting an Achieving Best Evidence (ABE) interview of a deaf complainant or witness, must ensure that the signing of both the witness and the interpreter is clearly recorded by the cameras. If this is not done, then the defence may apply to exclude it. In the event of a successful application, it will either need to be re-recorded or the witness will have to give evidence-in-chief live.

Ascertaining Capacity (see Chapter 14) and assessing mental health or cognitive needs

When representing a deaf defendant, it is important to ascertain his or her fitness to plead and stand trial as:
- (a) set out under the test in R v. Pritchard (1836) 7 C. & P. 303
- (b) interpreted in M (John) [2003] EWCA Crim 3452 at [22] and [23] namely, can the defendant enter a plea, instruct legal advisers, follow the evidence, give evidence on his or her own behalf and challenge a juror.

Inability to do any one of these things, will result in unfitness to plead. If a defendant is fit to plead, effective participation should nevertheless be considered[4]. Being able to effectively participate at trial means being able to; understand what defences are available, give instructions and follow the evidence. If a defendant is unable to fulfil any of these criteria, then consideration should be given to whether there are any special measures that will assist their effective participation.

A deaf defendant may well have additional needs that are best identified by specialist psychiatrists and psychologists **who are used to working with deaf people and who are BSL conversant.**

A psychological assessment will complement or augment a psychiatric assessment by testing the defendant's level of understanding, competence and effective participation. Psychologists and psychiatrists

---

[4] Courts are expected to make reasonable adjustments to remove barriers for people with disabilities (Equal Treatment Bench Book 2021 411-414). In preparation for trial, the court must take every reasonable step to facilitate the participation of any person, including the defendant (Criminal Procedure Rules 2020, rule 3.9(4)(a) and (b)). Further, see Practice Direction and case law on vulnerable defendants; all possible steps should be taken by the court to assist a vulnerable defendant to comprehend the proceedings and to engage fully with his defence adapting the ordinary trial process, as necessary.

without knowledge of BSL can make erroneous assumptions leading to misdiagnosis and incorrect capacity assessments.

Where language or learning deprivation is the issue, clear, jargon-free explanation and extra time for questions and explanation will be needed. Once communication problems are resolved the defendant will be able to give instructions, follow the evidence and participate effectively in the proceedings.

If a defendant is fit to plead, notwithstanding any diagnosis that may be made, then advice should be sought as to the deployment of relevant special measures.

Applying for prior authority from the Legal Aid Agency
Use Form CRM/4. Experts who are experienced in working with deaf people are likely to charge in excess of the allowed rates and solicitors will therefore have to justify the choice of expert on application. Counsel's advice should be included in the application and it is also worth citing the factors stated in the introduction to this chapter. In short, it can be argued that deaf cases are unique and enhanced rates are justifiable.

Guidance for prosecutors who seek to rely on the evidence of a deaf complainant/witness
If the defence seek to displace the presumption of competence, then the competence test provided by s.53(3) Youth Justice and Criminal Evidence Act 1999 requires that a witness be able to understand questions and give answers that can be understood. The witness's level of understanding should be assessed by a psychologist with expertise in BSL. The court should not be too quick to find that a witness is not competent (see, R v. F (JR) [2013] 2 Cr. App.R.13).

A psychologist can also be instructed to assist in adapting questions to the cognitive ability of the witness. It is not necessarily the case that an intermediary can fulfil this role just as well as a psychologist - although a deaf intermediary can comment on understanding, only an expert psychologist can comment on the cause of a lack of understanding.

Deaf intermediaries for prosecution witnesses are available under the Ministry of Justice Witness Intermediary Scheme. See Chapter 18 for more information.

Defence application for a Deaf Intermediary
Use of intermediaries by defendants is governed by common law because s. 104 of Coroners and Justice Act 2009[5] has not been brought into force. The courts now tend to restrict the use of intermediaries for defendants (see, R v Rashid [2017] 1 Cr. App. R. 25 - held that the trial judge had been right to restrict the use of an intermediary to the defendant's evidence). However, none of these cases are concerned with deaf intermediaries who, arguably, perform a function that is not readily apparent to the hearing court. The arguments in support of having the assistance of a deaf intermediary throughout the trial, as opposed to during the extent of the defendant's evidence, should cite the importance of context in bi-modal communication and the need for familiarity with idiosyncratic signs.

A CRM/4 Application should be made (as for the experts) for prior authority for an assessment by a deaf intermediary and thereafter, an application to the court for the granting of an intermediary under the Criminal Procedure Rules.

Issues that can arise when an intermediary is used
If a deaf intermediary is used, then this will be in addition to the use of interpreters. As this entails introducing another person into the chain of interpretation, this is likely to involve additional linguistic changes between the source and target language and it will also lengthen the time estimate of the proceedings.

Deaf Relays (see Chapter D4)
A deaf defendant who has been diagnosed with a learning disability or language deprivation, but who is nevertheless considered fit to plead, will benefit from the services of a Deaf Relay. This is a deaf person who is used to working with deaf people who have additional needs. The Deaf Relay will work with interpreters to assist communication by adding clarifying information. If this is to be done, then any additions will need to be sanctioned by the court at the time of communication.

Written communication
Where the case depends on written documentation, it may be necessary

---

[5] Which inserts ss.33BA and 33BB into the Youth Justice and Criminal Evidence Act 1999 thereby bringing about parity of special measures between witnesses and defendants.

to have these documents translated into BSL and video recorded, so that the translation is available for the defendant to view when giving instructions.

This will require prior authority for costs in excess of £100 and so a CRM/4 will need to be submitted. Those matters stated in the introduction to this chapter should be included in the application.

Visual recording of court proceedings
Court proceedings, and specifically evidence given, is audio recorded. This audio recording of the voice over is not the original evidence or an exact replication of that evidence.

Where defendants or witnesses are profoundly deaf, there is no accurate audio recording of evidence given in BSL. If there are disputes about what was signed or how it was signed, the court cannot return to the evidence to check it. Likewise, there can be no proper peer review of, for example, disagreements between the interpreters and/or the intermediary.

Consideration should therefore be given to video recording the deaf witness/defendant's evidence. This has been achieved in at least one case, R v H and another at Snaresbrook Crown Court June 2014. This case involved deaf witnesses and deaf defendants as well as the translation from ASL into BSL. A deaf media company provided a camera man who filmed the evidence in the court room. At the end of each day the recordings were downloaded and stored securely on the court file. Funding was provided by the court[6]. If it is proposed to record any part of the evidence, then this should be raised with the court at the Plea and Trial Preparation Hearing (PTPH).

Links to resources
See The Advocate's Gateway - https://www.theadvocatesgateway.org/
Toolkit 11 of the Advocates Gateway concerns 'Planning to question someone who is deaf'.

---

[6] For further discussion see "Making Special Measures Special: Reasonable Adjustments for Deaf Witnesses and Defendants "Dr Sue O'Rourke and Clare Wade in Addressing Vulnerability in Justice Systems eds. Penny Cooper and Linda Hunting Wildy Simmonds and Hill Publishing 2016.

17 Safeguarding vulnerable adults
Asher Woodman-Worrell

Terminology
I will be using the term 'deaf' to refer to all deaf, deafblind and hard of hearing people irrespective of their identity, cultural and language experience for the purpose of the brevity for readers. There are multiple elements in this chapter that are applicable for safeguarding work with deafblind people but this area will not be covered in depth as this is a specialist field best written by an expert in that field.

Introduction
Whilst the information in this chapter should support the reader in safeguarding work with deaf people, this knowledge is ultimately gained through years of practical work within the deaf communities. Therefore, this information will need to be supplemented by the reader's professional judgement, organisational policies, and ethical practice. Where possible, co-working with deaf specialist services is strongly recommended. Links to supportive information or agencies are included throughout the chapter.

This chapter will be discussing deaf people who are unable to protect themselves in the eyes of Care Act (2014), either because they have care/support needs, or because they have differing life experiences associated with their deafness.

However, it is important to understand that deaf people are diverse, just like the mainstream society, and have differing composition of traits that form their identities. This means the work with deaf people should be person centred with recognition that not all deaf people are the same and with an understanding that there are many capacitous deaf people who are capable of being involved in their decision making, rather than to be seen as vulnerable because they are deaf.

Risk factors
Power balance/dependence
The socio-historical relationship between deaf people and their hearing peers is an important factor to note, particularly in safeguarding work with the elderly deaf population. Historically, deaf communities have been

supported by hearing missionaries, social workers or teachers. These senior figures, in positions of power, were often the only source of information, thus creating unequal relationships.

As a result of this disempowerment, some deaf people may become dependent on their support network (family, friends or professionals), believing that hearing people (or even deaf people in positions of power) 'know best' and must be listened to. Well-meaning family or friends can unintentionally impede a deaf person's views and wishes by being a point of contact for them, putting forward their collective views without offering opportunities for the deaf person to do the same. However, this can also be consciously exploited in varying manners:
- abuser-victim relationship in domestic violence scenarios
- relationships between people in senior care professions controlling the information that the deaf client can access
- 'carers' using their privileges to groom victims
- 'carers' promoting themselves as the deaf client's 'point of contact' or 'interpreter', thus preventing the client disclosing abuse

An abuser's belief that their victims' vulnerability prevents them from disclosing abuse, tends to increase the scale of the abuse. Even if the deaf person has managed to leave the unequal power relationship or to take steps to address the power balance, they may subsequent have a distorted understanding of healthy relationship boundaries which may increase their vulnerability for future relationship abuse.

Institutional abuse within Deaf schools has been well documented (see Chapter F2). Whether the deaf person has experienced abuse as a child or an adult, it is important to understand the circumstances of this, in order to take preventative actions and reduce the risk of future abuse.

Poor education provision/delayed language acquisition (see Chapters C6 & B1)
It is sadly not uncommon that deaf children do not get appropriate levels of support or language input. This can negatively impact their developmental milestones, including cognitive aspects of development such as critical thinking, information processing and problem solving; language aspects such as comprehension, communication, reading and writing; and aspects of emotional literacy that affects both their self-care and their awareness of other's needs or motivations.

In the context of vulnerability this may result in some deaf children, young people and adults being unable to understand or weigh up information. They are then exposed to risks, or make risky and unwise decisions, that see them potentially embroiled in safeguarding situations.

Communication barriers

Your deaf client may use signed language, such as British Sign Language (BSL) (see Chapter C8). They may combine lipreading, residual hearing, and speaking (see Chapter D10), or use one of the deafblind communication systems (see chapter D11).

You may need to work alongside an interpreter (Chapter D2), a lip speaker (Chapter D9) or a relay interpreter (Chapter D4). You will definitely need to adapt your own communication style to meet the needs of your deaf client (see Chapters D10 and D14).

For a deaf person in a predominantly hearing world, they may have difficulties accessing educational information to help them stay safe or report concerns (whether for themselves or others). A deaf person who is already vulnerable can be made more vulnerable because their pathway to requesting help is not clear. Even once a safeguarding process has been initiated, if appropriate communication adaptions are not put in place, communication breakdown can prevent effective information sharing.

The majority of safeguarding resources (leaflets, websites, helplines) are not 'deaf friendly'. Educational information for deaf people to identify signs of abuse, especially for emerging forms of abuse such as Female Genital Mutilation, Hate Crime or Honour Based Violence, will need to be translated (in BSL, captions, Easyread etc.) and provided to the deaf communities in places where they will access them (e.g. deaf TV channels, deaf websites, deaf clubs, deaf schools etc.).

When considering the communication needs of your deaf client, consider also whether they have concurrent communication needs associated with: Autistic Spectrum Disorder (see Chapters E4 & E5); Intellectual Disability (see Chapter E3); mental health issues (see Section F); language deprivation (see Chapter B1); or as a non-native BSL user (Chapter D13).

Isolation v interconnected nature of deaf communities

Many deaf people live in isolation, often being the only deaf person in their family, school, or town (see Chapter F1), making it difficult to share information or support. However, for those members of the signing Deaf community, their relatively small population size, results in a degree of interconnectedness, that is only known to the hearing population in island or frontier communities.

Deaf people from a wide geographical area can know each other from schools, social clubs, sport teams or working for deaf organisations. This effect is magnified for deaf people living the same region.

This can become a significant factor in safeguarding work. The disclosure process can be a difficult and anxious experience if the perpetrator(s) are well-known in the local deaf community, or if the offence is committed by people or systems within deaf organisations. Professionals who have special deaf knowledge are valuable in terms of communication and cultural knowledge but governance or confidentiality can be compromised if professionals involved in the Safeguarding are also known to the service user on a recreational basis. Similarly, this can be difficult for interpreters who may have worked with the service user in other settings.

To maximise confidentiality, managers should check with the professionals, before the case allocation, to determine whether they know the service user. The service users should be consulted to confirm that they are comfortable with the allocated professionals. Where timing and safety allows, the service users should also be consulted about their interpreter preferences and this should be fed back to the interpreting agencies in an anonymous manner during the bookings.

Example: A deaf client who had disclosed abuse, did not want to work with face to face interpreters, who would be based locally to her, as she was concerned they may have worked with her previously at her college course. It was agreed that an online interpreter from well out of the client's area would be booked.

The professionals working in safeguarding situations with deaf people may need extra training and supervision to manage the challenges of ethical working in such small communities and to disclose and manage confidentiality issues.

Good practice in safeguarding work with deaf people
Deaf/sensory professionals

Where possible reach out to sensory teams and deaf professionals working in social/health care. Whilst some information can be shared through supervision or training, other information is so nuanced that only joint working with someone who has years of experience working with deaf people will suffice.

Example: A sensory social worker was jointly working with a mainstream childrens' social worker, on a case involving a deaf child and a hearing parent. During a home visit, the mainstream social worker was concerned that the child appeared to repeatedly look across to the parent. The social worker flagged a potential concern, hypothesising that the child was scared of the parent and was checking for permission before answering. However, the sensory social worker's deaf awareness helped him realise that the child was actually lipreading the parent and needed to look at them. This avoided the potential escalation of a sensitive situation.

If there are no deaf or sensory professionals in your organisation, then it would be wise to engage immediate deaf awareness training and to consider the recruitment of deaf/sensory professionals.

Independent advocates

The Care Act (2014) requires the Local Authorities to support vulnerable people to express their views and feelings, and to involve them in decision making, including individuals who have substantial difficulty in being involved and do not have any appropriate individuals to support them.

The appointment of independent Advocates provides the client with a neutral medium who can support them in information provision and decision making. Their role is not that of an interpreter but to support the information sharing process: ensuring information is fully understood by all parties; working with deaf individuals outside of meetings to support information comprehension; ensuring the deaf individual's views are heard during the proceedings.

Where the deaf client has supportive family or friends, but there are concerns about interdependence or power imbalance, the Advocate can enable the deaf client to have greater autonomy. There are several deaf organisations/charities that can provide trained Care Act Advocates:

https://royaldeaf.org.uk/services/for-professionals/advocacy/
https://www.deafplus.org/advocacy/
https://signhealth.org.uk/for-professionals/advocacy/

Alternative deaf organisations, local to you, may be able to offer this service or signpost to those that can.

Technology resources

Advances in technology are a useful resource in safeguarding work. EmergencySMS is a texting services that enables service users to contact emergency services over text. TapSOS is a similar service, allowing service users to contact emergency services with pictorial aids to compose their text messages.

Contact the local Telecare/Careline services that are relevant to your client to enquire whether they have email/texting facilities in place, and to request they note your client's needs. Police services are also able to designate target priority response for deaf service users.

Video Interpreting Relay Service providers connect two parties in two separate locations via a remote video call with a sign language interpreter. Check that your regional police department is using this facility.

There are also accessible helplines for deaf service users to contact if they wish to report or discuss safeguarding concerns. Both adults and children can contact Childline online via live chat, text or Video Relay Service: https://www.childline.org.uk/get-support/contacting-childline/#BSL-counselling

Shout and Crisis Text Line also offer 24/7 texting facility for deaf service users experiencing crisis:
https://signhealth.org.uk/with-deaf-people/crisis-text-service/#:~:text=If%20you%20need%20immediate%20support,information%20you%20feel%20comfortable%20with

RelayUK is a specialist software that offers text relay for deaf service users to conduct telephone conversations either by typing or speaking on the phone so the operator can type responses: https://www.relayuk.bt.com/

There are charities that have developed accessible educational videos about safeguarding abuse in BSL format. SignHealth have developed a series of informative videos in the domestic abuse section of their website. NSPCC has developed the Underwear Rule campaign video which educates children on how to stay safe from sexual abuse:
https://www.nspcc.org.uk/keeping-children-safe/support-for-parents/pants-underwear-rule/

ThinkUKnow and Childline have developed a series of videos for young children on staying safe online and from bullying:
https://www.thinkuknow.co.uk/parents/jessie-and-friends-BSL/
https://www.childline.org.uk/info-advice/bullying-abuse-safety/deaf-zone/bsl-videos/

British Deaf Association, North Yorkshire Police, Derbyshire Police and Zebra Uno have also published videos to raise awareness around hate crime:
https://bda.org.uk/project/hate-crime-project/
https://www.zebra-access.com/projects/hate-crime-bsl-project
https://northyorkshire.police.uk/news/north-yorkshire-police-release-british-sign-language-video-about-hate-crime/

Conclusion

Deaf people may become involved in safeguarding proceedings for all the same reasons as hearing people. For some, they may experience additional risks due to being exposed to different cultural factors linked to their deafness. The improvement in your team's deaf awareness, co-working with deaf/sensory specialist services and making full use of technological resources will support and empower deaf people's autonomy and Safeguarding teams' functioning.

18 Deaf Registered Intermediaries for vulnerable deaf clients
Louise Harte, Craig Flynn and Chris Bojas

The many stages of the Criminal Justice System (CJS) process can be stressful and confusing. Registered Intermediaries are specialists in communication, provided for children and vulnerable adults to maximise their engagement with the CJS. They are registered with, and employed by, the Ministry of Justice (MOJ) Service and follow a Code of Conduct.

Intermediaries work to promote the equality of access to justice for vulnerable people. Their services are obtained either by the police, the Crown Prosecution Service or the family court and can be provided to victims, witnesses and defendants, for the prosecution and defence.

The MOJ code of practice for Registered Intermediaries states:
"The primary responsibility of the intermediary is to enable complete, coherent and accurate communication to take place between a witness who requires special measures and the court" (point 1)

Intermediaries were first endorsed as a result of the Speaking Up for Justice report in 1998, which gave rise to the Youth Justice and Criminal Evidence Act (1999). The intention is to increase both the number of witnesses able to give evidence and the validity of the evidence given – as well as increasing general confidence in the CJS.

An intermediary will be involved throughout the whole process, from the initial investigation to the trial or hearing. They use their expertise in communication to assess the client's communication needs and skills. Their report is used as the basis for a meeting with the Judge and barristers, or magistrates in a court case. It sets out clearly how the vulnerable witness will be assisted, what strategies will be used, and how any difficulties (like needing breaks or not being able to answer a question) will be dealt with. This is called a Ground Rules Hearing.

The report includes advice and recommendations for the police and court officials, covering areas such as:
- how to phrase questions in a way that will be easily understood.
- how to assist the vulnerable person to give as much detail as possible
- what adaptations and resources will the client need to convey their message

The intermediary works with the client to:
- provide strategies so that the client can give evidence and explain what happened clearly and coherently
- assist them in understanding the trial or tribunal, to follow its actions, and to understand any judgements that are made
- to make informed choices and make their opinions known

The intermediary, having taken the intermediary oath, assists the client during the giving of evidence. They sit alongside the witness in the live link room (or stand next to them if they are giving evidence in court) to continually monitor the two-way communication. The intermediary is empowered to intervene during questioning, to assert the ground rules and recommendations of their report.

There are numerous types of communication specialist who work as intermediaries. Some are Speech and Language Therapists, some are experts in working with people with learning disabilities and others from mental health or other clinical backgrounds.

Deaf Registered Intermediaries
There are currently 4 Deaf Registered Intermediaries who are fluent in sign language. Where the client is a sign language user, working with a linguistic and cultural match is of huge benefit.

British Sign Language (BSL) is a visual, gestural language which differs in structure to spoken and written English. As such the role of the intermediary can involve some cultural and linguistic mediation if this assists the deaf person to understand what is being asked of them. If the deaf witness has an idiosyncratic style of sign language, then this linguistic mediation will be required to a greater degree.

It is important to recognise the difference between an MOJ intermediary, a British Sign Language (BSL) Interpreter (Chapter D1) and a Deaf Relay Interpreter (Chapter D4). The roles are fundamentally different. The parameters that an intermediary works within are much wider.

Intermediaries will advise which interpreters are most suitable to meet the deaf person's needs. When the deaf person is giving evidence, they will often recommend that all communication goes through them.

The intermediary will be very familiar with the background of the case and the level of understanding the deaf person has. The boundary of their role allows them to engage with the court and the deaf person in the way that a BSL interpreter or a Deaf Relay Interpreter cannot.

Information will be conveyed in a way that is meaningful to the deaf person by taking account any limitations or gaps in their knowledge (see Chapter B4), understanding (particularly of legal knowledge), and life experiences. If the deaf person does not fully understand information or questions put to them, the intermediary can rephrase and explain further.

It may be assumed that Deaf Registered Intermediaries are only able to work with clients who use BSL or other visual forms of communication. However, due to the common 'deaf experience', the personal understanding of communication barriers, and the visual platform, Deaf Registered Intermediaries can create an effective working relationship with clients who have a degree of hearing loss and who use spoken English and/or lip reading.

Further information is available on the Ministry of Justice website.
https://www.gov.uk/guidance/ministry-of-justice-witness-intermediary-scheme

I9 Discrimination laws
Abigail Gorman

"The purpose of the present Convention is to promote, protect and ensure the full and equal enjoyment of all human rights and fundamental freedoms by all persons with disabilities, and to promote respect for their inherent dignity. Persons with disabilities include those who have long-term physical, mental, intellectual or sensory impairments which in interaction with various barriers may hinder their full and effective participation in society on an equal basis with others" UNCPRD - Article 1

The United Nations Regional Centre for Peace and Disarmament (UNRCPD) is an international treaty, ratified by 182 states, and has 9 signatories[7]. The UK ratified the UNRCPD treaty in 2009, agreeing to work towards creating a society where disabled people are treated with the same dignity and respect as non-disabled citizens.

For the Deaf community, achieving this would be evidenced by improved outcomes for Deaf people in the following areas of their lives:
- health
- education
- employment
- access to justice
- personal security
- independent living
- access to information

However, the 2017 shadow report submitted by Disability Rights UK, Disability Wales and Inclusion Scotland highlighted the ongoing issues faced by disabled people in the UK, many of whom were not seeing any material change in their day to day lives. As a result, the shadow report listed a summary of twenty significant areas of concern, with the expectation that the government should be held accountable for improving outcomes for disabled people.

The wide reaching consequences of not doing so can be seen across every aspect of disabled people's lives, as referrals to front line support services have increased and resource availability has been reduced.

---

[7] Indicators.ohchr.org

The report can be found at: https://www.disabilityrightsuk.org/sites/default/files/pdf/GBUNCRPD30Feb2017.pdf

Public sector legal duties

All public authorities have a legal responsibility to give due regard to the Public Sector Equality Duty (PSED) of the Equality Act 2010. One of the key principles is promoting equality and working actively to reduce inequalities. It is not enough to simply consider this duty; you are required to evidence your compliance by demonstrating that you have been able to implement positive changes. Non-compliance puts you at an increased risk of legal action.

https://assets.publishing.service.gov.uk/government/uploads/system/uploads/attachment_data/file/85041/equality-duty.pdf

Internal audits are a useful tool to highlight areas where those bodies can work to eliminate discrimination, harassment and victimisation. This in turn helps to build positive relationships with people who have relevant protected characteristics. You can do this by ensuring that you are following a robust equalities policy and that all staff have received appropriate training. Working in this way helps to close the gap on health care inequality, giving patients better access to care and treatment, which will optimise healthcare outcomes.

Deaf people and social inequality

Deaf people are a part of mainstream society, whilst also inhabiting a culture that is distinct. Over the years, many Deaf people have experienced early years language deprivation (see Chapter B1). Consequently, as adults they may not have acquired the requisite tools to navigate a hearing world with ease.

Deaf people often face systemic barriers throughout their lives, and complaints resulting from audism (see Chapter C10) often arise.

Audism is a form of discrimination that is based on the idea that because a person is Deaf, they either: do not have the same capacity to make informed decisions as a hearing person would; or, their life is somehow less worthy because they are Deaf. Audism is also present when professionals do not adequately meet the needs of the Deaf person.

For instance, spoken language is a more prevalent method of communication for the majority of professionals, whereas interactions in sign language may be less frequent and seem incidental by comparison. Because members of the deaf community have discreet cultural needs, professionals may not initially be aware of their own training requirements and may struggle to adequately meet the needs of the Deaf person that they are working with. That lack of professional knowledge can result in well intentioned professional decisions being made, that ultimately put deaf people at a substantial disadvantage because provision is modelled on the support needs of a hearing population.

Examples:
- *A Deaf patient who is experiencing mental health difficulties is placed in a ward where no one is able to use sign language. This may exacerbate already poor mental health because of reduced access to information, no peer support and an increased risk of misdiagnosis.*
- *A court case involving a Deaf person may collapse if it goes ahead without an appropriately qualified and experienced interpreter being booked; or worse, a miscarriage of justice may occur.*

When working with Deaf people, service providers need to consider not just the person's deafness, but any other associated health (Chapter G1), mental health (Chapter G2) cognitive (Chapter E2) or literacy issues (Chapter B3), they may have, in order to get the best outcome.

In the eyes of the law, a failure to make reasonable adjustments based on a protected characteristic is considered 'Direct Discrimination' as stated in the Equality Act 2010.

Equality Act: Section 20 - Duty to make adjustments
https://www.legislation.gov.uk/ukpga/2010/15/section/20

There are three requirements under this section.
1. To ensure that your provision, criteria or practice does not place a disabled person at a substantial disadvantage and to take steps to avoid this from happening.

Example - Barrier from provision, criteria or practice: Ensure you have a communication plan in place. Identify the language requirements of the Deaf person. Create a list of agencies or local language service professionals you can contact should you require communication support.

2. If a physical feature prevents a person from accessing your service, steps must be taken to rectify this.

Example - Make sure that Deaf people can access your service by ensuring that your staff are familiar with Relay UK, a text relay service; as well as providing access via a Video Relay Service (Chapter D7), making it easier for Deaf sign language users to contact you directly. It should also be taken into consideration that Relay UK may not be suitable for some deaf people due to literacy skills. Any resources that you release into the public domain should have an in-vision sign language interpreter included as standard. All verbal announcements made should have an equivalent display, which includes visual announcements. Examples can include visual queuing systems or health and safety information.

3. Where the first or third requirement relates to the provision of information, you must enable access via an 'auxiliary aid' (e.g. qualified sign language interpreter) to ensure that the disabled person is not substantially disadvantaged.

Example - Interpreters should be appropriately qualified and experienced, and registered with a regulatory body (see Chapter D1). Interpreters are required to be impartial. It is not appropriate to rely on friends or family to relay information because you cannot assess accuracy. If you use a friend or family member for acquiring informed consent, you run the risk of a medical negligence claim. In instances where the deaf person has idiosyncratic language or BSL is not their first language, you will need to book an interpreting team that consists of a Deaf relay interpreter (Chapter D4) as well as a sign language interpreter - they will work together to get the best outcome.

It should also be noted that a person who is required to provide the service cannot expect the disabled person to financially contribute to access adjustments. As a service provider, refusing to provide a service because of a client's specific needs is unlawful discrimination. A service provider is not allowed to treat a person in a way that leads to a disproportionately worse experience. By doing so, this places the person at a substantial disadvantage when compared to other clients, based on protected characteristics.

Service providers are expected to comply with the law and provide a reasonable adjustment, unless they can evidence that the requirement is deemed unreasonable.

Accessible Information Standard and Disability laws
SignHealth's 'Sick Of It' report (see Chapter G1) was cited by Lord Howe as instrumental in helping to shape the Accessible Information Standard (AIS).

https://www.england.nhs.uk/ourwork/accessibleinfo/

As of 2016, organisations providing NHS care and/or publicly funded adult social care are legally required to follow the Accessible Information Standard. This includes establishing an individual's communication preferences from the outset.

When dealing with Deaf patients, it is important to take into consideration that there are varying levels of deafness; one size does not fit all. The Deaf community is diverse, and you cannot assume that just because a person is deaf, they will have the same needs.

Summary
Following these steps will ensure that you are complying with laws related to discrimination through service provision. Ensuring correct access, at the time it is needed, supports cost efficacy and relieves the burden on other services. It will help to reduce complaints regarding poor treatment and care and avoid financial repercussions for your service and CCG. Most importantly, it will ensure that your client is treated with respect and dignity. Failure to meet the needs of deaf people can leave you vulnerable to litigation, not just for discrimination, but also for professional negligence.

Section J

The future of services for deaf and Hard of Hearing people
Dr Sally Austen and Dr Ben Holmes

Whilst this book will have made some impact on access to services for deaf and Hard of Hearing (HOH) people, there is still much to do. And it needs to be done on a much, much wider scale.

Preventable conditions

It is appalling that, despite living in a wealthy country, with a highly prized health and education system, language deprivation is still allowed to persist. We have the knowledge and resources to prevent this. Greater co-working is needed so that people are not caused to suffer unnecessarily.

Discrimination

Despite the Equality Act (2010) and Accessible Information Standard (2016), deaf and HOH people are still treated unequally: in the health system, the legal system, in education, the workplace and in everyday life. Much greater awareness and action to eliminate this is needed.

Diversity

It has been difficult to do justice, even in an 84-chapter book, to the diversity of deaf and HOH people. Whilst it is easier to share knowledge that is categorised, we are (and should remain) aware that each person is uniquely formed by their own bio-psycho-social experiences.

We really hope the reader now understands that their services must be adapted to each person's differing communication, cultural and cognitive strengths, and needs.

Research

Where we had thought research in this field was limited by quantity, we now realise its limitation is that it is siloed.

To truly learn, and therefore benefit our clients, we must strive to gather and share data through multidisciplinary and multi-system approaches: deaf and HOH researchers, experts by experience, health, education, social care, commissioners and policy makers etc., until we are sufficiently informed to provide the best service for our clients.

Economies of scale
Whilst providing accessible services for HOH people (one in five of the population) should undoubtedly be expected of all service providers, there are more difficult planning issues to consider for less numerate groups, (e.g. older sign language users who require nursing home care or deaf children who need inpatient mental health services).

The predominant commissioning focus on economies of scale blights service access for people whose needs are different to the majority. Implicit competition that is encouraged between services only creates gaps that increase access difficulties. Further consideration of this is needed to determine more appropriate forms of service provision.

Continuing Professional Development (CPD)
Most often, we do not know what we do not know. Thus, requests for vital training in areas covered by this book might be limited.

Generic services are unlikely to commission training in how to work with deaf and HOH people and most likely to choose CPD topics that affect the greatest number of their clients.

Deaf specialists are mostly employed with specific remits (e.g. a particular client cohort or a specific geographical region). The conveyance of knowledge thus often falls to volunteers, which is both unfair and un-audited. Formalising funding and evaluation of the provision of such education is therefore crucial and should be centrally coordinated.

Co-working
The term 'deaf specialist' rightly refers to brilliant providers of services to deaf and HOH clients by professionals who themselves may be deaf, HOH, or hearing. However, a referral to a 'deaf specialist' does not replace the need for co-working.

Deaf specialists cannot replicate or replace **every** skill that **you the readers** have in **every** part of the country to **every** potential client. Whilst we consider ourselves good all-round clinicians, it would be unprofessional of us to work alone with deaf clients whose difficulties we are less skilled in supporting (e.g. eating disorders or perinatal psychosis). Likewise, our contributing authors include some of the best deaf clinicians and researchers in the country (if not the world) but you wouldn't want them to lead the treatment for your deaf client's burst appendix!

Commissioning and resource difficulties appear to be fuelling a belief that making a referral means moving the client from team A to team B, releasing team A from any responsibility for the client. However, a client with a presentation of multiple factors will be best served by the skills of multiple teams. Attempting to move the client into someone else's service can delay or reduce the help the client receives.

It is only through co-working that these gaps in access can be filled.

Conclusion
We very much hope this book will benefit you, your service and the people that access your service, so that we can all work together to improve the experience for deaf and HOH clients.

Section K

Working with a deaf or hard of hearing (DHH) young person in CAMHS
Dr Constanza Moreno

Working with a deaf or hard of hearing (DHH) young person in CAMHS
In addition to using strategies for effective communication (also known as 'deaf awareness'), when working with a young person with a hearing loss, we need to be aware of differences in:
- Communication
- Incidental learning
- Awareness of one's own communication needs
- Identity

It is unlikely that you will be able to cover all the work that you would typically cover with a hearing young person in a session.

The following information is provided to help guide you in your interactions with any deaf young people you may meet. You are welcome to copy and use this handout in your appointments.

Communication

The DHH young person may have a limited vocabulary, such as for emotions or synonyms of emotions. Sometimes, phrases are used differently (e.g. 'blackmail' is used to mean 'threaten' physically by some young deaf people):
- Check the young person has understood the concepts you use
- Check you have understood their use of language

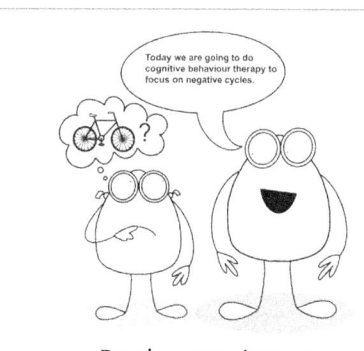

Don't ... use jargon	Do ... use clear language

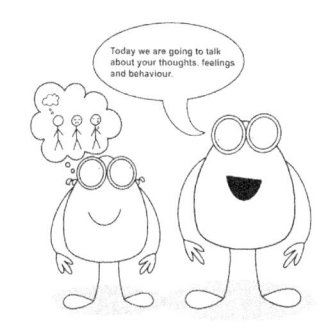

Literacy may be less developed in DHH young people than the typically developing young person. Some **_hate_** writing:
- Be aware of this if you set 'homework' tasks in therapy
- Setting writing and / or reading tasks could impact a lot on the therapeutic engagement

Check how the young person feels about writing, and how this may impact on self-esteem and their views of themselves as learners.

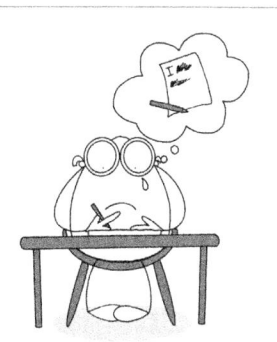

Don't ... make assumptions about literacy ability in homework	Do ... set homework tasks that the young person feels able to do

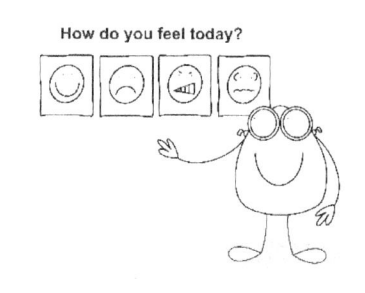

Created by Dr Constanza Moreno at National Deaf CAMHS (London team) & illustrations by Ms Shanée Buxton

Incidental learning

Emotional literacy is often less developed in DHH people, specifically: the ability to name and label emotions in self and others; the realisation that there is a range of intensity within each emotion; and this can lead to frustration and result in aggressive and / or externalising behaviour:
- Encourage the family to label emotional states and explain why people are behaving the way they are
- Model and role play different emotional states and range in session
- Express problem solving strategies (i.e. say thinking 'out loud' so the young person can see your thinking)
- Include direct teaching and modelling about what to do in different emotional situations (e.g. what to do / say when a person is upset)
- Discuss emotions, reactions and consequences to behaviours from TV story lines or real situations

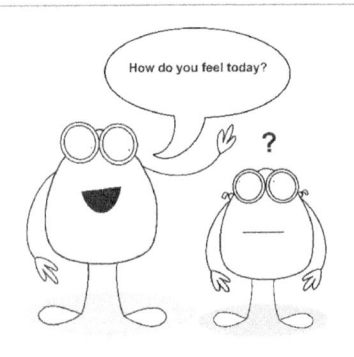

Don't ... assume the young person has same emotional literacy development as a hearing peer	Do ... use lots of different ways to talk / teach / model emotions

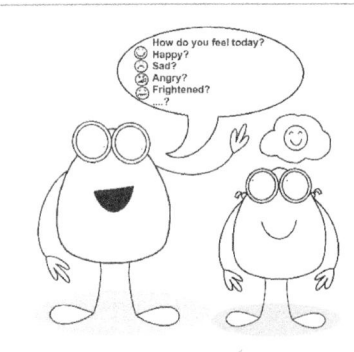

The young person cannot access surrounding sound and conversation with their hearing aids / cochlear implants in the same way a hearing person can. Lots of information about the world is missed.
- Check the young person is a part of all the conversations about care and future plans

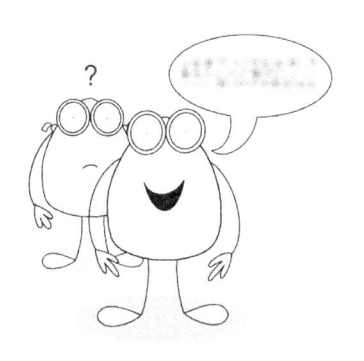

Don't... have 'corridor' conversations, lip reading and walking at the same time is tricky	Do... make sure the DHH young person can see you when you're talking

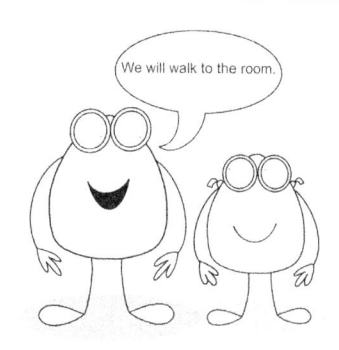

The young person may have 'patchy knowledge' about the world so although they seem to know about some age appropriate topics (e.g. Harry Potter or the latest films or games), they lack knowledge about topics that appear more simple (e.g. family structures or names of their relatives) or emotions that are required to fully understand the more complex information
- Check background concepts (e.g. in explaining therapeutic models in psycho-education)
- Help the family understand this lack of knowledge and how to compensate for this by explicit teaching and providing a 'running commentary' on what is happening

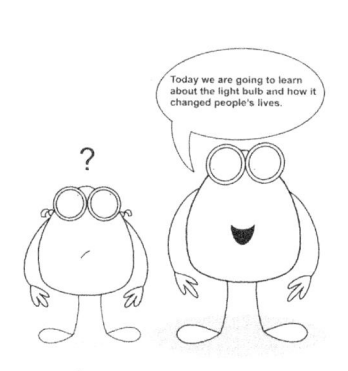

Don't ... assume person understands topics fully	Do ... check understanding of topics and explicitly teach to any gaps

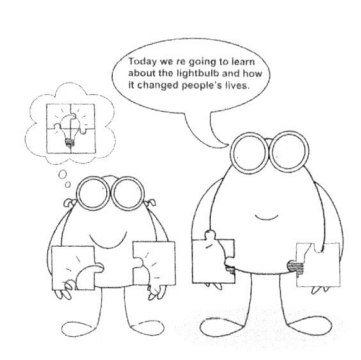

The young person may not know society's rules or norms that others pick up through over-hearing and observing.
- Check that the rules are clear
- Check assumed knowledge has been made explicit
- Teach the young person explicitly how to teach games

Teach the young person explicitly what to expect in different situations (e.g. at the hairdresssers, shops etc.)

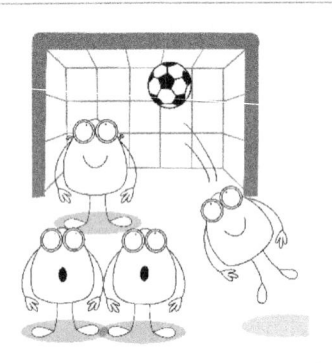

Don't ... assume knowledge of norms or laws	Do ... make the rules / norms / expectations clear

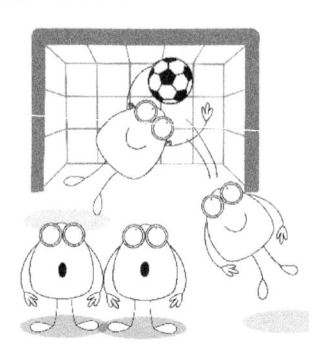

Awareness of one's own communication needs

Lip reading is tiring but the young person may not realise that they rely on lip reading
- Don't always wait for the young person to tell you they are tired. They may not realise the reason for feeling tired, or feel too embarrassed to say

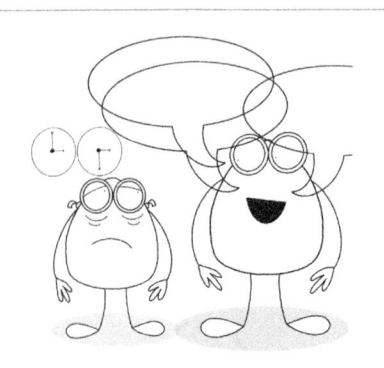

Don't ... rely on the young person to tell you they are tired/need a break	Do ... factor in lots of breaks

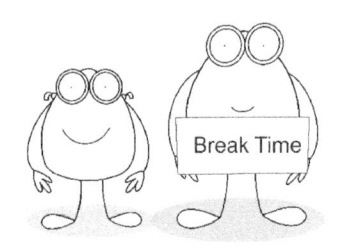

Hearing aids can break, batteries can run out, environmental noises vary, people's accents vary, the loudness of peoples' voices vary, 'acoustic friendliness' (e.g. whether sound echoes etc.) varies. Levels of tiredness and frustration vary.
- A DHH person has to learn about lots of factors that can impact on their ability to understand, this can take time and an acceptance of their level of hearing / deaf identity.
- Don't assume that the young person has already understood and accepted all of the above

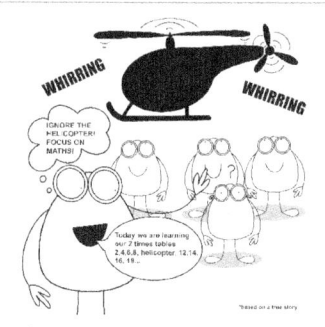

Don't … assume that DHH young person knows all about and can manage their deafness	Do … think about the environment you are having your sessions in – background noise? Think about shorter sessions

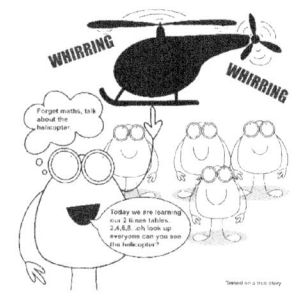

A young person may not be used to managing their own communication. Their parents and teachers may make many decisions on their behalf.
- Be explicit and support the young person to make choices (e.g. "Can you see my face well if I sit here?", "Tell me if my voice is too loud or quiet", "Shall I use more pictures to explain this?"
- Encourage the young person to explore what may help in different contexts (e.g. subtitles, drawings, notetakers)

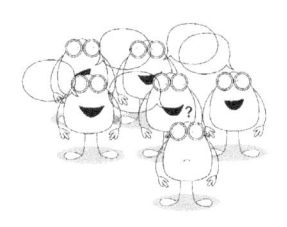

Don't … wait for the DHH young person to tell you if they are struggling to understand	Do … ask clear questions about your communication

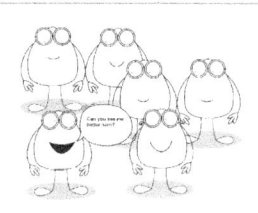

Identity

To develop our identity we need to meet other people who are like us. Lots of young people with a hearing loss don't meet others who they identify as like them. Providing opportunities to meet other DHH young people can facilitate this. For example,
- Accessing deaf events (e.g. National deaf Children's Society organised events)
- Contacting UK Deaf Sport for local organisations
- Drama companies (including Deafinitely theatre)

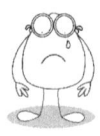

Don't ... underestimate the loneliness of not ever meeting or knowing anybody who is 'like you'	Do ... encourage activities with other DHH young people

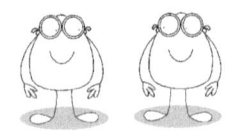

Use technology and visual aids to facilitate inclusion and communication
- Use photos as conversation starters and to share information
- Texts can also be used within social networks and to practise communicating with adults who agree to this
- Most people now use tablets and internet technology to communicate and participate in social groups
- Facilitate and ensure the young person is able to use this technology in a safe way with explicit teaching

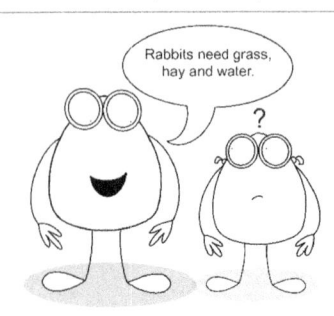

Don't ... be shy about using technology and visual aids	Do ... use visual aids and technology to communicate and teach appropriate use

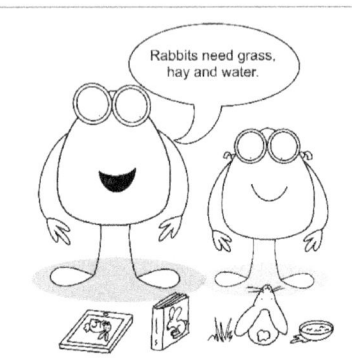

Section L

Index

1880 Milan conference 66, 71
abstract thinking 23-24, 42,45, 101, 201, 228, 357
abuse 20, 53, 67, 78, 98, 134, 180, 198-203, 210, 225, 235-236, 251, 253, 265, 304, 324, 327, 341, 345, 369-375
Access to Work (ATW) 78, 109, 127, 129
Accessible Information Standard (2016) 33, 109, 141, 383, 386
acoustic(s) 32, 122, 124-125, 306, 395
acquired hearing loss 176, 205-206, 332
adjustment
  of communication 100, 103, 106, 123, 169, 225
  to hearing loss 204, 208-209
  and identity 330
  reasonable adjustments 79, 247, 265, 268, 381-382
advocate 80, 250-251, 343, 358-359, 361, 373
All About Me: Care Program 249
Alport's syndrome 304, 321-322
anger 23, 86, 156, 178, 203, 253, 257-260, 262, 265, 310, 326
anxiety 117, 134, 156, 164, 174, 188, 192, 206-208, 213, 223-224, 279, 294-296, 308-309, 312,
arrest 257, 263, 336-337
ASD/autism 27, 37, 160-171, 330
assistance dog 129
Assistive Listening Devices (ALD)s 123, 125-126
attachment 58, 71, 157, 200, 349, 352
audiology/audiologist/audiological 57-58, 79, 125-126, 154, 206, 280, 308-309, 317, 320-321,
audism 18, 84-85, 291, 380
auditory neuropathy (AN) 323
Automated Auditory Brainstem Response (AABR) 56, 323
bi-modal communication 367
bipolar disorder 210, 223
bilingual 52, 60-61, 63-64, 73-75, 275, 350

Bluetooth/wireless 126-127
boarding school 67-69, 180, 201
Body Integrity Identity Disorder 329
Bone Anchored Hearing Aids 126
boundaries 43, 110, 198, 245, 307, 352, 370
Branchio-oto-renal syndrome (BOR) 304, 322
broker/brokering 61-63, 180, 279
capacity 177-178, 338, 355-359, 362, 365-366, 380
cardiology 322
Cerebral palsy 131, 303, 306, 316
challenging behaviour 23, 26, 70, 98, 146, 156-157, 168, 178, 252-256, 267, 345
CHARGE syndrome 131, 160,
cochlear implants 21, 55, 57, 65-66, 73-74, 80, 124-127, 131, 142, 164, 174, 265, 279-280, 305, 316, 321, 328, 334, 392
CODA 51, 60-64, 277, 279
cognitive behavioural 206-207, 227
cognitive decline 149, 178-180
cognitive functioning 147-153, 155, 172, 178, 180, 183-189
cognitive impairment 42, 53, 344
commissioning of services 65, 158, 212, 229, 271, 274, 276-277, 280, 282-284, 294, 347, 387-388
confidentiality 93, 110, 140, 141, 186-187, 226, 237, 372
conflicted role 45, 62
conflict of interest 140
congenital rubella 81, 131, 160, 217, 241, 254, 303, 322
consanguineous marriages 320
consent 66, 79, 177, 185-186, 263, 344, 346, 358-359, 362, 382
conversion disorder 323-325, 327
court 118, 124, 147, 338-341, 348, 352-353, 361, 363-368, 376-378,
Covid-19 35, 79, 112, 118, 123, 148, 177, 183-184, 188, 232, 234, 361
criminal justice system 97, 201, 254, 256, 336, 342, 363, 376
'Crossing the Bridge' 329
cued speech 77

398

cytomegalovirus (CMV) 160, 241, 303
Deaf club 195, 213, 268, 371, 381
Deaf Parenting UK 64
deaf professionals 22, 27, 45, 58-59, 72, 78, 80, 92, 96, 108, 109, 158, 161, 169, 178, 186, 214, 232, 259, 265, 268, 275, 358-359, 373
Deaf Relay Interpreter (DRI) 24-25, 41, 92, 99, 105-108, 114, 139, 233, 247, 293-294, 338, 353, 357, 360, 362, 367-368
deafblind manual 130, 132
delayed discharge 287-288
delusion(s) 210, 212-213, 217
depression 27, 192-197, 206, 210, 244, 270, 293, 295-296, 232-234
desistance 347
diagnostic overshadowing 146, 170, 173, 253
dialect 52, 77, 96, 110, 113, 150-151, 181
discrimination 18, 30, 46, 203, 205, 253, 257, 271, 347, 379-383, 386
Down's Syndrome 14, 304, 316, 320, 322
duration of untreated psychosis (DUP) 211
EMDR 202
empathy 37, 40, 42, 71, 77, 160, 252, 347
endocrinologist 322
ENT (Ear, Nose and Throat) 309, 316-317, 320-321
Equality Act (2010) 79, 109, 141, 249, 380-381, 386
eugenics 319
exclusion 157-158, 192-195, 203, 265, 347
executive functioning 22, 43, 71, 74, 147, 152, 173, 252, 254-255
Expert Witness 183, 348
Expert Lipreader 118
eye break 124
eye contact 54-55, 94, 117, 143, 187, 202, 224, 258, 261, 264
Fabricated and Induced Illness (FII) 331
facial hair, impact on communication 115

facial expressions 50, 54, 76, 94, 120, 123, 134, 158, 160, 188, 215, 239, 241, 262, 266, 294
factitious deafness 323, 325
feigned deafness, 323, 325, 330-331
fetish 325, 331
forensic services 38, 342-347
fund of information 26, 34-36, 110, 232, 246, 258, 356-357
genetic cause of deafness 16, 131, 180, 302-303, 306, 319, 320
gesture 50, 54, 55, 74, 76, 115, 119, 120, 130, 151, 156, 158, 160, 358
graceful recovery 327
hallucination 210, 212-213, 217-222, 313
hands-on sign 130, 132
hearing aids 17, 21, 54, 56-57, 65, 70, 124-128, 131, 142, 154, 174, 176-177, 206, 231, 265, 307, 311, 321, 324-325, 329, 331, 334, 392, 395
Hearing Impaired Resource Bases (HIRB) 69
heart health 206, 317, 322
heritage signers 51, 60-64
heterogeneity of need 69, 149, 273, 289, 302
HMFD 60
identity 15-16, 50-51, 60-61, 63-64, 67, 84, 176, 194, 200, 205, 208, 221, 222, 272, 276-277, 279-280, 319, 322, 327, 369, 390, 395-396
idiosyncratic communication 101, 104-105, 114, 133, 259, 367, 377, 382,
inpatient admission 247-249, 251, 274-276, 280-281, 284-285, 287-288, 298-300, 387
integration 65, 69-70, 74, 79, 181, 277
intellectual disability; see learning disability
intermediary 103-104, 337-340, 343, 349, 350, 353, 355, 357, 366-368, 376-378
International Sign 77-78, 140
intralingual, deaf relay 92, 105, 107, 139

isolation 26-27, 38, 65, 134,
    156-158, 161, 163, 170, 176-179,
    192, 194, 203, 204, 206, 208,
    210, 248-249, 252, 255, 275,
    287, 341, 347, 352, 371
Lipspeaker 91-92, 118, 120-121,
    179, 243, 364
locus of control (LoC) 46-47, 228
loneliness 208, 326, 330, 396
loop system 14, 70, 125-128
mainstream school 69, 80, 151,
    279-280
Makaton 76, 77, 130, 156
malingering 333-335
Menieres disease 318
meningitis 31, 205, 254, 280, 303
    305-306, 320
Mental Health Act (MHA) 358, 360
misdiagnosis 27, 29, 138, 146, 155,
    161, 164, 169, 173, 177-178,
    211, 217, 287, 366, 381
motivation 38, 153, 193, 195, 210,
    252, 291, 293, 324-327, 370
Munchausen syndrome 325, 331
narcissism 326, 330
nephrologist 322
NHS England 263, 280, 284
nightmares 312
nodding 29-30, 44, 224, 242
non-verbal communication 50,
    134-135, 228, 257, 261
note taker 92, 232
obsessive 164
occupational therapist 78, 164, 169,
    276, 284, 321
ophthalmology 321
older deaf people 15, 18, 21, 67, 77,
    167, 170, 176-182, 240, 316,
    367, 387
Otoacoustic Emissions (OAE) 56, 323
otolaryngologist 321
ototoxic 240, 241, 303, 307
Paget Gorman 76-77
palantypists 92
paranoia 86, 196, 213, 218, 261, 266
partial hearing unit 69
peer group 63, 65, 67, 69, 70, 163,
    170, 226, 345
Pendred's Syndrome 322
perseveration 215

personal space 94, 260
personality disorder 86, 169, 174,
    281, 325, 331
pharmacist/pharmacology 173-174,
    244, 350
pre-therapy 40, 229-230, 232
premature 14, 81, 253, 346
presbycusis 16, 176
pressure of speech 215, 223-224
primary care 196, 283, 296
prison 14, 30, 231, 255, 262-265,
    267, 340-341
probation 38, 288, 338, 341
prosody 215
psychopath 331
psychosis 27, 29, 86, 104, 134, 169,
    171, 210-215, 287, 288, 323
PTSD 199, 201-202
refugee 78, 114, 356
residual hearing 68, 120, 122-125,
    206, 213, 231, 240, 313,
    327-329, 355, 371
risk assessment 186, 260, 276,
    343-344, 347
role shift 25, 103, 351
role-play 100-103, 106, 200, 350,
    358, 392
schizophrenia 209, 213, 216, 218
secondary care 294
secondary symptoms 215
seizure 241, 322
sensory deprivation 85, 134, 210
sensory loss 16, 130, 134
side effect 239-40, 244, 247, 313,
    316
social reasoning 22
special school 70, 71
Speech and Language Therapist
    (SALT) 56, 64, 77-79, 327, 169,
    172, 284, 321, 350, 377
speech to text 92, 123
standardised assessment 155, 164,
    169, 292-294
Stickler Syndrome 322
stigma 63, 122, 138, 176, 205
Teacher of the Deaf (ToD) 79, 279,
    290
tertiary services 171, 283-284

The National Register of
    Communication Professionals
    (NRCPD) 90-92, 107, 120, 138-9,
    364
Theory of Mind (ToM) 22, 37-38,
    40-42, 63, 75, 105, 161, 166,
    227,-278, 254, 330, 347, 351
thought disorder 33, 210, 214
thyroid 206, 215, 241, 322
timelines 39, 44, 183
tinnitus 206, 213, 240, 308, 311,
    314, 332-334
tracking 130-132, 202, 306
translators 139
Treacher-Collins syndrome 304
unpacking concepts 101
Ushers syndrome 131, 303-4, 317,
    321
vestibular 303, 307, 316-318,
    320-321
video conference/conferencing 116,
    118, 177, 232
Video Remote Interpreting (VRI)
    112-113
Video Relay Services (VRS) 32, 79,
    112-113, 248, 374, 382
voices 86, 158, 213-222, 308,
    312-313, 395

NB Some terms (e.g. trauma, language deprivation, language acquisition, language delay, literacy) that might be expected in this index occur so frequently throughout the book that to include a list of where to find them would provide no benefit. The absence of these words is in no way reflective of their perceived importance.

Printed in Great Britain
by Amazon